SYNAPZ
The Complete Final MBBS Manual

SYNAPZ
The Complete Final MBBS Manual

Editors

McEnroe D Mordom MBBS
Government Medical College
Calicut, Kerala, India

Mridulal A MBBS
Government Medical College
Calicut, Kerala, India

Randeep AM MBBS
Government Medical College
Calicut, Kerala, India

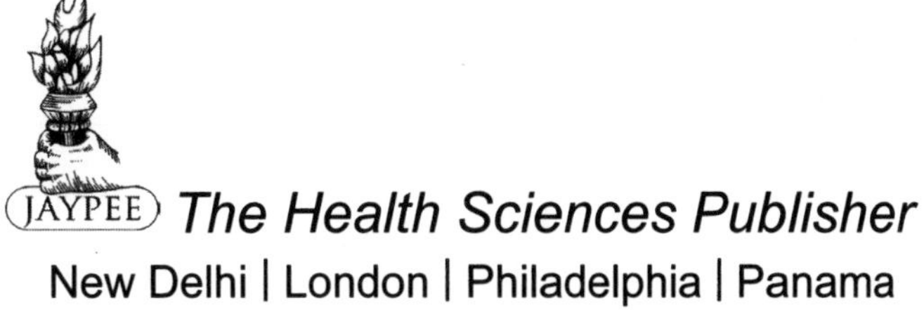

The Health Sciences Publisher
New Delhi | London | Philadelphia | Panama

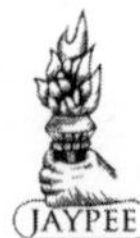

Jaypee Brothers Medical Publishers (P) Ltd.

Headquarters
Jaypee Brothers Medical Publishers (P) Ltd.
4838/24, Ansari Road, Daryaganj
New Delhi 110 002, India
Phone: +91-11-43574357
Fax: +91-11-43574314
E-mail: jaypee@jaypeebrothers.com

Overseas Offices

J.P. Medical Ltd.
83, Victoria Street, London
SW1H 0HW (UK)
Phone: +44-20 3170 8910
Fax: +44(0)20 3008 6180
E-mail: info@jpmedpub.com

Jaypee-Highlights Medical Publishers Inc.
City of Knowledge, Bld. 237, Clayton
Panama City, Panama
Phone: +1 507-301-0496
Fax: +1 507-301-0499
E-mail: cservice@jphmedical.com

Jaypee Medical Inc.
The Bourse
111, South Independence Mall East
Suite 835, Philadelphia, PA 19106, USA
Phone: +1 267-519-9789
E-mail: jpmed.us@gmail.com

Jaypee Brothers Medical Publishers (P) Ltd.
17/1-B, Babar Road, Block-B, Shaymali
Mohammadpur, Dhaka-1207
Bangladesh
Mobile: +08801912003485
E-mail: jaypeedhaka@gmail.com

Jaypee Brothers Medical Publishers (P) Ltd.
Bhotahity, Kathmandu, Nepal
Phone: +977-9741283608
E-mail: kathmandu@jaypeebrothers.com

Website: www.jaypeebrothers.com
Website: www.jaypeedigital.com

SYNAPZ—The Complete Final MBBS Manual

First Edition: 2008

Second Edition: **2015**

ISBN: 978-93-5152-890-6

Printed at Rajkamal Electric Press, Plot No. 2, Phase-IV, Kundli, Haryana.

Dedicated to

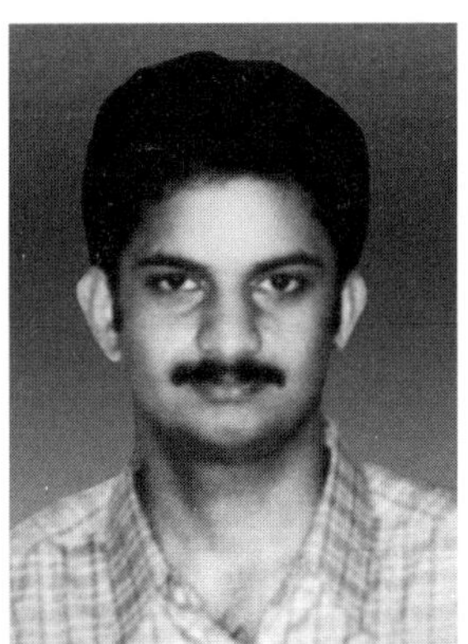

Late Dr Saju P

On a fateful January 26th, 2001 he embarked on a journey with a noble cause as a part of National Service Scheme–Mathrubhumi medical team to provide relief to the earthquake stricken people of Gujarat, India. On February 2nd, putting duty before life, he left this world serving humanity to his last breath; his soul shines eternally as a guiding light for everyone..............

Contributors

MEDICINE

Mukund A Prabhu
Alumni, Government Medical College
Calicut, Kerala, India

P Sandeep
Alumni, Government Medical College
Calicut, Kerala, India

SURGERY

Sreejith Nair
Alumni, Government Medical College
Calicut, Kerala, India

Jayan
Alumni, Government Medical College
Calicut, Kerala, India

ORTHOPEDICS

Rejith Valsalan
Alumni, Government Medical College
Calicut, Kerala, India

C Anoop
Alumni, Government Medical College
Calicut, Kerala, India

Nikhil
Alumni, Government Medical College
Calicut, Kerala, India

OBSTETRICS AND GYNECOLOGY

Anjali Prem
Alumni, Government Medical College
Calicut, Kerala, India

Geovin Ranji
Alumni, Government Medical College
Calicut, Kerala, India

PEDIATRICS

Arun Abhilash
Alumni, Government Medical College
Calicut, Kerala, India

Preface to the Second Edition

It is our pleasure to introduce the second edition of *SYNAPZ—The Complete Final MBBS Manual*. This book is designed to provide a concise summary of subjects taught in your final year MBBS. In the second edition, the entire book has been revised, with a view to eliminating errors, incorporating suggestions of readers, updating concepts, and discarding material that is no longer relevant. In this way, the book has been kept concise while remaining as up-to-date and accurate as possible. In keeping with the current trend of postgraduate entrance examinations, all topics are updated. Key points and comparisons are given in boxes for greater emphasis.

In shaping and revising this latest edition, we have committed ourselves to making the manual an invaluable resource for students.

We have revised the outline format used in last edition hoping to organize information in a logical and readily accessible format. In our quest to polish the second edition of the manual, we have sought to retain the virtues that have made the work a success. Each session has case-taking format followed by concise discussion of relevant topics. Alongside format modifications, we have carefully updated the contents of the manual to reflect advancing medicine. We added a section for objective structured clinical examination (OSCE), hoping it will be useful in exam preparation. We hope you will be benefited by the chest X-ray section with basics in chest radiology. We hope the collection of frequently asked questions will make your exam preparation easy. Operative procedures are briefly narrated for rapid recollection. Mnemonics sections are elaborated and definitions are added at end of sections in view of students' special interest.

We are greatly indebted to the many individuals who helped with the preparation of the book. Those who have really helpful in preparation of this edition including Dr Mukund A Prabhu, Dr Aquil Kalanad, Dr Sreejith Nair, Dr Jayan, Dr Rejith Valsalan, Dr Anjali Prem, Dr Geovin Ranji and Dr Arun Abhilash.

The book will not be complete without mention of the Students, Interns, Residents and Teachers of Calicut Medical College. We are inspired daily by their brilliance, compassion and dedication.

We thank our families for their support and inspiration.

Finally, we would like to thank M/s Jaypee Brothers Medical Publishers (P) Ltd., New Delhi, India, for giving us this greatest opportunity.

McEnroe D Mordom
Mridulal A
Randeep AM

Preface to the First Edition

SYNAPZ is an attempt of academic cooperation and self-help.

We know that final MBBS examination is too hard a nut to crack for an average medical student who does not have adequate dexterity familiarity with the examination pattern and frequently asked questions. It is obvious that along with a thorough theoretical knowledge, we need a sufficiently tactical approach based on common sense, which is an essential prerequisite for a sure success in the examinations especially for the practical sessions.

SYNAPZ is envisaged as a simple epistemological tool capable of bringing about a delightful compromise between the vast academic curriculum and the strictly constrained time period to tackle it. This is not supposed to replace the textbook, but can be used as a tool for effective exploration of the syllabus with a sense of sequential importance.

SYNAPZ consists of a collection of frequently asked questions, case format for all subjects, case discussion, mnemonics, practical examination tips, objective structured clinical examination (OSCE), diagram, surgical procedure and normal values.

McEnroe D Mordom
Mridulal A

Acknowledgments

Our heartfelt gratitude to Dr C Raveendran, Principal, Government Medical College, Calicut; Dr PK Sasidharan, Professor and Head, Department of General Medicine, Government Medical College, Calicut; Dr MP Sasi, Professor and Head, Department of Surgery, Government Medical College, Calicut; Dr Jyodish, Professor and Head, Department of Orthopedics, Government Medical College, Calicut; Dr Umadevi, Professor and Head, Department of Obstetrics and Gynecology, Government Medical College, Calicut; Dr Khadeeja Mumthaz, Professor, Department of Obstetrics and Gynecology, Government Medical College, Calicut; Dr Riyas A, Professor and Head, Department of Pediatrics, Government Medical College, Calicut; Dr Balraj G, Associate Professor, Department of Pediatrics, Government Medical College, Calicut; Dr Johnson Marion, Department of ENT, Nirmala Hospital, Calicut; Dr Premu Vensor, Consultant Gynecologist, Asian Reproductive Medicine Centre (ARMC), Calicut; Dr A Shibulal, SCTIMST, Thiruvananthapuram; Dr Seena S Lal, Assistant Professor, Department of Physiology, Government Medical College, Thrissur; Dr Bishara M Lal, Department of Physiology, Medical College, Thrissur; Dr Akhil Pushkar, Alumni, Amrita Institute of Medical Sciences, Kochi; Dr Lal Antony and Dr Shreeja Lal, Alumni, Medical College, Calicut; Dr Madhusudanan ES, Department of Anesthesiology, Government Medical College, Thrissur; Dr Ashok SK, Alumni, Government Medical College, Calicut; Dr Rohan Raj, Alumni, Government Medical College, Calicut; Dr Unniraja, Alumni, Government Medical College, Calicut; Dr Ushabhayi C, Department of Pharmacology, Academy of Medical Sciences, Pariyaram; Dr Nabil A and Dr Jinu Annie Jose, Alumni, Government Medical College, Calicut; Dr Firoz Khan V and Dr Fathima, Alumni, Government Medical College, Calicut; Dr Nishanth MN, Alumni, Government Medical College, Calicut; Dr Namitha, Alumni, Academy of Medical Sciences, Pariyaram; Dr Prasoon Thomas Joseph and Dr Sayooj KM, Alumni, Government Medical College, Calicut; Dr Mithun S and Dr Minu S, Alumni, Government Medical College, Calicut; Dr Keerthi Mohan, Alumni, Amrita Institute of Medical Sciences, Kochi; Dr Pramod R Pillai, Alumni, Amrita Institute of Medical Sciences, Kochi; Dr Nisha Kumari, Alumni, Amrita Institute of Medical Sciences, Kochi; Dr Deepa Dinesh, Alumni, Amrita Institute of Medical Sciences, Kochi; Dr Emil Joseph Eliston, Alumni, Amrita Institute of Medical Sciences, Kochi; Dr Arjun Krishnan, Alumni, Amrita Institute of Medical Sciences, Kochi; Dr P Raju and Dr Lakshmi, Alumni, Government Medical College, Calicut; Dr U Faizal and Dr Noufira, Alumni, Medical College, Calicut; Dr Mahesh Kumar D and Dr Khayas EK, Alumni, Government Medical College, Calicut; Dr Manoj Kumar E and Dr Vijun, Alumni, Government Medical College, Calicut; Dr Jithesh AK and Dr Suneesh Kumar K, Alumni, Government Medical College, Calicut; Dr Praveen TM and Dr Rimsy P, Alumni, Government Medical College, Calicut; Dr Jyothish Hari and Dr Anup Ahmed, Alumni, Government Medical College, Calicut; Dr Shabeerali K and Dr Abdusammad T, Alumni, Government Medical College, Calicut; Dr Aneesh George and Dr Anish Mohan, Alumni, Government Medical College, Calicut; Dr Mithun Vasudevan and Dr Febin P, Alumni, Government Medical College, Calicut; Dr Wales T George, Alumni, Government Medical College, Calicut; Dr Aslam Farooq ZA and Amjad Farooq ZA, Alumni, Government Medical College, Calicut; Dr Byju P, Alumni, Government Medical College, Calicut; Dr Jayesh Narayanan and Dr Anas N, Alumni, Government Medical College, Calicut; Dr Alex M and Dr Badira, Alumni, Government Medical College, Calicut; Dr Anish KP and Dr Anugunu, Alumni, Government Medical College, Calicut; Dr Sreehari GK, Alumni, Government Medical College, Calicut; Dr Sameeha Saidalavi, Alumni, Government Medical College, Calicut; Dr Santhosh Kumar N and Dr Jimil Francis, Alumni, Government Medical College, Calicut; Dr Vivek Raju, Alumni, Government Medical College, Calicut; Dr Sreekanth P and Dr Rohini, Alumni, Government Medical College, Calicut; Dr Aneesh KP, Alumni, Government Medical College, Calicut; Dr Rahul Raveendran, Alumni, Medical College, Calicut; Dr Anish KA and Dr Mathews Vergese Maret, Alumni, Government Medical College, Calicut; Dr Abdu Raheem Kapoor and Dr Sarath MB, Alumni, Government Medical College, Calicut; Dr Abhilash B and Dr Divya CK, Alumni, Government Medical College, Calicut; Dr Subheesh P, Alumni, Government Medical College, Calicut; Dr Thamizharasi A, General Duty Medical Officer, PHC, Thirubhuvanai, Puducherry; Dr Davidson Devasia, Alumni, Jubilee Mission Medical College, Thrissur; Dr Manjunath PS, Alumni, Jubilee Mission Medical College, Thrissur, Dr Abin Sooraj, Alumni, MES Medical College, Perinthalmanna; Dr Percy Mathew, Alumni, Amala Medical College, Thrissur; Dr Rahees Abdulla, Alumni, Amala Medical College, Thrissur; Dr Anoob PT and Dr Praveen, Government Medical College, Calicut; Mr Praveen Raj and Rani, Alumni, College of Pharmaceutical Sciences, Calicut; Benita Francis and Felina Francis, MBBS Students, Gokulam Medical College, Trivandrum, Kerala, India.

We acknowledge our sincere gratitude to our parents, teachers and also to 44th (2000) and 48th (2004) Batch MBBS Government Medical College, Calicut, Kerala, India.

We thank to Balesh and Sandeep, Associates, Government Medical College, Calicut; Mr Selvaraj PS, Artist, Department of Anatomy, Government Medical College, Calicut; Raju PG, 50th Batch MBBS Student, Government Medical College, Calicut; Anand Krishnan, Nithin Akkal, Navaneeth SB, Rajesh IR, 52nd Batch MBBS Students, Medical College, Calicut; Mr Niyesh, "Samagra", Calicut; Mr Sanoj, "Printers Fort", Calicut; Adv Shijo, Legal Advisor, Calicut; CAMPUS PULSE, Government Medical College, Calicut, Kerala, India.

Contents

1 CHAPTER

Medicine

CARDIOVASCULAR SYSTEM

Mitral Stenosis (MS)

1. Most common rheumatic heart disease
2. More common in females
3. Normal area of mitral valve orifice—4-6 cm^2
4. Mild MS—1.5-2.5 cm^2
5. Moderate MS—1.0-1.5 cm^2
6. Severe MS—<1.0 cm^2.

Causes

1. Almost all MS are due to rheumatic heart disease (RHD)
2. Lutembacher's syndrome—acquired mitral stenosis with atrial septal defect
3. Congenital mitral stenosis—rare
4. Calcification and fibrosis of the valve, valve ring and subvalvular apparatus (*Chordae tendineae*)—elderly
5. Carcinoid tumors metastasizing to the lung, or primary bronchial carcinoid.

Key Symptoms and Signs

1. **Symptoms:** Progressive dyspnea on exertion, orthopnea, PND, hemoptysis, embolic phenomenon
2. **Signs:** Mitral facies, tapping apex beat, apical diastolic thrill, loud S1, MDM, opening snap
3. **Mitral facies or malar flush:** Bilateral, cyanotic or dusky pink discoloration over the upper cheeks that is due to arteriovenous anastomoses and vascular stasis
4. **Hemoptysis in MS:** Due to pulmonary apoplexy, pulmonary edema, pulmonary infarction and effects of anticoagulant therapy.

Case Taking

Symptoms

1. Breathlessness
2. Paroxysmal nocturnal dyspnea (PND)
3. Hemoptysis.

Signs

1. **Pulse**
   a. Low volume, regular
   b. Rate—78/min.
2. **Blood pressure:** Low systolic
3. **Apex beat**
   a. Tapping in character
   b. Normal in position
   c. Presence of diastolic thrill best palpable in left lateral position and in expiration
   d. S1 palpable.

4. **Other features**
   a. Diastolic shock (palpable P2) present
   b. Left parasternal heave present
   c. JVP absent
   d. Epigastric pulsations absent.
5. **Auscultation**
   a. S1—short, sharp, accentuated and loud snapping S1
   b. S2—normally split with accentuated P2
   c. S3 or S4—not audible
   d. Opening snap audible just after S2
   e. Murmur—low pitched, mid diastolic rumbling murmur with presystolic accentuation of grade 4 intensity in mitral area without radiation
   f. Best audible with the bell of the stethoscope in left lateral position at the height of expiration and after doing mild exercise.
6. **Differential diagnosis (D/D) of murmur**
   a. Carey Coomb's murmur—active rheumatic valvulitis
   b. Functional MDM in VSD or PDA
   c. Left atrial myxoma
   d. Ball valve thrombus
   e. Conducted murmur of AI
   f. Cor triatriatum.
7. **Complications**
   a. A/c left atrial failure and A/c pulmonary edema
   b. Pulmonary hypertension
   c. Right ventricular failure
   d. Atrial fibrillation, atrial flutter
   e. Embolic manifestations
   f. Hemoptysis
   g. Infective endocarditis.
8. **Rationality of nervous system**
   a. Embolic stroke
   b. Sydenham's chorea
   c. Fundoscopy—Roth's sport.
9. **Rationality of respiratory system**
   a. Tachypnea, orthopnea
   b. Hydrothorax
   c. Creps at lung bases—in failure.
10. **Rationality of gastrointestinal system**
    a. Liver soft and tender
    b. Spleen palpable in SBE
    c. Ascites.
11. **Management**
    a. Investigations
       i. *Chest X-ray*: Straightening of left border of cardiac silhouette
          Right ventricular hypertrophy (RVH)
          Prominence of main pulmonary artery
          Dilation of upper lobe pulmonary vessels
          Kerley B lines
       ii. ECG-wide and notched P-wave, left atrial dilatation, RVH, AF (can occur)
       iii. ECHO-chamber enlargement, value pathology, mitral orifice, flow gradient.
    b. Treatment
       i. Percutaneous balloon mitral valvuloplasty
       ii. Valvotomy or commissurotomy
       iii. Mitral valve reconstruction
       iv. Valve replacement or prosthesis
       v. Medical treatment with diuretics, penicillin prophylaxis, digoxin, anticoagulants, salt restriction.

Hemodynamic Changes

MS→↓LV filling→low output state→↑LA pressure→↑Pulmonary venous pressure→PAH→RVH→RV failure

Severity assessment criteria

1. Presence of pulmonary hypertension—loud P2, signs of right heart failure—edema and hepatomegaly
2. The closeness of opening snap (OS) to S2 is proportional to the severity
3. The length of the mid-diastolic murmur is proportional to the severity

4. Softening of loud S1 and disappearance of OS—valve cusps becomes immobile
5. Mitral diastolic murmur becomes quieter—reduction of cardiac output (Pulmonary HTN).

Graham-Steell murmur: Pulmonary hypertension results in pulmonary valvular regurgitation that causes an early diastolic murmur in the pulmonary area.

Mitral Regurgitation (MR)

Causes

1. Acute rheumatic fever
2. Myocarditis
3. Dilated and hypertrophic cardiomyopathy
4. Hypertensive heart disease
5. Ischemic heart disease
6. Infective endocarditis
7. Connective tissue disorders—SLE
8. Collagen abnormalities—Marfan's syndrome and Ehlers-Danlos syndrome
9. Degeneration or mitral annular calcification
10. Rupture of the *Chordae tendineae* (myocardial infarction, infective endocarditis or trauma).

Key Symptoms and Signs

1. *Symptoms*
   a. Palpitation and dyspnea on exertion
   b. Orthopnea, PND, hemoptysis—LV dysfunction
2. *Signs*: Hyperdynamic (forcible) apex beat, apical systolic thrill, soft S1, PSM.

Case Taking

Symptoms

1. Palpitation
2. Exertional dyspnea
3. Rheumatic fever past history.

Signs

1. **Pulse**
   a. Jerky, good volume
   b. Rate—110/min.
2. **Blood pressure**
   Within normal limits.
3. **Apex beat**
   a. Left 7th ICS outside left MCL
   b. Forcible in character
   c. Systolic thrill best palpable in left lateral position and in expiration.
4. **Other pulsations**
   a. JVP engorged and pulsatile
   b. Epigastric pulsations present.
5. **Auscultation**
   a. S1 is soft
   b. S2—audible
   c. S3 or S4 in LVF
   d. Murmur—high pitched soft blowing PSM of grade 4 intensity with radiation towards left axilla and inferior angle of scapula best audible with the diaphragm of the stethoscope in left lateral position and at the height of expiration.
6. **Differential diagnosis of murmur**
   a. Functional murmur
   b. Ventricular septal defect—childhood
   c. Tricuspid incompetence—positive
   d. Carvallo's sign—increase in intensity of murmur with inspiration.

7. **Complications**
   a. A/c left ventricular failure
   b. Infective endocarditis
   c. Congestive cardiac failure
   d. *Arrhythmias*: Ventricular ectopics, atrial fibrillation
   e. Pressure symptoms due to giant left atrium.
8. **Rationality of RS**
   a. Vesicular breath sounds
   b. Rhonchi + no added sound
   c. No hydrothorax.
9. **Rationality of GIT**
   a. Liver soft and tender
   b. Spleen—not palpable
   c. Ascites—absent.
10. **Management**
    a. **Investigations**
       i. Chest X-ray-LAH+RVH
       ii. ECG- LAH+RVH (50%) biventricular hypertrophy
       iii. ECHO-giant or aneurysmal left atrium.
    b. **Treatment**
       i. Medical treatment
       ii. Surgical treatment—implantation of prosthesis, mitral valvuloplasty and annuloplasty.
11. Mitral valve prolapse
    a. Also known as Barlow's syndrome, billowing mitral valve syndrome, floppy valve syndrome
    b. Most common in young females
    c. Autosomal dominant inheritance
    d. Patients usually asymptomatic
    e. *On examination*: Systolic clicks often multiple. Late systolic murmur can occur accentuation of findings on Valsalva and standing
    f. *Investigation of choice*: Echocardiography
    g. *Complications*: MR, TIA, arrhythmia, IE, sudden death.

Aortic Stenosis (AS)

1. Normal aortic valve area 2.5–3.5 cm^2
2. Mild AS 1.5–2.0 cm^2
3. Moderate AS 1.0–1.5 cm^2
4. Severe AS 0.5–1.0 cm^2
5. Critical AS < 0.5 cm^2.

Causes

1. Rheumatic
2. Congenital—bicuspid aortic valve
3. Calcific degeneration
4. Associated with familial hypercholesterolemia, MPS
5. Functional—AI, thyrotoxicosis, anemia.

Key Symptoms and Signs

1. *Symptoms*: Angina on exertion, exertional syncope, dyspnea on exertion—classical triad
2. *Signs*: Low pulse pressure, heaving apex beat, systolic thrill in aortic area, paradoxical split, ESM, ejection click.

Case Taking

Symptoms

1. Chest pain
2. Exertional dyspnea
3. Occasional blackouts
4. Past history of rheumatic fever.

Signs

1. Pulse
   a. 72/min, low volume, regular
   b. Carotid shudder, anacrotic.
2. *Blood pressure*: Low with low pulse pressure
3. *Apex beat*: Normal position, heaving
4. *Aortic area*: Systolic thrill

5. Auscultation
   a. S1—audible
   b. S2—muffled
   c. Ejection click present.
6. *Murmur*: Harsh, midsystolic ejection murmur of grade 5 with direction towards carotids best audible in sitting and leaning forward and with the diaphragm of the stethoscope in full expiration.

Gallavardin Phenomenon

Aortic stenosis murmur is transmitted to apex
Ejection click
Valvular aortic stenosis.

Differential diagnosis

1. Subvalvular aortic stenosis
2. Supravalvular aortic stenosis.

Complications

a. A/c LVF
b. CCF
c. Infective endocarditis
d. Tachy and bradyarrhythmias
e. Complete heart block—sudden death.

Investigations

a. *Chest X-ray*: LVH or normal calcification of aortic valve
b. ECG-LVH, LAH, primary heart block, LBBB
c. ECHO-calcified valve, LVH.

Treatment

a. Aortic valve prosthesis
b. Aortic valvotomy
c. Medical treatment.

Severity Assessment

1. Symptomatic patients have severe AS
2. Narrow pulse pressure—severe AS
3. Lengthy ESM with late peaking
4. Paradoxical split of S2
5. Presence of S4
6. Presence of S3 indicates CHF
7. *ECG*: ST and T changes
8. CXR-cardiac enlargement
9. *ECHO*: Valve area < 0.75 cm^2, transvalvular pressure gradient > 50 mm Hg.

Aortic Regurgitation (AR)

Causes

Valvular

1. Congenital (bicuspid aortic valve)
2. Endocarditis
3. Rheumatic fever
4. Myxomatous (prolapse)
5. Traumatic
6. Syphilis
7. Ankylosing spondylitis.

Root Disease

1. Aortic dissection
2. Cystic medial degeneration
3. Marfan syndrome
4. Bicuspid aortic valve
5. Nonsyndromic familial aneurysm
6. Aortitis
7. Hypertension.

Key Symptoms and Signs

1. *Symptoms*: Palpitation on exertion, dyspnea on exertion
2. *Signs*: Wide pulse pressure, forcible apex beat, EDM.

Peripheral Signs of Aortic Regurgitation

1. Prominent digital artery pulsations
2. High volume collapsing pulse/Corrigan pulse
3. Wide pulse pressure with low diastolic pressure
4. Pulsation in suprasternal notch
5. **de Musset's sign:** A head nob occurring with each heart beat

6. **Traube's sign:** A pistol shot pulse (systolic and diastolic sounds) heard over the femoral arteries
7. **Duroziez's sign:** A systolic and diastolic bruit heard when the femoral artery is partially compressed
8. **Quincke's pulses:** Capillary pulsations in the fingertips or lips
9. **Muller's sign:** Systolic pulsations of the uvula
10. **Becker's sign:** Visible pulsations of the retinal arteries and pupils
11. **Hill's sign:** Popliteal cuff systolic pressure exceeding brachial pressure by more than 60 mm Hg
12. **Mayne's sign:** More than a 15 mm Hg decrease in diastolic blood pressure with arm elevation from the value obtained with the arm in the standard position
13. **Rosenbach's sign:** Systolic pulsations of the liver
14. **Gerhard's sign:** Systolic pulsations of the spleen
15. **Landolfi's sign:** Changes in pupil size
16. **Light house sign:** Alternate flushing and blanching of forehead.

Case Taking

Symptoms

1. Palpitation
2. Pulsatile or throbbing
3. Chest pain
4. Dyspnea
5. Edema-PND-(LVF or CCF).

Signs

1. Pulse
   a. 80/min high volume, regular
   b. Water hammer type.
2. **Blood pressure:** Wide pulse pressure
3. **Apex beat:** Diffuse hyperdynamic
4. **Aortic area:** No thrill
5. **Auscultation**
   a. S1-audible
   b. S2-muffled.
6. **Murmur:** High pitched soft blowing early diastolic decrescendo murmur of grade 3 intensity with radiation towards apex. Best audible in sitting and leaning forward position in the neoaortic area in full expiration and with the diaphragm of stethoscope.

Differential diagnosis

a. PDA, coronary arteriovenous fistula
b. Ruptured sinuses of Valsalva, wide pulse pressure
c. *Graham steel murmur*: Diastolic murmur.

Complications

a. A/c LVF
b. CCF
c. Infective endocarditis
d. Arrhythmias
e. Heart block.

Management

a. **Investigations**
   i. Chest X-ray—cardiomegaly, aortic root dilatation, aortic valve calcification
   ii. ECG-LVH and conduction defects
   iii. ECHO-LVH, calcified aortic valve.
b. **Treatment**
   i. Aortic valve prosthesis
   ii. Medical treatment—LVF and CCF
   iii. Prophylaxis of rheumatic fever and SBE.

Comparison between MS, MR, AS and AR

Features	MS	MR	AS	AR
Symptoms	DOE PND Hemoptysis	POE DOE	Angina Syncope DOE	POE

Contd...

Contd ...

Signs pulse	Low volume Irregular-AF	Good volume	Low volume	High volume Water hammer
Blood pressure **Apex beat**	Low systolic Tapping Diastolic thrill S1 palpable	Normal Hyperdynamic Systolic thrill	Low pulse pressure Heaving Systolic thrill	Wide Hyperdynamic No thrill
Aortic area auscultation	Loud S1 S2-normal Opening snap Low pitched MDM	S1 is soft S2-audible S3 or S4 in LVF No opening snap High pitched PSM	S1-N S2-muffled Ejection click Low pitched ESM	S1-N S2-muffled High EDM

1. DOE–Dyspnea on exertion
2. POE–Palpitation on exertion
3. PND–Paroxysmal nocturnal dyspnea
4. AF–Atrial fibrillation
5. S1–First heart sound
6. S2–Second heart sound
7. S3–Third heart sound
8. S4–Fourth heart sound
9. LVF–Left ventricular failure
10. RVF–Right ventricular failure
11. MDM–Mid-diastolic murmur
12. PSM–Pan systolic murmur
13. ESM–Ejection systolic murmur
14. EDM–Early diastolic murmur.

Pulse

The rhythmical dilatation of an artery produced by the increased volume of blood thrown into the vessel by the contraction of the heart. The method of palpation of pulse is called trisection.

Rate-Radial Artery

1. Normal 60–100/min
2. Bradycardia <60/min
3. Tachycardia >100/min.

Causes of sinus bradycardia
1. **Physiological:** Atheletes, sleep
2. **Pathological:** Hypothyroidism, obstructive jaundice, raised ICT (Cushing reflex), sick sinus syndrome
3. **Drugs:** Beta blockers, digoxin.

Causes of sinus tachycardia
1. **Physiological:** Exercise, infants, emotion
2. **Pathological:** Fever, thyrotoxicosis, pheochromocytoma, CHF, pericardial disease, hypovolemic shock
3. **Drugs:** Beta agonists (salbutamol), anticholinergic (Atropine).

Rhythm

Regularity with which one beat follows the other:

Regularly irregular pulse
1. Regular extrasystole
2. Sinus arrhythmia.

Irregularly irregular pulse
1. Atrial fibrillation
2. Multiple extra systole.

Volume

Amplitude of expansile movement of vessel wall during passage of pulse wave.

Low volume
1. Hypovolemia
2. AS
3. Severe PAH
4. Pericardial effusion
5. Myocardial damage.

High volume
1. AR
2. PDA
3. AV fistula
4. Anemia, high fever, thyrotoxicosis.

Varying volume
1. Atrial fibrillation
2. Ventricular tachycardia
3. *Pulsus alternans*: Alternating small and large volume pulse in regular rhythm
4. Severe left ventricular dysfunction
5. *Pulsus paradoxus*: It is an exaggerated reduction in the strength of arterial pulse during normal inspiration or an exaggerated inspiratory fall in systolic pressure of more than 10 mm Hg during quiet breathing.

Physiological
1. Pregnancy
2. Obesity.

Pathological
1. Pericardial tamponade
2. Constrictive pericarditis
3. Airway obstruction—acute severe asthma/COPD
4. SVC obstruction
5. Pulmonary embolism
6. Hypovolemic shock.

Character

Wavy pattern of pulse is not felt normally. It is obliterated by normal vascular tone.

Collapsing Pulse (Water Hammer Pulse; Corrigan's Pulse)

It is a large volume pulse with rapid upstroke (high systolic pressure) and a rapid downstroke (low diastolic pressure).
1. Patent ductus arteriosus
2. Aortic regurgitation
3. Arteriovenous fistula
4. Rupture of sinus of Valsalva.

Other Pulses

Pulsus bisferiens: It is a single pulse wave with two peaks in systole:
1. Aortic stenosis and aortic regurgitation
2. Severe aortic regurgitation
3. Hypertrophic obstructive cardiomyopathy.

Anacrotic pulse (Parvus et tardus):
1. A low amplitude pulse with slow rising and late peak
2. Severe valvular aortic stenosis.

Dicrotic pulse is double peaked pulse due to the palpability of dicrotic wave. Hypotonia of vessel wall lead to appearance of dicrotic wave.
1. Enteric fever, malaria
2. Septicemia
3. Severe heart failure, hypovolemic shock, cardiac tamponade
4. Conditions associated with a decreased stroke volume and elevated systemic vascular resistance
5. During the immediate postoperative period following aortic valve replacement:
   a. Reversed pulses parodoxus is found in HOCM
   b. Double apical impulse is seen in aortic stenosis and HOCM
   c. Pulmonary capillary wedge pressure denotes left atrial pressure
   d. Pulmonary arterial pressure denotes right atrial pressure.

Pulsus bigeminus: Pulse wave with a normal beat followed by a premature beat and a compensatory pause, occurring in rapid succession resulting in alternation of strength of the pulse. It is a sign of digitalis toxicity.

Blood Pressure

The lateral force exerted by the blood column per unit area of the vascular wall that is expressed in mm Hg.

Korotkoff Sounds

Phase 1	The first appearance of the sounds marking systolic pressure
Phases 2 and 3	Increasingly loud sound

Phase 4 Abrupt muffling of the sounds
Phase 5 Disappearance of the sounds.

Jugular Venous Pulse

It is the reflection of phasic pressure changes in the right atrium and consists of 3 positive waves (a, c, v) and 2 negative troughs (x, y).

Normal JVP

1. **A wave:** Right atrial systole
2. **C wave:** Bulging of tricuspid valve into right atrium during RV isovolumetric contraction
3. **V wave:** Right atrial filling during ventricular systole
4. **A-X descent:** Right atrial relaxation with downward descent of tricuspid valve
5. **V-Y descent:** Tricuspid valve opening and flow of blood to right ventricle
6. **Large 'a' wave:** Forceful atrial contraction against a stenosed tricuspid valve, e.g. TS/PS/PHTN
7. **Absent 'a' waves:** Seen in atrial fibrillation
8. **Cannon 'a' wave:** Atrial systole against a closed atrial valve, e.g. complete heart block, VT
9. **Giant 'v' wave:** Is an important sign of tricuspid regurgitation
10. **Prominent x y descent:** Occurs in constrictive pericarditis
11. **Kussmaul's sign:** Is an inspiratory increase in JVP, e.g. cp, cardiac tamponade.

Apex

Apex is the lowermost and outermost point of the precordium where a definite cardiac impulse can be seen or felt.

1. **Palpitation:** An unpleasant awareness of forceful, rhythmic or rapid beating of the heart
2. **Thrill:** A palpable murmur
3. **Murmur:** It is a sound heard due to the turbulent flow of blood within the heart and great vessels.

Levine and Freeman's Grading of Murmurs

Grade 1 Very soft (heard in a quiet room)
Grade 2 Soft
Grade 3 Moderate
Grade 4 Loud with thrill
Grade 5 Very loud with thrill (heard with a stethoscope)
Grade 6 Very loud with thrill (heard even when stethoscope is slightly away from the chest wall).

Named murmurs

1. Gibson's murmur : Continuous murmur of PDA
2. Carey-Coomb's murmur : MDM of rheumatic valvulitis
3. Graham Steell murmur : EDM of pulmonary regurgitation
4. Austin Flint murmur : MDM of severe AR
5. Seagull murmur : SBE in MR causes murmur with musical quality
6. Cooing Dove murmur : Same as Seagull murmur.

Heart Sounds

First Heart Sound (S1)

Closure of atrioventricular valves.

Soft S1-causes	Loud S1	Variable S1
Mitral regurgitation	Mitral stenosis	Atrial fibrillation
Tricuspid regurgitation	Tricuspid stenosis	Extrasystole
Right or left ventricular dysfunction	Short PR interval	Complete heart block
Calcification of AV valves	Tachycardia	
First degree heart block	High output state	

Second Heart Sound (S2)

1. Closure of semilunar valves
2. Splitting of S2—normally seen in children and young adults in inspiration.

Wide variable split	Wide fixed split
MR and VSD (early A2)	Atrial septal defect
RBBB and left ventricular ectopics (late P2)	Right ventricular failure

Third Heart Sound/Ventricular Gallop (S3)

Produced by passive filling of the ventricles.

Causes

Physiological	Pathological
Children	High output states
Athletes	ASD, VSD, PDA
Pregnancy	Hypertrophic cardiomyopathy

Fourth Heart Sound/Atrial Gallop (S4)

Produced by rapid emptying of the atrium into noncompliant ventricle.

Pathological causes

1. Hypertrophic cardiomyopathy
2. Systemic hypertension
3. Coronary artery disease—angina, MI, ventricular aneurysm.

Opening snap

High pitched diastolic sound produced by the sudden halt of the opening process of diseased mitral/tricuspid valve.

Causes

Tricuspid area	Mitral area
Tricuspid stenosis	Mitral stenosis
ASD	VSD, PDA

Diastolic Sounds

1. Pericardial knock
   a. Heard in early diastole
   b. Occurs earlier than S3 and is usually higher pitched than S3
   c. Occurs in atrial myxoma.
2. **Tumor plop:** Heard after 80–120 ms after the aortic closure sound resembling an opening snap
3. **Quadruple rhythm:** A quadruple rhythm is said to occur when both S4 and S3 are present.
4. **Incomplete summation gallop:** When S4 and S3 occur together at a faster heart rate.

Theories of Paroxysmal Nocturnal Dyspnea

1. Venous return increases in recumbency
2. Mobilization of edema fluid from extravascular to intravascular compartment
3. Adrenergic drive is reduced during sleep
4. Heart rate increases during REM sleep
5. Reduction of vital capacity in supine position.

Cardinal signs of LVF	Cardinal signs of RVF
Pulmonary congestion	Systemic congestion
Gallop rhythm	Enlarged and pulsatile neck veins
Fine basal crepitations	Mildly enlarged and soft tender and rarely pulsatile liver
Pulses alternans	Dependent bipedal edema

Pulmonary Hypertension

Symptoms

1. Breathlessness
2. Chest pain
3. Early fatiguability
4. Cough
5. Dizziness
6. Hemoptysis
7. Syncope.

Signs

1. Pulse—low volume
2. Neck veins—a wave prominent.

Inspection

1. Pulmonary artery pulsations in left 2nd ICS
2. Epigastric pulsations in RVH.

Palpation

1. Apex goes outwards
2. P2 palpable
3. Diastolic shock
4. Left parasternal heave.

Auscultation

1. S1 audible
2. Pulmonary ejection click
3. Ejection systolic murmur
4. Close splitting of S2 with loud P2
5. Graham-Steell murmur
6. Right sided S3.

Features of Pancarditis

1. **Pericarditis**
   a. Pericardial rub
   b. Pericardial effusion.
2. **Myocarditis**
   a. Relative tachycardia
   b. S1 muffled or soft
   c. Congestive cardiac failure
   d. Conduction defects
   e. Tic-tac heart sounds
   f. S3 gallop rhythm
   g. Enlarged heart size
   h. Arrhythmia.
3. **Endocarditis**
   a. Appearance of soft systolic murmur due to MI
   b. Soft early diastolic murmur due to AI
   c. Carey Coomb's murmur.

Subacute Bacterial Endocarditis (SABE)

Most common cause of bacterial endocarditis:

1. **In native valve:** *Staphylococcus aureus* (35%)
2. **In prosthetic valve:** Coagulase negative *Staphylococcus* (33%)
3. **In IV drug abusers:** *Staphylococcus aureus.*

Symptoms

1. Fever with chills
2. Sweating
3. Anorexia
4. Loin pain
5. Arthralgia
6. Fatigue
7. Palpitation.

Signs

1. Anemia (café-au-lait pallor)
2. Elevated temperature
3. Tachycardia
4. Osler's node
5. Painful clubbing
6. Petechiae
7. Splinter hemorrhage
8. Pansystolic murmur (Seagull murmur)
9. Mild tender hepatomegaly with splenic rub
10. Splenomegaly
11. Tender renal angle
12. Arthritis
13. Roth spots
14. Microscopic hematuria.

Differential Diagnosis

1. Acute rheumatic fever
2. Left atrial myxoma
3. Marantic endocarditis
4. Systemic lupus endocarditis.

Management

1. *Investigation*
   Blood culture (Investigation of choice).
2. *Treatment of SABE*
   Streptococcus viridans and bovis—benzyl penicillin IV (1.2 gm 4th hourly)+- gentamycin IV (80 mg 12th hourly) 2 weeks for sensitive organisms and 4 weeks for others.

Organisms implicated in endocarditis

Organism	Typical source of infection	First choice antibiotics
Streptococcus viridans	Upper respiratory tract	Benzyl penicillin; gentamicin
Streptococcus faecalis	Bowel and urogenital tract	Ampicillin; gentamicin
Anaerobic streptococcus	Bowel	Ampicillin; gentamicin
Staphylococcus epidermidis	Skin	Flucloxacillin; gentamicin
Fungi: *Candida, Histoplasmosis*	Skin and mucous membranes	Amphotericin B; 5 flucytosine
Coxiella burnetii	Complication of Q fever	Chloramphenicol; tetracycline
Chlamydia psittaci	Contact with infected birds	Tetracycline and erythromycin
Staphylococcus aureus	Skin	Flucloxacillin; gentamicin
Streptococcus pneumoniae	Complication of pneumonia	Benzyl penicillin; gentamicin
Neisseria gonorrhoea	Venereal	Benzyl penicillin; gentamicin

Jones Criteria for Acute Rheumatic Fever

Major manifestations

1. Carditis
2. Polyarteritis nodosa
3. Subcutaneous nodules
4. Chorea
5. Erythema marginatum.

Minor manifestations

1. **Clinical**
   a. Fever
   b. Arthralgia
   c. Previous rheumatic fever or rheumatic heart disease.
2. **Laboratory**
   a. High ESR or positive creactive protein
   b. Increased PR interval in ECG.

Presence of 2 major or 1 major + 2 minor criteria strongly suggests rheumatic fever with essential criteria.

Essential criteria

1. History of recent onset scarlet fever
2. Positive throat culture for group A *Streptococcus*
3. Increased ASO (antistreptolysin O titer) or titer of other streptococcal antibodies.

Hypertrophic Obstructive Cardiomyopathy

Symptoms	Signs
Dyspnea	Jerky pulse
Angina	Double or triple apex (S3/S4)
Syncope	MID systolic murmur associated with MR
Palpitation	AF associated with MVP.
Sudden death	

Conditions Aggravating the Symptoms of HOCM

1. Factors that increase the myocardial contractility
   a. Exercise b. Sympathomimetic amines c. Digitalis glycosides.
2. Factors which decrease the ventricular volume
   a. Valsalva maneuver b. Sudden standing c. Nitroglycerine
   d. Amyl nitrate e. Tachycardia.

Management

1. Beta blocker for angina
2. Amiodarone for (arrhythymias)
3. Septal myectomy/myotomy
4. In C/c AF use anticoagulants.

Myocardial Infarction (MI)

Cardiac markers In myocardial infarction

Cardiac marker	Seen	Returns to normal	Features
CK MB	Within 2–4 hours	By 48–72 hours	Quite specific
Troponin-I	Within 4–8 hours	After 7–10 days	Cardiac specific
Troponin-T	Within 4–8 hours	After 10–14 days	Not detected in blood

ECG Changes in Acute Infarction

1. **Hyperacute phase**
   a. Elevation of ST segment b. Tall widened T wave c. Increased ventricular size.
2. **Fully evolved phase**
   a. Pathological Q wave b. Elevated ST segment c. Inverted symmetrical T wave.
3. **Old infarction**
   Pathological Q wave.

Types of Anterior Wall MI and Leads Involved

Type of MI	Leads involved
Extensive anterior wall MI	Standard lead 1, lead AVL and all precordial leads (V1–V6)
Anteroseptal wall MI	Leads V1–V4
Anterolateral wall MI	Standard lead 1, lead AVL and leads V4–V6
Apical wall MI	V5–V6
Inferior wall MI	Standard leads 2 and 3 and lead AVF

Electrophysiologic Conduction System of Heart

1. **P wave:** Atrial muscle depolarization
2. **PR interval:** The time required for the conduction of impulse through atria, AV node, common bundle and bundle branches up to the time of ventricular depolarization
3. **QRS interval:** The depolarization of muscle fibers in ventricles

4. **ST segment:** The pause between ventricular muscle firing and ventricular muscle repolarization
5. **T wave:** Stage of repolarization of ventricles
6. **QT interval:** The duration of ventricular electrical activity
7. **U wave:** Due to repolarization of the bundle branches and Purkinje fibers.

Normal Duration of ECG Intervals

ECG interval	Average(s)	Range(s)	ms
PR interval	0.18	0.12–0.20	120–200
QRS duration	0.08	0.10	100
QT interval	0.40	0.43	400–445
ST interval	0.32		320

Treatment of Hypertension with Coexisting Conditions

Concomitant condition	Drugs preferred	Drugs to be avoided
Angina	B blocker, CCB	Vasodilators
BHP	A blocker	
Diabetes and hyperlipidemia	ACEI, ARB, CCB, A blocker	B blocker, diuretics
Elderly and isolated systolic HTN	Diuretics, CCB	
Low renin hypertension	Diuretics, CCB	
High renin hypertension	ACEI, ARB, B blocker	
Asthma	CCB, diuretics, ACEI, ARB	B blocker
CHF	ACEI, diuretics	CCB
Post MI	B blocker, ACEI	
PVD	CCB, A blocker	B blocker
Thyrotoxicosis	B blocker	Vasodilators

Drug Treatment of Arrhythmias

Type of arrhythmia	Drugs for acute therapy	Drugs for chronic therapy
AF/AFL	Propanolol; esmolol	Ibutilide, digoxinamiodarone, verapamil
PSVT	Adenosine	Verapamil; sotalol, propranolol; amiodarone
Ventricular tachycardia	Lignocaine; magnesium	Sotalol; amiodarone, quinidine
Ventricular fibrillation	Lignocaine; bretylium	Amiodarone
WPW syndrome	Flecainide	Propranolol; amiodarone
Torsades de pointes	Mg (for cong and acquired)	Propranolol (only congenital)
Digitalis induced ventricular arrhythmia	Lignocaine, phenytoin	Propranolol

Note:
1. Amiodarone can be used for treatment of all arrhythmias except torsades de pointes and digitalis induced arrhythmia
2. Cardioversion is the treatment of choice in ventricular fibrillation
3. Laser ablation of aberrant pathway is the definitive treatment of WPW syndrome.

RESPIRATORY SYSTEM

Pleural Effusion

Symptoms

1. Evening rise of temperature
2. Dry cough with chest pain
3. Heaviness of chest
4. Respiratory distress.

Past history

1. Trauma
2. Tuberculosis
3. Asbestosis
4. Diabetes mellitus
5. Skin rash, joint pain and LNE
6. Edema all over body
7. Hemoptysis
8. Similar illness.

General Examination

Decubitus

Prefers to lie on diseased side.

Respiration

Tachypnea and less movement on affected side.

Lymph nodes

Slightly tender cervical lymph nodes may be palpable.

Temperature

Rise.

Inspection

1. Fullness of intercostals space on affected side
2. Diminished movements
3. Apical impulse not seen.

Palpation

1. Expansion is less
2. Trachea shifted to opposite side in large effusion
3. Vocal fremitus decreased
4. No tenderness.

Percussion

1. Stony dullness on affected side and does not change on posture
2. Shifting dullness absent
3. Normal resonance on opposite side.

Auscultation

1. Diminished vesicular breath sounds
2. Vocal resonance diminished
3. Adventitious sounds absent
4. Coin sound present.

Etiology

1. Exudative
   a. Pneumonia
   b. Tuberculosis
   c. Bronchogenic carcinoma
   d. Pulmonary infarction.
2. Transudative
   a. Nephritic syndrome
   b. CCF
   c. Cirrhosis of liver
   d. Nutritional edema.

Complications

1. Spread of infection to pericardium or peritoneum
2. Thickened pleura
3. Collapse followed by fibrosis
4. Acute pulmonary edema
5. Hydropneumothorax
6. Empyema thoracis.

Differential diagnosis

1. Pneumonic consolidation
2. Thickened pleura
3. Liver abscess
4. Fibrosis or collapse of lung
5. Empyema thoracis
6. Subphrenic abscess
7. Bronchogenic carcinoma
8. Pericardial effusion.

Examination of CVS

1. Pericardial effusion
2. Anasarca.

Examination of GIT

1. Hepatosplenomegaly—CCF
2. Ascites-hydrothorax
3. Hydrocele
4. Abdominal lump.

Examination of CNS

1. Neck rigidity/stiffness
2. Altered higher function.

Management

1. **Investigations**
   a. Blood-high ESR and mild lymphocytosis—in case of TB
   b. Chest X-ray
      i. Triangular homogenous opacity with curved upper border concave medially and extends to axilla
      ii. Obliteration of costophrenic angle
      iii. Displacement of mediastinum to opposite side.
   c. Pleural fluid aspiration—50 mL
   d. Confirmation, culture
   e. Smear examination
   f. Mantoux test and FNAC
   g. Sputum examination.
2. **Treatment**
   a. Rest with good nutritious diet
   b. NSAIDs to relieve pain
   c. Aspiration of pleural fluid
   d. Chest physiotherapy
   e. ATT and steroids in case of TB
   f. Rx of CCF and cirrhosis
   g. Repeated aspiration and pleurodesis-malignancy.

Differences between transudate and exudate

Test	Transudate	Exudate
Appearance	Clear or light yellow	Straw colored, cloudy, purulent, hemorrhagic
Protein	< 3 gm/100 mL	> 3 gm/100 mL
LDH	Low	High
Pleural fluid LDH	< 2/3rd of normal upper limit of serum LDH	> 2/3rd of normal upper limit of serum LDH
Pleural fluid/LDH ratio	< 0.6	> 0.6
Pleural fluid/Serum protein ratio	< 0.5	> 0.5
RBC	< 10000/mm^3	> 100000/mm^3
WBC	< 1000/mm^3	> 1000/mm^3 > 50% of lymphocytes—TB and CA > 50% of polymorphs—infection
Glucose	Same as blood concentration	↑ In infection and neoplasm

Light's Criteria

Pleural fluid is exudate if one or more:

1. *Pleural fluid protein*: Serum protein > 0.5
2. *Pleural fluid LDH*: Serum LDH > 0.6
3. Pleural fluid LDH > 2/3 upper limit nl serum LDH.

Causes of low glucose pleural fluid

1. Malignancy
2. Rheumatoid arthritis
3. Empyema
4. Hemothorax
5. Paragonimiasis
6. Churg-Strauss syndrome.
7. Lupus pleuritis.

Pneumothorax

Symptoms

1. Sudden respiratory distress
2. Sudden chest pain
3. Rise of temperature.

Past history
1. Respiratory distress
2. Tuberculosis
3. Hemoptysis
4. Trauma
5. Prolonged recumbency with calf pain
6. Similar illness
7. Chest pain—IHD.

General Examination

Decubitus: Prefers to lie on affected side and becomes breathless lying on other side.

Respiration: Tachypnea and less movement on affected side.

Lymph nodes: Not palpable.

Temperature: Rise.

Inspection
1. Fullness of intercostals space on affected side
2. Absence of intercostal suction
3. Apical impulse not seen.

Palpation
1. Expansion is less
2. Trachea shifted to opposite side in large pneumothorax
3. Vocal fremitus decreased
4. No tenderness.

Percussion
1. Tympanitic note on affected side
2. Shifting dullness absent
3. Normal resonance on opposite side.

Auscultation
1. Diminished vesicular breath sounds
2. Vocal resonance diminished
3. Adventitious sounds absent.

Etiology
1. Rupture of subpleural apical bleb
2. Rupture subpleural TB focus
3. Rupture subpleural emphysematous bullae
4. Staphylococcal lung abscess
5. Penetrating or nonpentrating trauma
6. Bronchogenic carcinoma
7. Pulmonary infarction.

Complications

1. Hydropneumothorax
2. Pyopneumothorax
3. Empyema thoracis
4. Hemopneumothorax
5. Thickened pleura
6. Circulatory collapse
7. Atelectasis of lung
8. Surgical emphysema
9. Pneumomediastinum.

Differential Diagnosis

1. Large emphysematous bullae
2. Pulmonary thromboembolism diagnosis
3. Lung cyst
4. Superficial big empty cavity
5. Sliding hiatal hernia
6. Acute MI.

Management

1. **Investigations**
   a. Blood—TB findings
   b. Chest X-ray
      i. Increased radiolucency with absence of lung markings
      ii. Costophrenic angles clear
      iii. Displacement of mediastinum to opposite side.
   c. Mantoux test
   d. Sputum examination
   e. Lung function tests.

2. **Treatment**
   a. Small pneumothorax—conservative treatment
   b. Large or tension pneumothorax—O_2 inhalation and propped up position, water seal drainage
   c. Recurrent pneumothorax—chemical pleurodesis
   d. ATT
   e. Surgery—thoracoscopy, pleurectomy
   f. Decortication.

Hydropneumothorax

Symptoms

1. Dyspnea
2. Chest pain
3. Heaviness of chest
4. Pyrexia.

Test to Confirm (5S)

1. Shifting dullness
2. Succussion splash (below scapula and axilla)
3. Straight line dullness
4. Shifting of mediastinum
5. Sound of coin.

Etiology	Investigations
Rupture of subpleural TB focus	Chest X-ray PA view: 1. Horizontal fluid level 2. Increased radiolucency above horizontal level 3. Homogenous opacity below horizontal level 4. Shifting of trachea and cardiac shadow towards opposite side.
Rupture of subpleural lung abscess	Blood routine examination
Chest injury	Mantoux test
A/c pulmonary infarction	
Following cardiac surgery	
During aspiration of fluid in pleural effusion	
Secondary infection of pneumothorax	

Differential diagnosis	Treatment
Pyopneumothorax	Water seal drainage
Pleural effusion	Antituberculosis chemotherapy
Herniation of stomach in thorax	Proper antibiotics
Large lung abscess partially filled by exudates	Surgery in resistant cases

Features	Pleural effusion	Hydropneumothorax
Percussion note above fluid level	Skodaic resonance	Tympanitic
Shifting dullness	Absent	Present
Coin sound in upper chest	Absent	May be present
Succussion splash	Absent	Present
Horizontal fluid level on percussion	Absent	Present
Upper border of fluid level	Bronchial breath sound Bronchophony and whispering pectoriloquy may be heard	Diminished vocal resonance + Vesicular breath sounds

Pyopneumothorax

Clinical Features

1. Toxic and prostrated
2. Hectic rise of temperature with rigor and chills
3. Development of clubbing
4. Tachycardia
5. Intercostals tenderness
6. Signs of hydropneumothorax.

Treatment

Aspiration of pus by a wide bore needle through intercostal space over the area of maximum dullness.

Consolidation

Symptoms

1. High fever with chills and rigor
2. Malaise and headache
3. Pain on left side of the chest and dyspnea
4. Cough with purulent sputum.

General Examination

1. Patient looks toxic and ill
2. Decubitus—propped up at 45°
3. Cyanosis—absent
4. *Pulse*: Respiration—2:1
5. Herpes labialis present.

Inspection

1. Diminished movements on affected side (lower part and lateral aspect of chest)
2. No fullness or flattening of chest
3. Absence of intercostal suction
4. Accessory muscles working.

Palpation

1. Restricted movement on affected side towards the affected side
2. Trachea and apex beat-N
3. Vocal fremitus increased
4. Friction fremitus—lower back.

Percussion

Woody dullness on affected side.

Auscultation

1. Tubular breath sounds
2. Increased vocal resonance
3. Egophony
4. Pleural rub
5. Absence of rhonchi and creps.

Management

1. **Investigations**
   a. Blood examination
   b. Sputum examination
   c. Blood culture
   d. X-ray chest PA and lateral view
   e. Serological test
   f. Nose and throat swab
   g. Pleural fluid
   h. Blood gas analysis
   i. CT scan of thorax
   j. Bronchoscopy
   k. Lung biopsy.
2. **Treatment**
   a. Rest and nutritious diet
   b. Antibiotics after C and S
   c. Oxygen inhalation
   d. Cough suppression by methadone, pholcodine
   e. Hydrocortisone.

Differential Diagnosis of Consolidation

1. Pleural effusion
2. Collapse of lung
3. Bronchogenic carcinoma
4. Pulmonary tuberculosis
5. Pulmonary infarction.

Complications of Consolidation

1. Delayed resolution
2. Lung abscess
3. Pleural effusion
4. Empyema thoracis
5. Pyopneumothorax
6. Pneumatocele
7. Fibrosis of lung
8. Respiratory failure.

Neurological complications	CVS complications
Meningism	Myocarditis
Meningitis	Endocarditis
Cerebral abscess	Pericarditis
	Peripheral circulatory failure

Collapse

Symptoms

General examination

1. Dyspnea, orthopnea
2. Central cyanosis
3. Clubbing
4. Tachypnea.

Inspection

1. Flattening of chest and supraspinatus area
2. Crowding of ribs
3. Restricted movements on affected side
4. Drooping of shoulder
5. Shifting of apical impulse
6. Kyphoscoliosis resulting from fibrosis.

Palpation

1. Shifting of trachea and apex beat
2. Movement of chest diminished
3. Vocal fremitus—diminished.

Percussion

Impaired resonance or dull note.

Auscultation

1. Collapse with obstructed bronchus or fibrosis
   a. Diminished vesicular breath sounds
   b. Decreased vocal resonance
   c. Fine creps and rhonci in fibrosis
   d. Rhonchi and creps are absent in collapse with obstructed bronchus
2. Collapse with patent bronchus
   a. Tubular breath sounds
   b. Bronchophony with whispering pectoriloquy
   c. Coarse crepitations.

Management

1. **Investigations**
   a. Blood examination
   b. Chest X-ray
   c. Lung function test
   d. Bronchoscopy
   e. Lung biopsy.
2. **Treatment**
   a. IV fluids
   b. Assisted ventilation in respiratory failure
   c. Analgesics for pleural pain
   d. Postural drainage and chest physiotherapy.

Etiology of Collapse

Upper lobe fibrosis (SSARRP)

1. Silicosis
2. Sarcoidosis
3. Ankylosing spondylitis
4. Radiation
5. Rheumatoid arthritis
6. Pulmonary tuberculosis.

Lower lobe fibrosis (BLAF)

1. Bronchiectasis
2. Loeffler's syndrome
3. Asbestosis
4. Fibrosing alveolitis.

Bronchiectasis

Persistent and irreversible dilatation and distortion of medium sized bronchi (5th - 9th generation) more than 2 mm.

Symptoms

1. Cough with sputum, hemoptysis, pleuritic pain, dyspnea, recurrent pneumonias
2. Systemic symptoms—fever, weight loss, anemia
3. O/E—pallor +, clubbing +, febrile.

Examination of Chest

1. Vesicular breath sounds
2. B/l basal coarse leathery crepitations.

Management

1. **Investigations**
   a. Blood picture—anemia, raised ESR
   b. Urine examination—proteinuria with amyloidosis
   c. ABG—respiratory alkalosis or hypoxemia.

Complications

a. Hemoptysis
b. Pneumonia
c. Lung abscess
d. Empyema
e. Septicemia
f. Osteomylitis
g. Amylodosis
h. Brain abscess
i. Aspergillosis
j. Cor pulmonale
k. Respiratory failure
l. Hypoproteinemia.

2. **Treatment**
   a. Postural drainage
   b. Antibiotic therapy, surgical treatment (Rx)
   c. Bronchiectasis sicca—hemoptysis without sputum production. Seen in upper lobe TB.

Bronchogenic Carcinoma

Lung Carcinoma

1. MC variety of lung carcinoma in India - Squamous cell carcinoma
2. MC variety in the world - Adenocarcinoma
3. MC variety in young patients - Adenocarcinoma
4. Histological variety that cavitates - Squamous cell carcinoma
5. MC histological variety to metastasize - Small cell carcinoma
6. Ca which metastasize to opposite lung - Adenocarcinoma
7. Clubbing is least common in - Small cell carcinoma
8. Gynecomastia is seen in - Large cell carcinoma
9. Most common site for metastasis from ca lung - Brain
10. Variety most responsive to chemo and RT - Small cell carcinoma
11. Variety that is central in location - Squamous cell and small cell carcinoma

12. Variety which is peripheral in location - Adenocarcinoma
13. Variety with best prognosis - Squamous cell carcinoma.

Common Types

1. Squamous cell carcinoma or epidermoid
2. Small cell carcinoma or oat cell carcinoma
3. Large cell carcinoma
4. Adenocarcinoma.

Predisposing Factors

1. Smoking
2. Asbestos exposure
3. Occupational hazards
4. Air pollution
5. Familial predisposition
6. History of COPD, diffuse pulmonary fibrosis, scleroderma, sarcoidosis.

Clinical Features

1. Cough
2. Hemoptysis
3. Dyspnea
4. Pancoast tumor
5. Symptoms due to SVC obstruction
6. Recurrent laryngeal nerve palsy
7. Dysphagia.

Investigations

Specific

1. *X-ray chest*: Hilar enlargement, collapse, pleural effusion, mediastinal widening
2. Bronchoscopy
3. *Sputum cytology*: Malignant cells
4. *Biopsy and histopathological examination*: Parenchymal biopsy by bronchoscopy, pleural biopsy in pleural effusion and lymph node biopsy.

Nonspecific

1. LFT
2. USG abdomen
3. CT -brain, abdomen, thorax.

Treatment (Depend Upon the Stage)

Surgery/chemotherapy/radiotherapy.

Ectopic hormones produced by lung carcinoma

Hormones produced	Type of cancer	Symptoms produced
ACTH	Small cell carcinoma	Cushing syndrome and hypokalemia is the most common symptom
SIADH or atrial natriuretic peptide	Small cell carcinoma	Induces hyponatremia
Parathyroid hormone or PTH related peptide	Squamous cell carcinoma	Induces hypercalcemia and hypophosphatemia
Calcitonin	Small cell carcinoma	Hypocalcemia
Gonadotropins	Small cell carcinoma	Gynecomastia

Adenocarcinoma is not related to smoking.

Differentiating features in certain lung diseases

Conditions	Percussion	Breath sound	Voice transmission	Adventitious sound
Normal	Resonant	Vesicular lung base	Normal	Absent
Foreign body aspiration	Hyper-resonant	Decreased		
Aspiration pneumonia	Dull	Decreased	Decreased	Absent
Asthma	Hyper-resonant	Vesicular	Normal	Wheezing
Pleural effusion	Dull	Decreased	Decreased	Absent or pleural rub
Pneumothorax	Hyper-resonant	Decreased	Decreased	Absent or pleural rub
Emphysema	Hyper-resonant	Decreased	Decreased	Absent or wheezing
Interstitial lung disease	resonant	Vascular	Normal	Crackles

Accessory Muscles of Respiration (PASS SALT)

1. **P**ectoralis major
2. **A**lae nasae
3. **S**ternomastoid
4. **S**calene
5. **S**erratus anterior
6. **A**bdominal muscles
7. **L**atissimus dorsi
8. **T**rapezius.

Cyanosis: A dark bluish or purplish discolouration of the skin or/and mucous membrane due to deficient oxygenation of the blood which becomes evident when reduced Hb in the blood exceeds 5 gm/100 mL.

Clubbing: It is selective bulbous enlargement of the distal segment of a digit due to soft tissue proliferation.

Wheeze: The sound made by air passing through the fauces, glottis or narrowed tracheobronchial airways in difficult breathing.

Stridor: A high pitched noisy respiration like the blowing of wind due to respiratory obstruction in the trachea or larynx.

Hemoptysis

It is the expectoration of blood or bloody sputum.

Types of hemoptysis

1. Frank hemoptysis—is the expectoration of blood only. Massive and fatal blood loss may occur. Frank hemoptysis daily suggests bronchogenic carcinoma
2. Hemoptysis in suppurative lung disease—large quantities of foul smelling sputum and blood suggests suppurative lung disease
3. Spurious hemoptysis—hemoptysis present secondary to upper respiratory tract infection, above the level of larynx
4. Pseudohemoptysis—is due to pigment prodigiosin produced by gram-negative organism (*Serratia marcescens*)
5. Endemic hemoptysis—present in infections with *Paragonimus westermani.*

Severity of hemoptysis

Mild	:	< 100 mL blood loss per day
Moderate	:	100 to 150 mL blood loss per day
Severe	:	Up to 200 mL blood loss per day
Massive	:	> 500 mL blood loss per day (or) rate of blood loss > 150 mL/hr (or) 100 mL blood loss per day for more than 3 days.

Dyspnea

It is defined as the undue awareness of respiratory effort or of the need to increase the effort.

Grading of dyspnea

Grade 1	:	No limitation of activities with ordinary physical work, i.e. asymptomatic though the patient is suffering from organic heart disease.
Grade 2	:	No limitation under resting condition but symptoms appear on ordinary activity.
Grade 3	:	Limitation of activities on mild exertion or less than ordinary activity.
Grade 4	:	Limitation of activities at rest, restricting the patient to bed or chair.

Breath Sounds

1. **Normal—vesicular:** Produced by airflow in the large airways and larynx and altered by passage through the small airways before reaching the stethoscope. Often described as rustling. Heard especially well in inspiration and early expiration
2. **Bronchial breathing:** It is caused by an increased density of matter in the peripheral lung allowing sound from the larynx to the stethoscope unchanged. Has a hollow, blowing quality, heard equally in inspiration and expiration, often with a brief pause between
3. **Conditions:** Consolidation, lung abscess, dense fibrosis and at the upper border of a pleural effusion.

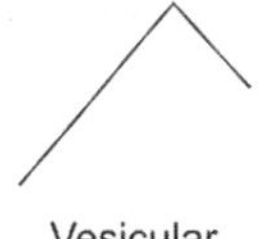

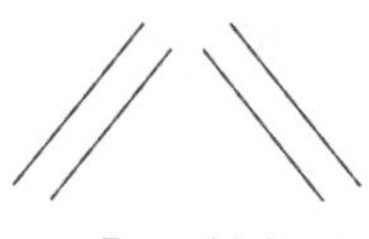

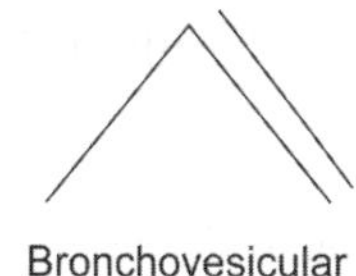

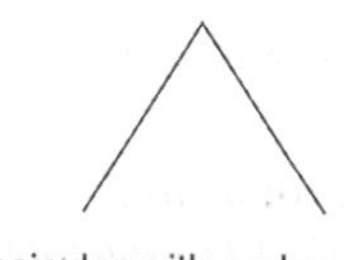

Breath sounds

Types

1. **Tubular:** High pitched. Consolidation, partial collapse and above the level of pleural effusion.
2. **Cavernous:** Low pitched. Cavity.
3. **Amphoric:** Low pitched with high pitched overtone. Thin walled cavity, tension pneumothorax.

Added Sounds

Wheeze (Rhonchi): Musical whistling sounds caused by narrowed airways.

Heard easier in expiration.

Different caliber airways = different pitch note as asthma and COPD can cause a chorus of notes termed **polyphonic wheeze**.

Monophonic wheeze indicates a single airway is narrowed, usually by a foreign body or carcinoma.

Crackles (Crepitations, rales): Caused by air entering collapsed airways and alveoli producing an opening snap. Heard in inspiration.
Coarse crackles made by larger airways opening and sound like the snap and pop of a certain breakfast cereal.

Causes: Fluid or infection.
Fine crackles occur later in inspiration. The sounds can be reproduced by rolling the hair at your temples between the thumb and forefinger.

Causes: Fluid, infection or fibrosis (particularly at lung bases).
Crackles are often a normal finding at the lung bases, If so, they will clear after asking the patient to cough.

Rub: Creaking sound likened to the bending of new leather. Heard at the height of inspiration. Caused by inflamed pleural surfaces rubbing against each other.

Causes: Pneumonia, pulmonary embolism with infarction.

Differences between pleural rub and crepitation

Pleural rub	Crepitation
Continuous	Interrupted
Do not disappear with cough	May disappear with cough
Superficial	Deep
Scratchy leathery char	Bubbling character
Throughout cycle	During inspiration mainly
Localized	Not localized
Associated with pain	Not usually associated with pain

Bronchophony: The loud sound appears to be produced at the ear piece of the stethoscope, e.g. consolidation, above the level of pleural effusion, cavity communicating with bronchus
Whispering pectoriloquy: Whispered voice is transmitted without distortion so that the individual syllables are recognized clearly, e.g. pneumonic consolidation
Egophony: Voice sound has nasal quality due to high pitch, e.g. consolidation, above the level of pleural effusion, cavity.

Pancoast Syndrome

It is caused by either a superior sulcus tumor or superior sulcus infiltrative disorder, e.g. upper lobe pulmonary tuberculosis.

Components of the syndrome are:
1. Compression of C8, T1, T2 nerve roots resulting in shoulder and arm pain
2. Compression of the cervical sympathetic chain and stellate ganglion producing Horner's syndrome
3. Erosion of adjacent ribs and vertebrae producing a constant chest pain.

External Manifestations of Respiratory Disease

1. **Asterixis (flapping tremor):** Respiratory failure
2. **Halitosis:** Suppurative lung disease
3. **Gynecomastia:** INH, digoxin, bronchogenic carcinoma
4. **Horner's syndrome:** Pancoast tumor
5. **Small muscle wasting:** Pancoast tumor
6. External markers of tuberculosis
   a. Tinea versicolor
   b. Lupus vulgaris
   c. Erythema nodosum
   d. Scrofuloderma
   e. Epididymo-orchitis.
7. External markers of cor pulmonale
   a. Raised jugular venous pressure
   b. Pedal edema
   c. Ascites
   d. Liver enlargement.

Dermatological Manifestations of Tuberculosis

1. Erythema nodosum
2. Scrofuloderma
3. Lupus vulgaris
4. Phlycten
5. Choroid tubercles
6. Tinea versicolor
7. Chemosis
8. Horner's syndrome
9. Bitot's spot
10. Poncet's arthritis.

Special Signs in a Cavity within a Lung

1. Post-tussive crepitations
2. Post-tussive suction
3. Cracked pot sound on percussion over empty cavity.

Traube's space (Boundaries)

Right - Left lobe of liver
Left - Spleen
Above - Left dome of diaphragm and left lung (6th rib)
Below - Left lower costal margin

Traube's space is dull in the following conditions

1. Carcinoma involving fundus of stomach
2. CA fundus of stomach
3. Massive spleen
4. Food in stomach
5. Left sided pleural effusion
6. Enlarged left lobe of liver
7. Situs inversus totalis
8. Achalasia cardia.

Types of respiratory failures

Type 1 respiratory failure	Type 2 respiratory failure
PaO_2: Low (<60 mm Hg)	PaO_2: Decreased(<60 mm Hg)
$PaCO_2$: Normal or low (<=49 mm Hg)	$PaCO_2$: Increased (>49 mm Hg)
$PA\text{-}aO_2$: Increased	$PA\text{-}aO_2$: Normal
This type is caused by conditions which affect diffusion like: 1. Parenchymal diseases (V-Q mismatch) 2. Disease of vasculature or shunt 3. Interstitial lung disease.	This type is caused by conditions causing hypoventilation as in: 1. Obstructive lung disease 2. Decreased central respiratory drive 3. Weakness of respiratory muscles

Pulmonary function tests in obstructive lung disease

Forced expiratory vital capacity (FEVc)	Normal to slightly decreased
Forced expiratory volume in 1 sec (FEV1)	Decrease out of proportion to FVC
FEV1/FVC	Decreased can be as low as 20–30%
Peak expiratory flow rate	Decreased
Total lung capacity	Increase
Residual volume	Increase
Functional residual capacity	Higher

Pulmonary function tests in restrictive lung disease

Forced vital capacity (FVC)	Decreased more than obstruction
Forced expiratory volume in 1 sec (FEV1)	Decreased in proportion to FVC
FEV1/FVC	Near normal or increased
Forced mid expiratory flow rate	Reduced
Total lung capacity	Decreased
Residual volume	Generally decreased
Functional residual capacity	Higher

Pulmonary embolism

Symptoms	Signs
Dyspnea (Most common)	Tachypnea (Most common)
Chest pain (2nd most common)	Cyanosis
Orthopnea	Hypotension
Fainting	Neck vein distention
Hemoptysis	Unilateral leg swelling
Cough	Fever, crackles, wheeze
Palpitations	Pleural friction rub

Diagnostic criteria of allergic bronchopulmonary aspergillosis

Main diagnostic criteria:

1. Bronchial asthma
2. Pulmonary infiltrates
3. Peripheral eosinophilia
4. Immediate wheal and flare response
5. Serum precipitins to A fumigates
6. Elevated serum IgE
7. Central bronchiectasis.

Other diagnostic criteria

1. History of brownish plugs in sputum
2. Culture of A fumigates from sputum
3. Elevated IgE and IgG class antibodies specific for A fumigates.

GASTROINTESTINAL SYSTEM

Presenting Complaint

1. Anorexia, nausea and vomiting
2. Jaundice
3. Pain abdomen
4. Hematemesis/melena
5. Diarrhea/constipation
6. Alteration in bowel habit
7. Abdominal distension/edema
8. Oliguria/hematuria
9. Neuropsychiatric manifestation in a case of liver disease.

History of Present Illness

1. Acute/insidious in onset
2. Associated-chills, headache, nausea, vomiting
3. Abdominal pain, malaise, anorexia, loose stools
4. Yellow discoloration of urine and normal color of stools
5. Itching and symptoms of obstructive jaundice during the cholestatic phase
6. Bleeding tendencies
7. Features of portal hypertension.

Past History

History of contact, blood transfusion, drugs immunization dental extraction.

Personal History

1. Alcoholism-nature of drink, frequency, amount.
2. Diet.

Immunization History

Hepatitis vaccination.

Socioeconomic Status

Details of drinking water and sanitation.

Family History

1. Similar illness in the family
2. History of neurological deficits in family (Wilson's disease)
3. History of surgery following jaundice (to rule out HS)
4. History of contact.

General Examination

1. Jaundice
2. Signs of vitamin deficiency
3. Signs of liver failure
4. Signs of chronic liver disease
5. Fetor hepaticus.

Vital Signs

Bradycardia.

GIT

1. Mild-to-moderate abdominal distension
2. Tenderness in right hypochondrium
3. Tender soft to firm liver
4. Splenomegaly—in portal hypertension
5. Ascitis—shifting dullness/fluid thrill.

Respiratory System

1. Pleural effusion
2. **Cardiovascular system:** Myocarditis, pericarditis.

Diagnosis

1. Chronic liver disease
2. Compensated/decompensated
3. *Etiology*: Alcoholic, viral, NAFLD, metabolic, etc.
4. With or without complications—portal hypertension, hepatic encephalopathy, ascites, spontaneous bacterial peritonitis, hepatorenal syndrome, hematemesis.

Investigations

Routine investigations

Blood count and indices

1. *Leukopenia and thrombocytopenia*: Portal hypertension and hypersplenism
2. Leukocytosis may occur with cholangitis, alcoholic hepatitis and hepatic abscesses

3. *Erythrocytosis*: Hepatocellular carcinoma—ectopic secretion of erythropoietin—paraneoplastic
4. *High MCV*: Alcoholic liver disease
5. *Thrombocytosis*: Active gastrointestinal hemorrhage and with hepatocellular carcinoma.

Peripheral smear
1. Normochromic normocytic anemia—gastrointestinal hemorrhage
2. Hypochromic microcytic anemia secondary iron deficiency due to chronic blood loss
3. Atypical lymphocytes are seen in infectious mononucleosis, complicated by an acute hepatitis.

Urine: Bile salts, bile pigments, urobilinogen.

Specific Investigations

Liver function test
1. Bilirubin, enzymes (ALT-liver specific, AST, ALP, GGT, albumin, globulin, total protein)
2. Alcoholic liver disease AST/ALT=2:1; ALT synthesis is inhibited by pyridoxine deficiency.

Serum markers of hepatitis
HbsAg, HBeAg for hepatitis B, HCV RNA for hepatitis C.

Ceruloplasmin: Low in Wilson's disease

Prothrombin time and INR

Diagnostic paracentesis
1. Total albumin (Plus serum albumin)
2. Amylase
3. White cell count (>250N-SBP)
4. Cytology
5. Microscopy and culture.

Liver biopsy
1. *Wilson's disease*: Dry copper weight
2. Hemochromatosis.

Imaging studies
1. Ultrasonogram
2. CT/MRI
3. MRCP/ERCP.

Chronic Liver Disease

Clinical Features

1. Sunken eyes
2. Frontal balding
3. Gynecomastia in males
4. Spider nevi
5. Testicular atrophy
6. Hollowed out temporal bone
7. Abscence of hair in chest, axilla
8. Breast atrophy in females
9. Abdomen-ascites
10. Diffuse hyperpigmentation.

Features in hand—terry's nails, clubbing, white nails, palmar erythema (liver palm), Dupuytren's contracture.

Clinical Features Specific to Alcoholic Liver Disease

1. Parotidomegaly
2. Duputyren's contracture
3. Gynecomastia
4. Testicular atrophy.

Pathological Features of Alcoholic Liver Disease

1. Alcoholic hepatitis
2. Neutrophil infiltration
3. Pericellular fibrosis
4. Fibrosis and cirrhosis
5. Lipogranuloma
6. Mallory's hyaline
7. Macrovesicular steatosis
8. Central hyaline sclerosis.

Clinical Syndromes of Alcoholic Liver Disease

Fatty liver
1. Asymptomatic abnormal liver biochemistry
2. Normal/large liver.

Alcoholic hepatitis

1. Jaundice
2. Malnutrition
3. Hepatomegaly
4. Features of portal hypertension (e.g. ascites, encephalopathy).

Cirrhosis stigmata of chronic liver disease

1. Large, normal or small liver
2. Ascites/varices/encephalopathy
3. Hepatocellular carcinoma.

Eye Signs in Liver Disease

1. **K**ayser-Fleischer rings
2. **I**cterus
3. **S**ubconjunctival hemorrhage
4. **S**unflower cataract.

Common Causes of Elevated Serum Transaminases

Minor elevation (< 100 U/l)

1. Chronic hepatitis C
2. Chronic hepatitis B
3. Hemochromatosis
4. Fatty liver disease.

Moderate elevation (100–300 U/l)

1. Causes of minor elevation
2. Alcoholic hepatitis
3. Nonalcoholic steatohepatitis (NASH)
4. Autoimmune hepatitis
5. Wilson's disease.

Major elevation (> 300 U/l) drug toxicity

1. Paracetamol overdose
2. Acute viral hepatitis
3. Autoimmune liver disease
4. Ischemic liver
5. Toxins, e.g. amanita phalloides poisoning.

Causes of Ascites

Common causes

1. Malignant disease
   a. Hepatic
   b. Peritoneal.
2. Cardiac failure.
3. Hepatic cirrhosis.

Other causes

1. Hypoproteinemia
   a. Nephrotic syndrome
   b. Protein-losing enteropathy
   c. Malnutrition.
2. Hepatic venous occlusion
   a. Budd-Chiari syndrome
   b. Veno-occlusive disease.
3. Pancreatitis
4. Lymphatic obstruction
5. Infection
   a. Tuberculosis
   b. Spontaneous bacterial peritonitis.

Rare causes

1. Meigs' syndrome
2. Vasculitis
3. Hypothyroidism
4. Renal dialysis.

Grading of Ascites

+	Detectable only by careful examination
++	Easily detectable but of relatively small volume
+++	Obvious ascites but not tense
++++	Tense ascites

Fluid thrill	> 1200 mL
Shifting dullness	> 500 mL
Puddle's sign	120 mL
USG abdomen	30 mL

Ascitic fluid: Appearance and analysis

Cause	Appearance
Cirrhosis	Clear, straw-colored or light green
Malignant disease	Bloody
Infection	Cloudy
Biliary communication	Heavy bile staining
Lymphatic obstruction	Milky-white (Chylous)

Management of Ascites

1. Sodium and water restriction
2. **Diuretic drugs:** Spironolactone (100–400 mg/day) is the drug of choice, loop diuretics, e.g. furosemide
3. **Paracentesis:** Large-volume paracentesis with intravenous albumin or another plasma expander
4. **Peritoneovenous (LeVeen) shunt:** The peritoneovenous shunt is a long tube with a nonreturn valve running subcutaneously from the peritoneum to the internal jugular vein in the neck, which allows ascitic fluid to pass directly into the systemic circulation
5. Transjugular intrahepatic portosystemic stent shunt (TIPSS).

Spontaneous Bacterial Peritonitis (SBP)

SBP presents with abdominal pain, rebound tenderness, absent bowel sounds and fever in a patient with obvious features of cirrhosis and ascites.
Ascitic fluid—cloudy fluid, neutrophil count > 250 × 106/L.

Treatment
1. Broad-spectrum antibiotics, such as cefotaxime
2. Recurrence of SBP reduced by prophylactic quinolones such as norfloxacin (400 mg daily) or ciprofloxacin (250 mg daily).

Cirrhosis

Cirrhosis is defined as an irreversible chronic injury of the hepatic parenchyma and includes extensive fibrosis in association with the formation of regenerative nodules.

Morphological classification
1. Micronodular cirrhosis (Laënnec's cirrhosis)
2. Macronodular cirrhosis (postnecrotic or viral)
3. Mixed type.

Etiopathological classification
1. Alcoholic cirrhosis or Laennec's cirrhosis
2. Postnecrotic or postviral cirrhosis
3. Biliary cirrhosis
4. Cardiac cirrhosis
5. Metabolic cirrhosis
6. Miscellaneous.

Causes of Cirrhosis

1. Alcohol.
2. Chronic viral hepatitis (B or C) Nonalcoholic fatty liver disease.

Immune
1. Primary sclerosing cholangitis
2. Autoimmune liver disease.

Biliary
1. Primary biliary cirrhosis
2. Cystic fibrosis.

Genetic
1. Hemochromatosis
2. α1-antitrypsin deficiency
3. Wilson's disease.

Cryptogenic (Unknown)

Clinical Features of Hepatic Cirrhosis

1. Hepatomegaly (although liver may also be small)
2. Jaundice
3. Ascites.

Circulatory changes: Spider telangiectasia, palmar erythema, cyanosis.

Endocrine changes
1. Loss of libido, hair loss
2. *Men*: Gynecomastia, testicular atrophy, impotence
3. *Women*: Breast atrophy, irregular menses, amenorrhea.

Hemorrhagic tendency: Bruises, purpura, epistaxis, menorrhagia.

Portal hypertension
1. Splenomegaly, collateral vessels, variceal bleeding, fetor hepaticus
2. Hepatic (portosystemic) encephalopathy.

Other features: Pigmentation, digital clubbing.

Child-Pugh classification of prognosis in cirrhosis

Score	1	2	3
Encephalopathy	None	Mild	Marked
Bilirubin (μmol/L)	< 34 (2 mg/dL)	34–50 (2–3 mg/dL)	> 50 (3 mg/dL)
In primary biliary cirrhosis and sclerosing cholangitis	< 68	68-170	> 170
Albumin (g/L)	> 35	28–35	< 28
Prothrombin time (Prolonged)	< 4	4–6	> 6
Ascites	None	Mild	Marked

Add the individual scores: < 7 = Child's A; 7–9 = Child's B; > 9 = Child's C
* To convert bilirubin in μmoL/L to mg/dL, divide by 17.

Complications of Cirrhosis

1. Portal hypertension
2. Ascites
3. Hepatic encephalopathy
4. Spontaneous bacterial peritonitis
5. Hepatorenal syndrome
6. Hepatocellular carcinoma
7. Coagulopathy.

Treatment

1. Alcohol should be forbidden
2. Diet-enriched with protein and amino acids
3. Avoid hepatoxic drugs
4. Management of complications.

Portal Hypertension

Features

1. Splenomegaly
2. Ascites
3. Collateral formation-varices
4. Fetor hepaticus—mercaptans passing directly to lungs due to shunting.

Causes of Portal Hypertension

Extrahepatic postsinusoidal
Budd-Chiari syndrome.

Intrahepatic postsinusoidal

Veno-occlusive disease.

Sinusoidal

1. Cirrhosis
2. Cystic liver disease
3. Partial nodular transformation of the liver
4. Metastatic malignant disease.

Intrahepatic presinusoidal

1. Schistosomiasis
2. Sarcoidosis
3. Congenital hepatic fibrosis
4. Vinyl chloride
5. Drugs.

Extrahepatic presinusoidal

1. Portal vein thrombosis due to sepsis
2. Abdominal trauma, including surgery
3. Malignant disease of pancreas or liver
4. Pancreatitis
5. Congenital.

Complications of Portal Hypertension

1. Variceal bleeding esophageal, gastric, other (rare)
2. Congestive gastropathy
3. Hypersplenism
4. Ascites
5. Renal failure
6. Hepatic encephalopathy.

Major sites of collaterals

1. Esophageal and gastric varices (Left gastric vein and short gastric vein join with the intercostals, diaphragmatic, esophageal and azygous veins of the caval system)
2. Hemorrhoids (Superior hemorrhoidal vein of the portal system to middle and inferior hemorrhoidal veins of the caval system)
3. Caput medusae (Remnants of the umbilical circulation of the fetus present in the falciform ligament may form a large paraumbilical vein).

Hepatic Encephalopathy

Features

1. Altered sleep rhythm
2. Lack of family and social concern
3. Improper handwriting
4. Intellectual deterioration
5. Altered sensorium
6. Fetor hepaticus—pungent smell due to mercaptans
7. Flapping tremor
8. Contructional apraxia.

Differential Diagnosis of Hepatic Encephalopathy

1. Subdural hematoma
2. Drug or alcohol intoxication
3. Delirium tremens
4. Wernicke's encephalopathy
5. Primary psychiatric disorders
6. Hypoglycemia
7. Neurological Wilson's disease.

Clinical Grading of Hepatic Encephalopathy

Clinical grade	Clinical signs
Grade 1	Poor concentration, slurred speech, slow mentation, disordered sleep rhythm
Grade 2	Drowsy but easily rousable, occasional aggressive behavior, lethargic
Grade 3	Marked confusion, drowsy, sleepy but responds to pain and voice, gross disorientation
Grade 4	Unresponsive to voice, may or may not respond to painful stimuli, unconscious

Factors Precipitating Hepatic Encephalopathy

1. **A**lcohol, aspiration pneumonia
2. **B**leeding
3. **C**onstipation
4. **D**rugs, dehydration, diuretics
5. **E**xcessive protein
6. **F**luid paracentesis
7. **S**urgery
8. **H**ypokalemia
9. **I**nfection.

Management—Evacuation and Sterilize Bowel

1. Identify and remove the possible precipitating causes—drugs, constipation or electrolyte imbalance, diuretics
2. Give purgation and enemas to empty the bowels of nitrogenous substances. Lactulose and lactilol maintain nutrition with adequate calories
3. Do not restrict protein for more than 48 hours
4. Give antibiotics. Rifaximin is mainly unabsorbed and well tolerated long-term
5. Give intravenous fluids
6. Treat any infection
7. Increase protein in the diet to the limit of tolerance as the encephalopathy improves.

Viral Hepatitis

Signs and Symptoms

1. Anorexia, nausea and vomiting
2. Jaundice
3. HSM
4. Arthralgia, myalgia and malaise
5. Headache
6. Fever
7. Pharyngitis, cough and coryza
8. Fatigue
9. Dark urine and clay colored stools.

Investigations

1. Blood R/E—Hb, TC, DC, ESR
2. Liver function test—bilirubin total and direct, SGOT, SGPT, ALP, albumin and total protein, A:G ratio
3. Prothrombin time
4. Urine and stool examination
5. USG, CT abdomen
6. Liver biopsy, fundoscopy—KF ring-Wilson's disease.

Serological test

HbsAg - Hepatitis B
Anti-HAV - Hepatitis A
Anti-HCV - Hepatitis C

Order of appearance of antigens and antibodies (Sage with canes)
HbsAg; HbcAg; antibody C; antibody E; antibody S

Treatment

1. Bed rest—reassure the patient
2. Diet—low fat, high CHO, high caloric diet, plenty of oral fluids
3. Hepatoprotective drugs.

Symptomatic Rx

1. Antiemetics—domperidone
2. Vitamins—parenteral injection of vitamin K
3. Sever vomiting and fluid loss—10% dextrose drip
4. Cholestyramine for intense pruritus.

Differential Diagnosis

1. Hepatic amebiasis
2. Alcoholic hepatitis
3. Carcinoma of liver
4. Drug induced hepatitis
5. Hemolytic jaundice
6. Cirrhosis of liver
7. IMN
8. Weil's disease
9. Yellow fever.

Complications

1. Serum sickness syndrome
2. Fulminant hepatitis
3. Cholestatic viral hepatitis
4. Relapsing hepatitis
5. Posthepatitis syndrome
6. Cirrhosis of liver
7. Hepatocellular carcinoma
8. Polyarteritis nodosa.

Treatment of Hepatitis

1. *Hepatitis B treatment*: Lamivudine at 100 mg/day orally, adefovir dipivoxil, interferon alpha
2. *Hepatitis C treatment*: Antiviral therapy+Interferon
3. *Icterus*: Yellowish discoloration of skin, mucous membrane and sclerae due to increased levels of bile pigments in the blood.

Types of jaundice

1. Hepatocellular jaundice (hepatic)
2. Hemolytic (prehepatic)
3. Obstructive (posthepatic).

Types of congenital jaundice

1. Crigler-Najjar syndrome (type 1)
2. Crigler-Najjar syndrome (type 2)
3. Gilbert's syndrome
4. Dubin-Jonson syndrome
5. Rotor's syndrome.

Edema—an accumulation of excessive amount of fluid in the interstial fluid
Melena—the passage of dark colored tarry stools due to the presence of blood altered by the intestinal juices
Hematemesis—is defined as the vomiting of fresh blood, either bright red or of coffee ground character
Hematochezia—is the passage of red or maroon blood from the rectum. Usually signifies bleeding from a source distal to the ligament of treitz. It can also occur from massive upper GI bleed from esophagus, stomach and duodenum.

Causes of Hemochromatosis

Primary hemochromatosis

1. Hereditary hemochromatosis
2. Congenital aceruloplasminemia
3. Congenital atransferrinemia.

Secondary iron overload

1. Parenteral iron-loading (e.g. repeated blood transfusion)
2. Iron-loading anemia (Thalassemia, sideroblastic anemia, pyruvate kinase deficiency)
3. Liver disease
4. Dietary iron overload (Prolonged oral iron therapy).

Complex iron overload juvenile hemochromatosis

1. Neonatal hemochromatosis
2. Alcoholic liver disease
3. Porphyria cutanea tarda
4. African iron overload (Bantu siderosis).

Hepatosplenomegaly

Causes of Hepatosplenomegaly

HSM with recurrent fever

1. Typhoid
2. Leptospirosis/DHF
3. Brucellosis
4. IMN
5. Tuberculosis
6. Histiocytosis syndrome
7. Leukemia
8. HIV
9. Chronic hepatitis.

HSM with jaundice/recurrent jaundice

1. Chronic liver disease–chronic hepatitis
2. Cirrhosis with activity
3. Congenital hepatic fibrosis
4. Caroli's disease
5. Hemolytic jaundice.

HSM with petechiae and purpura

1. Leukemia
2. Septicemia with DIC.

HSM with recurrent GI bleed

Portal hypertension—EHPO, NCPF, cirrhosis.

HSM with Pallor

1. Hemoglobinopathies
2. Leukemias
3. Portal hypertension
4. Malaria
5. CLD
6. Hemolytic anemia
7. DHF.

HSM failure to thrive

1. HIV
2. Disseminated TB
3. Langerhans histiocytosis.

HSM with renal involvement

1. Wilson's disease
2. Tyrosinemia
3. Type B chronic liver disease
4. Leptospirosis
5. Leukemia
6. Hereditary fructose intolerance
7. Microhamartoma
8. Congenital hepatic fibrosis with PCKD.

HSM with generalized lymphadenopathy

1. Tuberculosis
2. HIV
3. Leukemia
4. Lymphoma
5. Tangier's disease
6. Histiocytosis syndrome
7. Chronic granulomatous disease.

HSM with neurological manifestations

1. Wilson's disease
2. GSD
3. Niemann-Pick
4. Gaucher's
5. Zellweger
6. Mucolipidosis
7. Alpert's.

HSM with ascites/+ (or)- pedal edema

1. Chronic liver disease
2. Subacute hepatic failure
3. Tuberculosis
4. Lymphoma
5. Portal hypertension
6. CML.

Causes of Painful Hepatomegaly

1. Congestive cardiac failure
2. Viral hepatitis
3. Hepatic amebiasis
4. Pyemic abscess
5. Hepatoma
6. Actinomycosis
7. Secondaries
8. Budd-Chiari syndrome.

Causes of Pulsatile Liver

1. Tricuspid regurgitation
2. Tricuspid stenosis
3. Aortic regurgitation.

Causes of splenomegaly

Mild (5 cm)	Moderate (5–8 cm)	Massive (> 8 cm)
Congestive cardiac failure	Viral hepatitis	Chronic myeloid leukemia
Acute malaria	Cirrhosis	Myeloid metaplasia
Typhoid	Lymphomas	Myelofibrosis
Infective endocarditis	Leukemias	Hairy cell leukemia
Septicemia	Infectious mononucleosis	Gaucher's disease
SLE	Hemolytic anemia	Niemann-Pick disease
Rheumatoid arthritis	Splenic infarcts	Sarcoidosis
	Splenic abscess	Thalassemia major
		Chronic malaria
		Kala azar

Infections

Leptospirosis

Clinical features

Incubation period: 1–2 weeks

Four main clinical syndromes:

1. *Bacteremic leptospirosis*: Nonspecific illness—high fever accompanied by weakness, muscle pain and tenderness (especially of the calf and back), intense headache, photophobia, conjunctival congestion, diarrhea and vomiting.
2. *Aseptic meningitis*: Conjunctival congestion, Neutrophil leucocytosis, abnormal LFTs, presence of albumin and casts in the urine.

3. *Icteric leptospirosis (Weil's disease)*: Characterized by fever, hemorrhages, jaundice and renal impairment. Hepatomegaly, conjunctival congestion, transient macular erythematous rash, oliguria or anuria.
   Severe cases–Epistaxis, hematemesis and melena, or bleeding into the pleural, pericardial or subarachnoid spaces. Due to thrombocytopenia.
   Others-myocarditis, encephalitis and aseptic meningitis. Uveitis and iritis.
4. *Pulmonary syndrome*: Hemoptysis, patchy lung infiltrates on chest X-ray, and respiratory failure. Fatal cases—total bilateral lung consolidation and ARDS.

Investigations

1. *Blood count*: Polymorphonuclear leukocytosis, thrombocytopenia
2. *Creatine phosphokinase*: Elevated in severe cases
3. *Liver function test*: Raised transaminases
4. *Prothrombin time*: Prolonged
5. *The CSF in leptospiral meningitis*: Variable cellular response, a moderately elevated protein level and a normal glucose content
6. *Blood culture*: Taken before the tenth day of illness
7. Serological investigation of choice is the microscopic agglutination test (MAT)
8. *PCR*: Detect leptospiral DNA in blood and urine.

Differential diagnoses: Dengue, malaria, typhoid fever.

Treatment

1. Doxycycline 100 mg 12-hourly for 1 week
2. Intravenous benzylpenicillin is administered as 1.5 mega-units 6-hourly for 1 week
3. Parenteral ceftriaxone 1 g daily—equally effective as penicillin
4. *Renal failure*: Peritoneal dialysis or hemodialysis—life-saving.

Typhoid Fever

Clinical features

First week : Fever, headache, myalgia, relative bradycardia, constipation, diarrhea, vomiting.
End of 1st week : Rose spots on trunk, splenomegaly, cough, abdominal distension, diarrhea.
End of 2nd week : Delirium, complications, then coma and death (if untreated).

Investigations

1. Blood count: Leukopenia
2. Blood culture
3. The Widal reaction detects antibodies.

Treatment

1. The fluoroquinolones remain the drugs of choice (Ciprofloxacin 500 mg 12-hourly) for 14 days
2. The chronic carrier should be treated for 4 weeks with ciprofloxacin
3. Cholecystectomy—some carriers.

Complications of typhoid fever

Bowel : Perforation, hemorrhage
Septicemic foci : Bone and joint infection, meningitis, cholecystitis
Toxic phenomena : Myocarditis, nephritis.

Infectious Mononucleosis (IMN)

Caused by the Epstein-Barr virus (EBV), a gamma herpes virus.

Clinical features

1. Lymphadenopathy, especially posterior cervical
2. Pharyngeal inflammation or exudates
3. Fever
4. Splenomegaly
5. Palatal petechiae
6. Periorbital edema
7. Clinical or biochemical evidence of hepatitis
8. Nonspecific rash.

Investigations

1. *Peripheral smear*: Lymphocytes must have an atypical morphology
2. Characteristic heterophile antibody detected by the classical Paul-Bunnell titration
3. Specific EBV serology (Immunofluorescence).

Acute infection is characterized by

1. Antiviral capsid (VCA) antibodies in the IgM class
2. Antibodies to EBV early antigen (EA)
3. Absent antibodies to EBV nuclear antigen (anti-EBNA).

Treatment

1. *Symptomatic*: Aspirin gargles for sore throat
2. *If throat culture*: β-hemolytic *Streptococcus*—a course of erythromycin
3. Amoxicillin and similar semisynthetic penicillins avoided—induce a maculopapular rash in patients with IMN
4. Severe pharyngeal edema—prednisolone 30 mg daily for 5 days.

Complications of infectious mononucleosis

Common	:	Severe pharyngeal edema, antibiotic-induced rash, chronic fatigue syndrome (10%).
Uncommon neurological	:	Cranial nerve palsies, polyneuritis, transverse myelitis, meningoencephalitis.
Hematological	:	Hemolytic anemia, thrombocytopenia.
Renal	:	Glomerulonephritis, interstitial nephritis.
Cardiac	:	Myocarditis, pericarditis.
Pulmonary	:	Interstitial pneumonitis.
Rare	:	Ruptured spleen, respiratory obstruction, arthritis, agranulocytosis.

Malaria (P. falciparum; P. vivax; P. ovale; P. malariae)

Malaria is transmitted by the bite of female anopheline mosquitoes.

Causes of anemia in malaria infection

1. Hemolysis of infected red cells
2. Hemolysis of non-infected red cells (blackwater fever)
3. Dyserythropoiesis
4. Splenomegaly and sequestration
5. Folate depletion.

Clinical features

Incubation period is 10 to 21 days:

1. Fever, with general malaise, headache, vomiting, or diarrhea accompanied by rigors and drenching sweats
2. *P. vivax or P. ovale infection*: Anemia develops slowly, tender hepatosplenomegaly
3. *P. malariae infection*: In children glomerulonephritis and nephrotic syndrome
4. *P. falciparum infection*: Cerebral malaria is marked by diminished consciousness, confusion, and convulsions, often progressing to coma and death.

Blackwater fever is due to widespread intravascular hemolysis, affecting both parasitized and unparasitized red cells, giving rise to dark urine.

Some Features of Severe Falciparum Malaria

CNS	:	Cerebral malaria (Coma convulsion)
Renal	:	Hemoglobinuria (Blackwater fever) Oliguria Uremia (Acute tubular necrosis)
Blood	:	Severe anemia (hemolysis and dyserythropoiesis) Disseminated intravascular coagulation (DIC)
Respiratory	:	Acute respiratory distress syndrome
Metabolic	:	Hypoglycemia (Particularly in children) Metabolic acidosis
Gastrointestinal/liver	:	Diarrhea Jaundice Splenic rupture
Other	:	Shock-hypotensive Hyperpyrexia

Hyper-reactive Malarial Splenomegaly [Tropical Splenomegaly Syndrome (TSS)]

This is seen in older children and adults in areas where malaria is hyperendemic. It is associated with an exaggerated immune response to repeated malaria infections, and is characterized by anemia, massive splenomegaly, and elevated IgM levels. Malaria parasites are scanty or absent. TSS usually responds to prolonged treatment with prophylactic antimalarial drugs.

Diagnosis

Thick or thin blood film.

Quantitative buffy coat analysis (QBC), in which the centrifuged buffy coat is stained with a fluorochrome which 'lights up' malarial parasites.

Treatment

1. The drug of choice chloroquine in sensitive organisms
2. Drug treatment of uncomplicated malaria in adults.

Type of malaria	Drug treatment
Plasmodium vivax, P. ovale	Chloroquine 600 mg
P. malariae, CQ-sensitive *P. falciparum*	300 mg 6 hours later
	300 mg 24 hours later
	300 mg 24 hours later
CQ-resistant, SP-sensitive *P. falciparum*	*Pyrimethamine/sulfadoxine (SP)*: 3 tablets as single dose
CQ- and SP-resistant *P. falciparum*	*Quinine*: 600 mg 3 times daily for 7 days plus *Tetracycline*: 500 mg 4 times daily for 7 days or SP: 3 tablets as single dose Alternative therapies *Mefloquine*: 20 mg/kg in 2 doses 8 hours apart or *Atovaquone/Proguanil*: 4 tablets daily for 3 days or *Artemether/Lumefantrine*: 4 tablets 12-hourly for 3 days or Chlorproguanil/Dapsone
CQ, chloroquine; SP-pyrimethamine/sulfadoxine	

Hematology

Presenting Complaint and History of Present Illness

1. Nonspecific symptoms—fatigue, fevers, weight loss
2. Symptoms relating to anemia, e.g. reduced exercise capacity, recent onset of breathlessness and nature of its onset, or worsening of angina, presence of ankle edema
3. Symptoms relating to neutropenia, e.g. recurrent oral ulceration, skin infections, oral sepsis
4. Evidence of compromised immunity, e.g. recurrent oropharyngeal infection
5. Details of potential hemostatic problems, e.g. easy bruising, bleeding episodes, rashes
6. Anatomical symptoms, e.g. abdominal discomfort (Splenic enlargement or pressure from enlarged lymph nodes), CNS symptoms (from spinal compression).

Past History

Previous surgical procedures—splenectomy.

Transfusion History

History of previous transfusion(s) and their timing.

Personal History

1. Alcoholism and smoking
2. History of travel–HIV infection.

Family History

Examination

General examination

1. Weight loss, pyrexia, pallor, jaundice, cyanosis or abnormal pigmentation or skin rashes.
2. *Oral cavity*: Ulceration, purpura, gum bleeding or infiltration, and teeth.
3. *Hands and nails*: Terry nails, clubbing, white nails, palmar erythema (liver palm), Duputyren's contracture.
4. Lymphadenopathy.

Abdominal examination

1. Hepatic and/or splenic enlargement.
2. Ascitis—shifting dullness/fluid thrill.
3. Bones and joints—hemarthrosis—hemophilia. In myeloma, areas of bony tenderness and deformity.

Neurological examination

1. Fluctuations of conscious level and confusion—hyperviscosity.
2. Isolated nerve palsies—acute leukemia of neurological involvement or disease relapse.
3. Peripheral neuropathy and long tract signs—B_{12} deficiency.

Leukemia

Classification of Leukemias

1. Acute myeloblastic leukemia
2. Acute lymphoblastic leukemia
3. Chronic lymphatic leukemia
4. Chronic myeloid leukemia.

Acute leukemias

1. Acute myeloid leukemia
2. Acute lymphoblastic leukemia.

AML (FAB classification)

M0 Minimally differentiated AML
M1 AML without maturation
M2 AML with maturation
M3 Promyelocytic
M4 Myelomonocytic
M5 Monocytic
M6 Erythroleukemia
M7 Megakaryocytic leukemia.

ALL (Working classification)

L1 Small round blasts with scanty cytoplasm
L2 Pleomorphic larger blasts with more cytoplasm and prominent nucleoli
L3 Vacuolated cytoplasm with vesicular nuclei.

Presenting Complaints

1. *Exertional dyspnea*: Excessive tiredness, weakness—anemia.
2. *Recurrent infections*: Leukopenia.
3. *Bleeding and bruising*: Thrombocytopenia.
4. *Bone pain*: Marrow infiltration.

Examination

1. Pallor
2. Fever
3. Petechiae, purpura, bruises, fundal hemorrhage
4. Lymphadenopathy, hepatosplenomegaly
5. Violaceous skin lesions
6. Testicular enlargement (acute lymphoblastic leukemia)
7. Cranial nerve palsies occasionally found (Acute lymphoblastic leukemia).

Investigations

1. *Blood count*: Hb low, WBC raised, platelets low.
2. *Blood film*: Blast cells almost invariably seen, lineage identified morphologically, confirmed with immunophenotyping.
3. *Bone marrow aspirate*: Increased cellularity, reduced erythropoiesis, reduced megakaryocytes, sometimes trilineage dysplasia. Blast cells > 20% (often approaching 100%). Lineage confirmation by immunophenotyping (FISH), cytogenetic and molecular genetics.
4. *Chest X-ray*: Mediastinal widening often present in T lymphoblastic leukemia.
   For planning therapy:
   a. *Biochemistry*: Serum uric acid, renal and liver function test
   b. *Cardiac function*: ECG, ECHO to assess left ventricular function.

Principles of Treatment

Palliative therapy: It includes both chemotherapy and irradiation in addition to blood product support.

Curative therapy: Supportive care and active therapy.

Supportive care
1. Correct anemia (keep hemoglobin > 10 g/dL)—repeated transfusion of packed red cells.
2. Prevention or control of bleeding-platelet transfusions.
3. *Treatment of infection*: (a) Prophylaxis. Education of patients, relatives and staff about handwashing and isolation facilities. The use of selected antibiotics and antifungals; (b) Therapeutic management of fever with protocol/algorithm of antibiotic and antifungal combinations.
4. Control of hyperuricemia with hydration, prophylactic allopurinol and very occasionally rasburicase.

Specific treatment
1. Induction chemotherapy
2. Successful remission induction is always followed by consolidation
3. Stem cell transplantation.

Drugs commonly used in the treatment of acute leukemia

Phase	ALL	AML
Induction	Vincristine (IV)	Daunorubicin (IV)
	Prednisolone (Oral)	Cytarabine (IV)
	L-asparaginase (IM)	Etoposide (IV and oral)
	Daunorubicin (IV)	
	Methotrexate (Intrathecal)	
Consolidation	Daunorubicin (IV)	Cytarabine (IV)
	Cytarabine (IV)	Amsacrine (IV)
	Etoposide (IV)	Mitoxantrone (IV)
	Methotrexate (IV)	
Maintenance	Prednisolone (Oral)	
	Vincristine (IV)	
	Mercaptopurine (Oral)	
	Methotrexate (Oral)	

Good Prognostic Factors of A/c Leukemias
1. WBC count < 50,000/Ul
2. Female sex
3. Age between 2 and 10 years
4. Hyperdiploidy in the chromosome
5. L1 stage
6. Early remission within 4 weeks.

Poor Prognostic Factors of A/c Leukemias
1. High white cell count at presentation (> 100,000/mL)
2. Male sex
3. Age < 2 or > 10 years

4. Chromosomal abnormalities
   a. Philadelphia chromosome—poor prognosis
   b. Pre-B-cell ALL with t(1:19) translocation—poor prognosis
   c. Mature B-cell ALL with t(8:14) translocation—very poor prognosis.
5. CNS involvement
6. L2 and L3 stages.

Chronic Leukemias

Chronic myeloid leukemia (CML)

Presenting complaints

1. Exertional dyspnea due to anemia
2. Abdominal discomfort—splenomegaly
3. Weight loss
4. Fever, sweats, not due to infection
5. Headache—hyperleukocytosis
6. Bruising, bleeding (Uncommon).

Examination

1. Pallor
2. Splenomegaly, often massive
3. Lymphadenopathy, at times of blast crisis
4. Retinal hemorrhage due to leukostasis.

Investigations

1. *Blood count*: Hb low or normal, WBC raised, platelets low, normal or raised
2. *Blood film*: Neutrophilia with the whole spectrum of myeloid precursors including occasional blasts
3. *Bone marrow aspirate*: Increased cellularity, increased myeloid precursors. Cytogenetics reveals t(9;22) translocation (the Philadelphia chromosome)
4. Fluorescein—*in situ* hybridization (FISH), reverse transcriptase polymerase chain reaction (RT-PCR) or microarray expression may be needed to demonstrate the cytogenetic/molecular abnormality
5. LAP is usually reduced.

Treatment

1. Imatinib, a tyrosine kinase inhibitor that specifically blocks the enzymatic action of the BCR-ABL fusion protein is first-line treatment for the chronic phase
2. Imatinib can be continued indefinitely
3. Stem cell transplantation (SCT).

Chronic Lymphocytic Leukemia (CLL)

This is the most common leukemia, occurring predominantly in later life and increasing in frequency with advancing years.

Presenting complaints

1. Recurrent infection
2. Anemia
3. Painless lymphadenopathy
4. Splenic discomfort.

Examination

1. Pallor
2. Fever (due to infection)
3. Generalized lymphadenopathy
4. Hepatosplenomegaly, sometimes massive.

Investigations

1. *Blood count*: Hb normal or low; WBC raised, and may be very high; platelets normal or low
2. *Blood film*: Lymphocytes increased above 5×10^9/L
3. *Bone marrow*: Reflects peripheral blood, often very heavily infiltrated with lymphocytes
4. Immunophenotyping shows mainly CD19/20 + CD5+ B cells
5. *Coombs' test*: May be positive if there is hemolysis
6. *Immunoglobulins*: Low or normal.

Treatment

General/supportive treatment

1. Anemia due to hemolysis—steroids. Anemia refractory or recurrent/splenic discomfort—splenectomy
2. Anemia due to marrow infiltration—chemotherapy and blood transfusion/erythropoietin
3. Infection—antibiotics
4. Prophylactic antibiotics during chemotherapy
5. Allopurinol—hyperuricemia.

Specific treatment

1. Chlorambucil
2. Purine analogs—fludarabine, with/without cyclophosphamide or mitoxantrone (with or without steroids can induce complete or molecular complete remission
3. Rituximab in combination therapy
4. Myeloablative chemotherapy with autologous stem cell rescue and allogeneic stem cell under trial.

Hairy Cell Leukemia

Hairy cell leukemia (HCL) is a clonal proliferation of abnormal B (or very rarely T) cells which, as in CLL, accumulate in the bone marrow and spleen.
The bizarre name—due to the appearance of the cells on a blood film and in the bone marrow having an irregular outline owing to the presence of filament-like cytoplasmic projections.

Clinical features

1. Pallor
2. Fever and weight loss
3. Splenomegaly.

Blood count: Anemia, neutropenia, thrombocytopenia and low monocyte counts are found.

Treatment

1. The purine analogs 2-chloroadenosine acetate (2-CDA) (cladribine) and pentostatin specific
2. Rituximab—if no response to the above drugs.

Poor Prognostic Factors of Chronic Leukemia

1. Age > 60 years
2. Male sex
3. Persistent anemia or eosinophilia
4. Presence of additional chromosomal abnormalities (double ph, 8+, 17 q+)
5. Spleen > 10 cm below the costal margin
6. Platelets > 7 lakhs/Ul
7. Blasts > 3% in blood or > 5% in marrow
8. Basophils > 7% in blood or > 3% in marrow.

Clinicopathologic Forms of Myelodysplastic Syndrome

FAB subtypes

1. Refractory anemia (RA)/refractory cytopenia (RC)
2. Refractory anemia with ringed sideroblasts (RARS)
3. Refractory anemia with excess blasts (RAEB)
4. Refractory anemia with excess blasts in transformation (RAEBT)
5. Chronic myelomonocytic leukemia (CMML).

Lymphomas

The lymphomas are commoner than the leukemias.
There is abnormal proliferation of the lymphoid system, and occur at any site where lymphoid tissue is found.
The most common manifestation is the development of lymphadenopathy at single or multiple sites.
Lymphomas are classified into:

1. Hodgkin's lymphoma (HL)
2. Non-Hodgkin's lymphoma (NHL).

Hodgkin's Lymphoma (HL)

The hallmark of HL is the Reed-Sternberg cell.

Pathological classification of Hodgkin's lymphoma

1. Nodular lymphocyte—predominant Hodgkin's lymphoma
2. Classical Hodgkin's lymphoma
   a. Nodular sclerosis HL
   b. Lymphocyte-rich HL
   c. Mixed cellularity HL
   d. Lymphocyte-depleted HL.

Clinical features

1. Lymph node enlargement—painless and rubbery consistency
2. Enlargement of the spleen/liver
3. *'B' symptoms*: Fever, (25%) drenching night sweats, weight loss of > 10% bodyweight
4. Other constitutional symptoms, such as pruritus, fatigue, anorexia and, occasionally, alcohol-induced pain at the site of enlarged lymph nodes.

Investigations

1. *Blood count*: Normal/normochromic, normocytic anemia. Lymphopenia and eosinophilia
2. Erythrocyte sedimentation rate (ESR)—raised
3. Liver function test
4. Serum lactate dehydrogenase; raised level—adverse prognostic factor
5. *Serum uric acid*: Normal or raised
6. *Chest X-ray*: Mediastinal widening, with or without lung involvement
7. *CT scans*: Involvement of intrathoracic nodes in 70%, abdominal or pelvic lymph nodes are also found
8. CT is the investigation of choice for staging
9. PET scanning is increasingly being used
10. Bone marrow aspiration and trephine biopsy—not done. Unusually involved at initial presentation
11. Lymph node biopsy is required for a definitive diagnosis.

Treatment

Specific treatment is based on the anatomical distribution of disease, its 'bulk' and the presence or absence of 'B' symptoms.

Cotswolds modification of Ann Arbor staging classification

Stage	Description
Stage I	Involvement of a single lymph node region or lymphoid structure (e.g. spleen, thymus, Waldeyer's ring) or involvement of a single extralymphatic site
Stage II	Involvement of two or more lymph node regions on the same side of the diaphragm (hilar nodes, when involved on both sides, constitute stage II disease); localized contiguous involvement of only one extranodal organ or site and lymph-node region(s) on the same side of the diaphragm (IIE). The number of anatomic regions involved should be indicated by a subscript (e.g. II3)
Stage III	Involvement of lymph node regions on both sides of the diaphragm (III), which may also be accompanied by involvement of the spleen (IIIS) or by localized involvement of only one extranodal organ site (IIIE) or both (IIISE) III1 With or without involvement of splenic, hilar, coeliac, or portal nodes III2 With involvement of para-aortic, iliac, and mesenteric nodes
Stage IV	Diffuse or disseminated involvement of one or more extranodal organs or tissues, with or without associated lymph node involvement

Designations applicable to any disease state

A : No symptoms

B : Fever (temperature > 38°C), drenching night sweats, unexplained loss of more than 10% of body weight within the previous 6 months

X : Bulky disease (a widening of the mediastinum by more than one-third of the presence of a nodal mass with a maximal dimension greater than 10 cm)

E : Involvement of a singe extranodal site that is contiguous or proximal to the known nodal site.

'Early stage' (IA, IIA no bulk)

The treatment of choice—brief chemotherapy followed by involved field irradiation.

ABVD 2 to 4 cycles followed by involved field irradiation (20–30 Gy) has become standard care.

Advanced disease

The treatment of choice: Cyclical combination chemotherapy with or without irradiation to sites of 'bulk' disease is for all these patients.

The 'gold standard' combination is ABVD 6–8 cycles each month.
All patients with mediastinal bulk receive irradiation whether or not the CT scan returns to normal.
Infertility and second malignancy are much less common than following the previous gold standard therapy MOPP (or MVPP).
ABVD : Adriamycin, bleomycin, vinblastine, dacarbazine.
MOPP : Mustin, oncovin (vincristine), procarbazine, prednisolone
MVPP : Mustin, vinblastine, procarbazine, prednisolone.

Non-Hodgkin's Lymphoma (NHL)

These are malignant tumors of the lymphoid system classified separately from Hodgkin's lymphoma.

Classification
The WHO classification (2001) which is based on the Revised European American Lymphoma (REAL) system.

Clinical features
1. Peripheral lymphadenopathy
2. *Systemic symptoms (B symptoms)*: Fever, sweats, anorexia and weight loss
3. Extranodal presentation—more common than in HL and may involve GIT, lung, brain, testes, thyroid and skin
4. *Abdominal involvement*: Hepatosplenomegaly
5. *Skin involvement (T cell lymphomas)*: Mycosis fungoides and Sézary syndrome
6. Oropharyngeal involvement occurs rarely
7. HIV predisposes to NHL.

Investigations
1. *Complete blood count*: Normochromic, normocytic anemia, an elevated white cell count or neutropenia and thrombocytopenia are suggestive of bone marrow infiltration
2. ESR may be elevated
3. *Urea and electrolytes*: Renal impairment due to ureteric obstruction secondary to intra-abdominal or pelvic lymph node enlargement
4. Serum uric acid level may be raised
5. *Liver function test*: Abnormal if there is hepatic involvement
6. Serum lactate dehydrogenase and β2-microglobulin are prognostic indicators
7. *Serum immunoglobulins*: Decreased levels may occur with paraproteinemia
8. Chest X-ray, CT scans of chest, abdomen and pelvis. PET and gallium scans help in staging
9. Bone marrow aspirate and trephine biopsy are always performed
10. Lymph node biopsy (or Trucut needle biopsy, often under radiological guidance, in the case of surgically inaccessible nodes). Immunophenotyping and cytogenetic/molecular analysis (DNA microarray analysis), to distinguish type of NHL.

Treatment

I. **Low-grade NHL**

Indications for treatment
1. Marked systemic symptoms
2. Lymphadenopathy causing discomfort or disfigurement
3. Bone marrow failure or compression syndromes.

Radiotherapy: This can be used for localized stage I disease, which is rare.

Chemotherapy: Oral therapy with chlorambucil.

Monoclonal antibody therapy: The anti-CD20 antibody rituximab transplantation.

Studies of autologous stem cell transplantation are in progress.

II. **High-grade NHL**

Need treatment at initial presentation.

Chemotherapy: Intravenous combination chemotherapy. The CHOP regimen (Cyclophosphamide, doxorubicin, vincristine and prednisolone) remains the mainstay of therapy.

Radiotherapy: A few stage I patients without bulky disease.

Monoclonal antibody therapy: The combination of R-CHOP [CHOP chemotherapy+rituximab (R)] is currently recommended for those with stage II or greater diffuse large-cell lymphoma as first-line therapy.

Transplantation: Autologous stem cell transplantation benefits patients with relapsed chemosensitive disease.

NERVOUS SYSTEM

Hemiplegia

Paralysis of one side of body due to pyramidal tract lesion at any part from its origin up to C-5.

Types

1. Complete
2. Incomplete
3. Crossed.

Etiology

1. Congenital
2. Acquired
   a. Vascular
   b. Infective
   c. Neoplastic
   d. Demyelinating
   e. Traumatic
   f. Hysterical.

CVA/Stroke

Abrupt onset of nonconvulsive neurological deficit due to focal vascular lesions lasting longer than 24 hours.

Differential diagnosis of acute neurological deficits:

1. Todd's palsy
2. Hemiplegic migraine
3. Multiple sclerosis
4. Hypoglycemia.

Clinical Classification

1. Completed stroke
2. Stroke in evolution
3. TIA
4. RIND.

Pathophysiology

1. Infarct
   a. Opening of anastomotic channels
   b. Compensatory homeostatic changes.
   If both fails:
   a. Failure of electric functions
   b. Failure of ion pumps and cell death.
   Extent of ischemia depends on:
   a. Degree of collaterals
   b. Fever
   c. Location of occlusion
   d. BP
   e. High blood sugar.
2. Hemorrhage
   a. Toxic effect
   b. Mass effect.

Causes of thrombosis

1. Vessel wall
   a. Atherosclerosis
   b. Vasculitis.
2. Hypercoagulable states
   a. Polycythemia
   b. Thrombocytosis
   c. Apla
   d. Protein C deficiency.
3. Slow circulation
   a. Heart failure
   b. Shock.

Causes of embolism

1. Heart
   a. Nonrheumatic AF, MI, RHD
   b. Prosthetic valve
   c. Bacterial endocarditis.
2. Distal vessels
   a. Artery to artery
   b. Venous thrombosis
   c. Paradoxical emboli.
3. *Rare sources*: Lungs, bone, tumor, parasitic, amniotic fluid.

Causes of hemorrhage

1. *Intracerebral hemorrhage*: Hypertension
2. *Subarachnoid hemorrhage*: Aneurysm, arteriovenous malformation
3. *Subdural hemorrhage/Extradural hemorrhage*: Trauma.
   Major site of intra cerebral hemorrhage
   Putamen + caudate nucleus -> ganglionic hematoma

Presenting complaints

1. Weakness of one side of body
2. Facial deviation.

History of present illness

Sudden		Gradual
Embolism	– Seconds	Space occupying lesions
Hemorrhage	– Minutes to hours	
Thrombosis	– Hours	
Infective	– Hours to days	
Demyelinating	– Days to weeks	

Time of onset

1. *During sleep/soon after rising*: Thrombosis
2. *Exertion/activity*: Embolism
3. *Peak of emotion*: Hemorrhage.

Evolution and Progress

1. *Thrombosis*: Gradual/stuttering
2. *Embolic*: Maximum deficit at onset
   a. Stationary/resolve
   b. Hemorrhagic transformation.
3. *Hemorrhage*: Abrupt onset over minutes to hours
   a. Dramatic presentation
   b. Associatted with headache, convulsion, unconsciousness.

Risk factors

Nonmodifiable	: Modifiable
Age	: High BP
Gender	: Heart disease
Race	: DM
Heredity	: Hyperlipidemia
Prevention vascular events	: Smoking Alcoholism OCP

Past history

1. Similar attacks which recover completely—TIA, Todd's palsy, Hemiplegic migraine
2. HTN, DM
3. Rheumatic fever
4. TB
5. Bleeding tendency
6. Trauma
7. Intermittent claudication
8. Epilepsy.

Personal history

1. Addictions
2. Menstrual history.

Family history

1. Similar illness [in young individuals]
2. DM, HTN, migraine, epilepsy.

Drug history
OCP, aspirin, anticoagulants.

Examination
1. *Look for features of*: Atherosclerosis, infective endocarditis
2. *CVS*: Pulse, JVP, bruit, LVH, murmurs
3. *RESP*: Pulmonary edema, RESP infections
4. *GIT*: Splenomegaly in IE
5. Nervous system in detail.

Young stroke
< 40 years

Causes: Infants and children—congenital heart disease, AVM.

Young adults
1. Cardiovascular
2. Premature atherosclerosis
3. Arteritis
4. Homocystinuria
5. SLE, APLA
6. Mitochondrial cytopathy
7. Thrombophilia
8. Primary hemorrhage
9. Nephrotic syndrome
10. Cadasil.

	Thrombosis	Embolism	Hemorrhage
Age	Middle age/Elderly	Any age/Young females	> 40 years
Mode of onset	Hours	Seconds	Minutes-hours
Time of onset	During sleep/After waking	Exertion/Activity	Peak of emotion
Associated features	Mild headache, seizure, transient loss of consciousness	Convulsion	Headache, vomiting, unconsciousness
Risk factors	Atherosclerosis, HTN, cardiac insufficiency	Valvular heart disease, other sources	HTN
Evolution progress	Gradual recovery	Early complete recovery possible	Early recovery uncommon

Localization

1. Cortical
2. Subcortical
3. Internal capsule
4. Brain stem
5. Spinal cord.

Cortical

1. Frontal lobe
2. Parietal lobe (dominant)
3. Parietal lobe (nondominant)
4. Temporal lobe (dominant)
5. Temporal lobe (nondominant)
6. Occipital lobe.

Frontal lobe
1. Executive functions, movements and behavior
2. Motor area (Area 4)
3. Premotor area (Area 6)
4. Area of voluntary conjugate eye movements
5. Broca's area (Area 44)
6. Prefrontal Area
7. Paracentral lobule
8. *Prefrontal area*: Higher centre for mentality, personality and behaviour, inhibition of primitive reflexes
9. *Paracentral lobule*: Micturition control and bowel voiding
10. *Control of conjugate eye movement*: Voluntary conjugate eye movement to opp side
11. *Broca's area*: Dominant lobe, motor center for speech. Lesion—motor aphasia.

Frontal lobe lesion
1. Contralateral monoplegia, faciobrachial involvement, spastic hemiplegia (massive involvement)
2. Primitive reflexes may be present
3. Emotional lability
4. Impaired memory
5. Motor aphasia (dominant).

Parietal lobe

Concerned with:

1. *Intergration of sensory perception*: Somatosensory area (3, 2, 1)
2. *Language*: Supramarginal gyrus
3. Expression of ideas and concepts in language—angular gyrus
4. Calculation
5. Spatial awareness and orientation (nondominant)
6. Contructional skills (nondominant).

Sensory pathway lesions: Loss of sensation, absent pain, touch, temp; tingling; pins and needles.

Posterior column lesions:

1. Incoordination in dark, feeling of walking on cotton wool, exaggerated evening. It position, vibration and cortical senses. Romberg's sign (+).
2. Cortical sensation-tactile localization, 2 point discrimination, stereognosis, graphesthesia, sensory inattention
3. Sensory involvement, mild hemiparesis, homonymous inferior quadrantanopia.

Parietal dominant

1. *Acalculia, alexia, finger agnosia, right-left confusion*: Gerstmann syndrome
2. Ideomotor apraxia.

Nondominant parietal lobe

1. Constructional apraxia
2. Dressing apraxia
3. Sensory inattention.

Temporal lobe

1. Primary auditory and vestibular cortex
2. Olfactory cortex
3. Parahippocampal cortex—nonverbal memory
4. *Structures of limbic system*: Amygdala and hippocampus—processing memory and emotions
5. Wernicke's sensory aphasia (dominant)
6. Homonymous superior quadrantanopia.

Occipital lobe

1. Visual processing
2. Contralateral hemifield in primary cortex
3. Adjacent areas for visual submodalities.

Cortical lesion

1. Monoplegia, faciobrachial (UMN) contralateral side
2. Jacksonian convulsions, headache, coma
3. Cortical type of sensory loss
4. Aphasia and agraphia (dominant).

Subcortical lesion

1. Assymetrical involvement of hemiplegia
2. Involvement of thalamocortical fibers—postural sense, tactile localization, 2 point discrimination in affected limb.

Internal capsule lesion

1. Dense hemiplegia
2. Hemianesthesia
3. Homonymous hemianopia.

Brainstem lesion

1. Contralateral hemiplegia (crossed)
2. Gaze paralysis—vol eye movement towards lesion absent
3. Cranial nerve involvement—LMN
4. Midbrain (3, 4)
5. Pons (5, 6, 7, 8)
6. Medulla (9, 10, 11, 12).

Spinal cord

1. Between C1 and C5 segments, picture of Brown-Séquard syndrome
2. At level of lesion
   a. Ipsilateral motor LMN type
   b. Ipsilateral loss of all sensation.
3. Below the level of lesion
   a. Ipsilateral hemiplegia
   b. Ipsilateral deep sensory loss (postcolumn)
   c. Contralateral loss of pain and temperature
   d. Bilateral touch diminishes.

Investigations

Baseline

1. CBC, ESR
2. Blood glucose and lipid profile
3. Serum electrolytes and proteins
4. Chest X-ray
5. ECG and ECHO
6. Carotid Doppler.

Special

1. ANAs and lupus anticoagulant
2. Anticardiolipin antibodies
3. Protein C and S, antithrombin III
4. S. cholesterol
5. VDRL.

CT scan—to differentiate hemorrhagic stroke: Acute blood is white and CT detects intracerebral bleeds immediately.

Indications for immediate CT

1. On anticoagulants
2. Plan for thrombolysis/anticoagulation
3. Deteriorating conscious level/rapidly progressing defects
4. Suspected cerebellar hematoma.

Magnetic Resonance Imaging

Carotid angiography and CSF study

Management of stroke

1. General
2. Treatment of cerebral edema
3. Specific treatment
4. Physiotherapy.

General

1. Care of airway and respiration
2. Care of urinary bladder
3. Care of nutrition and fluid balance
4. Care of skin
5. Care of bowel.

Treatment of cerebral edema

1. Osmotherapy—20% mannitol 100 mL IV TDS and water restriction
2. Artificial ventilation
3. Hemicraniectomy
4. Suboccipital decompression in large cerebellar infarcts.

Specific Treatment

Ischemic stroke

1. Drugs to lower BP
   Indications
   a. BP > 185/110 mm Hg
   b. Malignant hypertension
   c. Myocardial ischemia
   d. Thrombolytic therapy.
2. Thrombolysis with r-tPA (recombinant tissue plasminogen activator)
   Indications
   a. Clinical diagnosis of stroke
   b. Onset of symptoms < 3 hours
   c. CT showing no hemorrhage
   d. Age > 18 years
   e. Dose—0.9 mg/kg IV, 10% as bolus and rest in 1 hour.
3. Antiplatelets
   a. Aspirin 300 mg
   b. Clopidogrel
   c. Ticlopidine 250 mg BD—skin rash, diarrhea, reversible neutropenia
   d. Dipyridamole—50 mg TID.
4. Anticoagulants in:
   a. Evolving stroke
   b. Cardiogenic embolic stroke
   c. Heparin—5000 IU/6th hourly.

Contraindicated in:

1. Hemorrhagic infarction
2. Bleeding disorder
3. SABE
4. Renal and hepatic failure.

Hemorrhagic stroke

1. General care
2. Antihypertensives
3. Osmotherapy and induced hyperventilation
4. Prothrombin complex, FFP, vitamin K in coagulopathy
5. Fresh platelets if thrombocytopenia
6. Surgical evacuation of hematoma.

Prevention of further stroke

1. Long-term antiplatelets
   a. Aspirin 75-300 mg daily
   b. Clopidogrel
   c. Aspirin + dipyridamole.
2. Anticoagulation in AF
3. BP lowering
4. Carotid endarterectomy in >70% stenosis or in carotid TIA.

Physiotherapy

1. Soon after neuronal shock
   a. Prevent contractures
   b. Prevent bed sores and edema
   c. Compression stockings—deep vein thrombosis (DVT)
   d. Chest physiotherapy.
2. Rehabilitation—speech and occupation therapy
3. Stroke centers.

Complications of Acute Stroke

1. Chest infection
2. Epileptic seizures
3. DVT/pulmonary embolism
4. Painful shoulder
5. Pressure sores
6. UTI
7. Constipation
8. Depression and anxiety.

Stroke

Cerebrovascular disease/stroke—rapidly evolving focal or global cerebral dysfunction of vascular origin lasting more than 24 hours or leading to death.

Major site of intracerebral hemorrhage

Putamen + caudate nucleus → Ganglionic hematoma.

Sites of Lacunar Infarcts

1. Internal capsule or the adjacent corona radiata—pure motor hemiplegia
2. Thalamus—pure hemisensory defect
3. Ventral pons—pure motor hemiplegia, dysarthria, clumsiness of hand
4. Midbrain pons—ataxia
5. Corticobulbar tract—pseudobulbar palsy.

Risk Factors

1. TIA
2. Hypertension
3. DM
4. Obesity
5. Smoking
6. History of previous stroke
7. History of CAD
8. Hyper lipidemia.

Complications

1. Death - HMGE > infaction
2. Vegetative state
3. Permanent disability
4. Infection - RSPY, urinary, bed sore
5. GI hemorrhage
6. Intracranial hemorrhage
7. Aphasia
8. Hydrocephalus.

Anatomical Localization

Muscle Diseases

1. Proximal symmetric weakness
2. No sensory loss but pain and cramping can occur
3. Normal size, no atrophy (exception—myotonic dystrophy) or fasciculation
4. Muscle tone normal or mildly decreased
5. Reflexes normal or mildly decreased.

Neuromuscular Junction

1. Fatiguability present
2. Proximal symmetric weakness increased by use
3. Waxing and waning
4. Involves face, eyes, jaw muscles more
5. Muscle normal in size no atrophy or fasciculation
6. Normal tone and DTR
7. Ankle jerk absent in Eaton-Lambert syndrome.

Peripheral Nerve Lesion

1. Distal weakness
2. Usually asymmetric
3. Atrophy and fasciculation seen
4. Negative (loss) and positive (numbness, tingling) sensory symptoms may be present
5. Autonomic nervous system involvement.

Root Diseases

1. Sharp shooting root pain along its distribution
2. Evidence of denervation
3. Myotomal distribution of weakness
4. SLR, neck rotation, straining increases the pain
5. Asymmetric weakness
6. Dermatomal sensory loss
7. Tone normal or decreased
8. DTR normal or decreased.

Spinal Cord

1. Sensory motor and reflex level present
2. Distal symmetric spatic weakness and flexor spasm
3. Sphincter disturbances (frequency, urgency and detrusor sphincter dyssynergia-UMN; retension with overflow incontinence-LMN)
4. Leg involvement more than arm
5. Loss of superficial reflexes
6. Involvement of extensor and antigravity muscles more than flexors
7. DTR +++, extensor plantar.

Brainstem

Deficits of various muscle groups

1. Combing hair - **Proximal** muscles of **UL**
2. Buttoning shirt and mixing food - **Distal** muscles of **UL**
3. Getting up from squatting, climbing stairs - **Proximal** muscles of **LL**
4. Slipping of footwears - **Distal** muscles of **LL**

Always crossed hemiplegia

1. Midbrain
   a. 3, 4 involvement
   b. History of drooping of eyelids, diplopia, difficulty in climbing stairs
   c. On examination dilated pupils, abnormality in range of eye movements.
2. Pons
   a. 5 (chief, sensory and motor), 6, 7 involvement
   b. History of decreased facial sensation, inability to chew and open mouth
   c. On examination convergent squint, gaze palsy, diplopia on looking laterally, LMN facial palsy.
3. Medulla
   a. 9, 10, 11, 12 involvement
   b. History of dysphagia, dysarthria, nasal intonation, regurgitation, inability to turn neck and shrug shoulder, difficulty in clearing mouth with tongue
   c. On examination palatal asymmetry, deviation of uvula, loss of palatal and gag reflexes, wasting and deviation of tongue, crossed sensory loss, Horner's syndrome.

	Medial	Lateral
Mid brain	3, 4	
Pons	6	5, 7, 8
Medulla	12	9, 10, 11

Lateral medullary syndrome (9, 10, 11)

Occlusion of

1. Vertebral artery
2. Posteroinferior cerebellar artery
3. Superior lateral medullary artery
4. Middle lateral medullary artery
5. Inferior lateral medullary artery.

Focal Vascular Syndromes of the Brainstem

Region	Syndrome	Vascular supply	Anatomical structure	Clinical features
Midbrain	Weber's syndrome	Branches of PCA and top of basilar artery	Oculomotor nerve fascicles	Ipsilateral 3rd nerve palsy
Midbrain tegmentum	Claude's syndrome	Branches of PCA and top of basilar artery	Cerebral peduncle; oculomotor nerve fascicles	Contralateral hemiparesis; ipsilateral 3rd nerve palsy
			Red nucleus, superior cerebellar peduncle fibers	Contralateral ataxia
Midbrain base and tegmentum	Benedikt's syndrome	Branches of PCA and top of basilar artery	Oculomotor nerve fascicles	Ipsilateral 3rd nerve palsy
			Cerebral peduncle, red nucleus, substantia nigra, superior cerebellar peduncular fibers	Contralateral hemiparesis, contralateral ataxia, tremor and involuntary movements
Medial pontine base and tegmentum	Foville's syndrome	Paramedian branches of basilar artery, ventral and dorsal territories	Corticospinal and corticobulbar tracts	Contralateral face, arm and leg weakness; dysarthria
			Facial colliculus	Ipsilateral face weakness; ipsilateral horizontal gaze palsy
Medial pontine base and tegmentum	Millard-Gubler syndrome	Paramedian branches of basilar artery, ventral and dorsal territories	Corticospinal and corticobulbar tracts, abducent fascicules, facial fascicules	Contralateral face, arm and leg weakness; dysarthria; I/L paresis of lateral rectus with diplopia; I/L paresis of upper and lower face

Cerebellum

1. History
   a. *Clumsiness of legs*: Drunken or wide based gait
   b. *Clumsiness of arms*: Targeting difficulties
   c. Scanning speech
   d. *Action*: Tremor
   e. Onset
   f. Symmetry
   g. Recurrent episodes/improving/static or worsening.
2. Etiology
   a. Alcoholism
   b. Family history
   c. Nutritional
   d. Collagen vascular diseases
   e. CNS infections
   f. Neoplasia
   g. Vaccination
   h. Toxins and drugs
   i. Hypothyroidism
   j. Raised ICT.
3. Characteristic syndromes
   a. *Flocculonodular syndrome*: Truncal ataxia and nystagmus, no intention tremor or limb ataxia
   b. *Anterior lobe syndrome*: Gait ataxia, decerebrate rigidity, UL relatively preserved, e.g. alcoholism
   c. *Post lobe syndrome*: Ipsilateral hypotonia and ataxia, dentate nucleus involvement—intention tremor.

Blood Supply of Cerebellum

1. **Posteroinferior cerebellar artery:** Intracranial branch of vertebral artery (PICA)
2. **Anteroinferior cerebellar artery:** Branch of basilar artery (AICA)
3. **Superior cerebellar artery:** Branch of basilar artery (SCA).

Angle lesions cerebellopontine

1. 5, 7, 8 CNS, SCA, AICA, superior petrosal vein territories
2. Decreased corneal reflex
3. Ataxia, vertigo, headache with diplopia, long tract signs and respiratory depression
4. Tinnitus, hearing loss, facial paresis.

Dense hemiplegia occurs at the site of merging of corticospinal tract internal capsule, peduncles, pyramid
Sensory modalities are appreciated at thalamic level, in cortical lesions, primary sensations are intact
Subcortical lesion: Patchy involvement and homonymous hemianopia, sometimes aphasia, no seizures.
Cortical lesion: Asymmetric paralysis with:

1. Aphasia
2. Cortical sensory loss
3. Apraxia
4. Convulsions
5. Agnosia and other such lobar syndromes.

Cerebral arterial occlusion

1. *ICA occlusion*: Dense hemiplegia – face + upper limb + lower limb, global aphasia
2. *MCA trunk*: Contralateral hemiplegia, hemianesthesia, global aphasia
3. *MCA upper division occlusion*: Contralateral hemiparesis, hemianesthesia, aphasia or hemineglect
4. *MCA lower division*: Wernicke's aphasia, behavioral disturbance, hemianopia
5. *ACA occlusion*: Main trunk occlusion depends on whether Hubner's artery is present or not
   a. Hubner's artery + in UMN facial, spastic upper limb, flaccid leg, motor and sensory loss
   b. No Hubner's artery – face and arm spared leg involved in flaccid paralysis with cortical sensory loss.

Combination of hemiplegia, hemianesthesia and hemianopia

1. MCA stem occlusion
2. Anterior choroidal artery occlusion
3. Hemorrhage into internal capsule.

Ataxic Hemiparesis

1. Muscle power should be > 3 to comment as ataxic hemiparesis due to involvement of frontopontocerebellar fibers
2. Site of lesion:
   a. Frontal cortex
   b. Anterior part of corona radiata
   c. Anterior limb of internal capsule.

Pure sensory stroke	Hemiplegia sparing face
PVL thalamus	Corona radiata lesion
Corona radiata	Post limb of internal capsule
Postlimb of internal capsule	Medullary pyramid

Lesions of anterior limb of internal capsule can cause

1. Pure motor hemiparesis
2. Ataxic hemiparesis
3. Speech and language disturbances
4. Confusion.

Loss of Consciousness with Stroke

Early: Vertebrobasilar stroke; CVAs associated with seizures; carotid stroke
Late: MCA striate infarct; frontotemporal infarct.

Aphasia–Analysis

Clinical features of aphasias

Aphasia	Comprehension	Repetition	Naming	Fluency
Wernicke's	Impaired	Impaired	Impaired	Preserved
Broca's	Preserved	Impaired	Impaired	Decreased
Global	Impaired	Impaired	Impaired	Decreased
Nonfluent transcortical	Preserved	Preserved	Impaired	Impaired
Fluent transcortical (sensory)	Impaired	Preserved	Impaired	Preserved

Intracerebral Hemorrhage at Various Sites

1. *Putaminocapsular hemorrhage*: Contralateral eyes deviate away from the site of the lesion, dysarthria
2. *Thalamic hemorrhage*: Contralateral hemiplegia, hemianesthesia, dysarthria, visual loss
3. *Pontine hemorrhage*: Deep coma, quadriplegia, pinpoint pupil, absent doll's, apneustic breathing, hypertension/hypotension, tachycardia
4. *Cerebellar hemorrhage*: Vomiting, ataxia, occipital headache, ipsilateral 6th and 7th nerve involvement, skew deviation, dysarthria, dysphagia and later brainstem compression
5. *Subarachnoid hemorrhage*: Causes—berry aneurysm, AVM rupture; history of sentinel headache +, neck stiffness, sudden onset of explosive headache, loss of consciousness.

Vessels involved in hemorrhages

1. Extradural hemorrhages caused by middle meningeal artery
2. Subdural hemorrhage caused by rupture of cortical bridging veins
3. Subarachnoid hemorrhage caused by rupture of berry aneurysm
4. Intracerebral hemorrhage caused by lenticulostriate branch of middle cerebral artery.

Ocular signs in intracerebral hemorrhage

1. *Putaminal hemorrhage*: Eyes are deviated to the side opposite the paralysis
2. *Thalamic hemorrhage*: Downward deviation of eyes; nonreactive pupil
3. *Pontine hemorrhage*: Eyeballs are fixed, pinpoint reactive pupil
4. *Cerebellar hemorrhage*: Eyes are deviated laterally to the side opposite the lesion; ocular blobbing may occur.

Disturbances of ocular movements

1. **Infranuclear lesions:** Sixth nerve palsy, third nerve palsy and fourth nerve palsy
2. **Supranuclear lesions:** Conjugate gaze palsies (Lateral gaze, upward gaze, downward gaze and internuclear gaze palsy) and complex supranuclear gaze palsies (convergence nystagmus)
3. **Cerebellar lesions:** Nystagmus
4. **Extrapyramidal lesions:** Slowed and interrupted smooth pursuit movements.

Common Causes of Facial Nerve Palsy

Unilateral UMN	Bilateral UMN
Usually vascular	Often vascular
Cerebral tumor	Motor neuron disease
Multiple sclerosis	

Unilateral LMN	Bilateral LMN
Bell's palsy	Guillain-Barre syndrome
Parotid tumor	Sarcoidosis uveoparotid fever
Head injuries	Leprosy
Skull base tumors	Leukemia/lymphoma
Diabetes	
Hypertension	

Difference between UMN and LMN lesions

Features	UMN	LMN
Movements	Paresis of movement of limb	Individual muscle/muscle glycogen phosphorylase affected
Muscle involvement	Diffuse distribution	Individual muscle
Tone	Hypertonia	Hypotonia
Musclar wasting	No wasting initially later disuse atrophy	Muscle wasting present
Deep tendon reflex	Brisk	Depressed or absent
Plantar response	Extensor	Flexor
Associated involuntary movement	Flexor spasms may be present	Fasciculation may be present

Motor Neuron Disease

1. Involvement of both UMN (corticospinal tract) and LMN (anterior horn cell)—amyotrophic lateral sclerosis
2. Predominantly UMN lesion—primary lateral sclerosis
3. Predominantly LMN lesion—spinal muscular atrophy.

Clinical features of dystonia and extrapyramidal disorders

1. Plastic or spastic increase in muscle tone
2. Abnormal postures
3. Involuntary movements and tremor
4. Loss of postural reflexes
5. Normal or increased tendon reflexes
6. Plantar responses normal or extensor.

Paraplegia

Causes

1. **UMN lesion**
   Cerebral
   Parasagittal meningioma
   Superior sagittal sinus thrombosis
   Bilateral anterior cerebral artery lesion
   Parasagittal trauma.
   Spinal cord
   Compressive myelopathy
   Extramedullary extradural: Spine secondaries, Pott's disease
   Extramedullary intradural: Neurofibroma, meningioma
   Intramedullary: Ependymoma
   Noncompressive myelopathy
   Congenital: Hereditary spastic paraplegia, syringomyelia
   Vascular: Anterior spinal artery occlussion, dissecting aneurism of aorta
   Traumatic
   Infection: Syphilis, epidural abscess, herpes, HIV, TB spine
   Demyelinating diseases: Primary (disseminated sclerosis), secondary (post/para infectious)
   Degenerative diseases: MND, hereditary ataxia
   Nutritional: Subacute combined degeneration, lathyrism, fluorosis
   Myelopathy in systemic diseases: SLE, Sjögren's, myelopathy in paraneoplastic syndrome
   Toxins and physiological agents: Nitrous oxide, radiation.
2. **LMN lesion**
   Anterior horn cell: Spinal muscular atrophy
   Anterior root: GBS
   Cauda equina: Neuropathy, IVDP, secondaries
   Lumbosacral plexus: Ischemic plexopathy of diabetes, traumatic
   Peripheral neuropathy

3. **Neuromuscular junction disease:** myasthenic syndrome
4. **Muscle disease:** polymyositis, muscular dystrophy
5. **Hysterical**
6. **Recurrent paraplegia:** demyelinating disease, dumbbell tumor, spinal arachnoid cyst.

5 Ts of Paraplegia (Most common causes)

1. Tuberculosis	2. Trauma	3. Tumor
4. Thrombosis	5. Transverse myelitis.	

Clinical Picture of Spinal Cord Lesion (Focal)

At the level of the lesion

Vertebral manifestations (if the cause is vertebral)
1. Localized pain and tenderness
2. Localized deformity or swelling.

Radicular manifestations (in extra-medullary cases)
1. Posterior root affection
   a. Early pain in the back referred to distribution of the affected root and described as 'girdle pain'. Increases on coughing, sneezing and/or straining
   b. Later on, there is hypoesthesia or anesthesia in the dermatome supplied by the affected root.
2. Anterior root affection
   Localized LMN weakness in muscles supplied by the affected root.

Below the level of the lesion

Motor manifestations
1. Acute cause (inflammatory, vascular or traumatic)
   a. Stage of Flaccidity due to neuronal shock
   b. Stage of Spasticity.
2. Gradual cause (neoplastic)
   Gradual progressive weakness of lower limbs with hypertonia and hyper-reflexia
3. *Weakness*: Distal > Proximal and Flexor > Extensor
4. Initially, only pyramidal tract is involved—paraplegia in extension is seen—hypertonia and hyper-reflexia affect extensors more than the flexors (i.e. antigravity > progravity)
5. With progression of lesion, extrapyramidal fibers are involved—paraplegia in flexion—hypertonia and hyper-reflexia will be more in flexors than extensors (Mass reflex may be seen in this stage).

Sensory manifestations
1. Extramedullary lesion
   a. Encroachment of ascending fibers results in diminished sensations below the level of the lesion
   b. Early loss of sensation in the saddle area (S3, 4, 5) as sacral fibers are outermost in the spinothalamic tract.
2. Intramedullary lesion
   a. Jacket sensory loss (hypoesthetic area with normal sensations above and below it)
   b. Sensory loss is of dissociated nature, i.e. pain and temp are lost but touch and deep sensations are preserved (due to interruption of decussating fibers)
   c. Sensations over saddle area preserved (sacral sparing).

Sphincteric manifestations
1. In acute lesion:
   a. Retention of urine in the shock stage
   b. Precipitancy of micturition in stage of spasticity.
2. In gradual lesion, precipitancy of micturition (which may terminate in autonomic bladder when complete transection of cord occurs).
3. These start late in extramedullary lesions and early in intramedullary lesions as pyramidal fibers controlling the bladder center lie medailly in the cord.

Clinical Picture of Cerebral Lesion

1. Extremely rare
2. History of Jacksonian fits and cortical sensory loss may be present
3. Spastic paraplegia in extension (may be flaccid in shock stage but never produces paraplegia in flexion)
4. Features of increased intracranial pressure may be present (headache, vomiting, convulsions)
5. Abnormalities in higher function, speech difficulty, cranial nerve affection may be present.

Investigations
1. Blood R/E—TC, DC, ESR, sugar, urea
2. Urine—Routine examination and culture-sensitivity test are done
3. Mantoux test
4. CXR—Exclude TB, Bronchogenic carcinoma, lymphoma or metastasis
5. X-ray spine (AP and lateral view)—Dx of caries spine, metastasis, fracture/dislocation of vertebra
6. CSF examination
   a. CSF pressure
      i. Markedly reduced in extramedullary lesion
      ii. Less markedly reduced in intramedullary lesion.
   b. Queckenstedt's test
      i. Bilateral jugular vein compression below the angle of mandible normally leads to rapid rise of CSF pressure in the manometer; release of the compression leads to rapid drop back to normal
      ii. Extramedullary compression—no change in CSF pressure (complete dynamic block) due to complete obstruction of the subarachnoid space
      iii. Intramedullary compression—Slower and lesser rise in CSF pressure (partial dynamic block) due to incomplete obstruction.
   c. CSF constituents
      i. Extramedullary—marked rise in proteins leading to spontaneous coagulation and yellowish discoloration (xanthochromia) without any rise in cell count (cytoalbuminous dissociation)
      ii. Intramedullary—no marked change.
7. Myelography
   a. A water soluble radiopaque substance (metrizamide/myodil) is injected into subarachnoid space and its movement is viewed on screen
   b. Normally, the dye moves freely through the subarachnoid space
   c. In extramedullary compression, there is complete block with short tails (saddle shape appearance)
   d. In intramedullary compression, there is increased width of cord with long tails (fusiform shape).
8. Miscellaneous
   a. Muscle biopsy
   b. Muscle enzymes
   c. Electromyography
   d. Blood for vitamin B_{12} estimation
   e. VDRL
   f. HIV.

N.B.: The association of xanthochromia, cytoalbuminous dissociation and spontaneous coagulation of CSF is called Froin's syndrome.

Common causes of xanthochromia
1. Old SAH (due to presence of old blood)
2. GB syndrome (due to high protein)
3. Acoustic neurofibroma (due to high protein)
4. Froin's syndrome (due to high protein)
5. Deep jaundice (due to high bilirubin)
6. Massive old intracerebral bleed or hemorrhagic infarction (due to presence of old blood).

Treatment
1. Nutritious diet
2. *Care of bowel, bladder and trophic ulcers*:
   a. Bladder—self-retaining catheter, change it every 2–3 weeks, bladder wash, antibiotics when necessary.
   b. Bowel—Treat constipation with laxatives.
   c. Skin—Reposition every 2 to 4 hours, keep skin dry and clean, soft bed coverings changed regularly, clean any bed sores with hydrogen peroxide.
3. Muscle spasms are treated with diazepam, baclofen, tizanidine.

4. Treat underlying cause
   a. Caries spine—Application of traction in the early stage. Later on, 'plaster jacket' is applied for immobilization. ATT is usually continued for 1 year
   b. Treatment of carcinoma or lymphoma by radiotherapy and/or chemotherapy
   c. Acute transverse myelitis—High dose corticosteroids (1 mg/kg/day) for 2 weeks with gradual tapering
   d. GB syndrome—High dose IV Ig (0.4 g/kg/day × 5 days), plasmapheresis, respiratory assistance.
5. Physiotherapy
   a. Massage to increase blood supply to the paralysed muscles
   b. Passive exercises to guard against fibrosis and stiffness
   c. Active exercises to strengthen muscles
   d. Paralysed limb is put in a position slightly opposite the hypertonia.
6. Surgery
   Drainage of cold abscess, laminectomy for caries spine, excision of extramedullary tumor.

Conditions causing paraplegia

1. Caries spine causing paraplegia
   a. Caries spine should be thought of as the first cause of paraplegia in India, irrespective of the age and sex of the patient
   b. Caries spine can cause paraplegia in the following ways:
      i. Compression of the spinal cord by cold abscess (extradural) - most common
      ii. Tuberculous myelitis (involvement of the spinal cord from the bone)
      iii. Pachymeningitis or arachnoiditis
      iv. Tuberculous arteritis or thrombosis of the radicular artery—responsible for the sudden onset of paraplegia or acute exacerbation of existing paraplegia
      v. Granulation tissue encircling the dura
      vi. Compression by sequestrated bone
      vii. Dislocation of vertebra—rare
      viii. Combination of multiple factors.
2. Anterior spinal artery occlusion
   Clinical picture is the same as that of transverse myelitis but there is sparing of deep sensations as posterior columns of spinal cord are supplied by the posterior spinal arteries.
3. Features of acute transverse myelitis
   a. Behaves like a compressive lesion (spastic)
   b. Very often follows a viral illness/post-vaccinal
   c. Onset is acute to subacute (evolves over several days to 2-3 weeks)
   d. Fever may be present before paralysis presents
   e. Early bladder involvement
   f. Though behaves like a compressive lesion, there is absence of root pain, spinal tenderness or spinal deformity
   g. Back pain and progressive paraparesis is most common presenting feature
   h. Extensor plantar response
   i. Complete or partial sensory loss with a definite upper level (in contrast to GB)
   j. Majority (70%) recover within 12 weeks.
4. Poliomyelitis
   a. Flaccid paralysis (acute and symmetrical)
   b. 24-36 hours from onset to full paralysis
   c. High fever always present at onset of flaccid paralysis, gone the following day
   d. Severe myalgia and backache
   e. No sensory changes
   f. Bladder dysfunction absent.
5. Guillain-Barre syndrome
   a. It is an acute polyradiculoneuropathy (i.e. inflammatory demyelination involving the spinal roots and peripheral nerves)
   b. Flaccid paralysis
   c. Association with Epstein-Barr virus, measles, campylobacter jejuni, HIV, CMV, postvaccinal and postsurgical events
   d. Hypothesis regarding pathology—immune reaction due to hypersensitivity

   e. Typical history
      i. Viral illness (respiratory catarrh)
      ii. 2 weeks later, paralysis with paraesthesia starts
      iii. Paralysis progresses for 3 wks and then stops
      iv. Paralysis is static for 2 weeks
      v. After 2 weeks, recovery starts, usually completed within 6 months.
   f. Acute ascending LMN type palsy
   g. No sensory abnormalities
   h. Plantar—flexor or no response
   i. Tendon reflexes absent
   j. Bowel and bladder not involved.
6. Subacute combined degeneration
   a. Due to vitamin B_{12} deficiency
   b. Presents with a triad of
      i. Anemia
      ii. GI manifestations—stomatitis, swollen tongue (beefy tongue), dyspepsia, nausea, vomiting, colic, diarrhea
      iii. Neurological manifestations.
   c. Pain and paraesthesia in limbs, followed by 'stocking/glove' sensory loss
   d. Weakness in limbs with +ve Babinski; however the tone and deep reflexes are diminished (due to peripheral nerve and postcolumn lesions)
   e. Sensory ataxia may be present (post column degeneration).
7. Syringomyelia
   a. Characterized by gliosis (proliferation of astrocytes in damaged areas) and cavitation around central canal in gray matter of spinal cord especially in lower cervical and upper thoracic segments
   b. Gradual onset with progressive course
   c. Paraplegia is a late manifestation—spastic paraplegia due to encroachment on the pyramidal tracts
   d. Jacket sensory loss of dissociated nature
   e. Autonomic—trophic ulcers of fingers, painless nail infection and vasomotor changes (Morvan's syndrome).
8. Neurosyphilis
   a. Meningeal syphilis
      i. Chronic meningitis—thickening of meninges results in compression of roots and cord
      ii. Causes spastic paraplegia with radicular limb pain.
   b. Tabes dorsalis
      i. 15 to 20 years after primary infection
      ii. Degeneration of postroots and post columns
      iii. Severe, knife-like, shooting pains followed by marked impairment of the superficial and deep sensations
      iv. Sensory ataxia present
      v. Tendon reflexes lost
      vi. Muscle tone diminished
      vii. Ulcers of foot and arthropathies or Charcot's joint are common.
9. Hereditary spastic paraplegia
   a. Broad group of genetically and clinically diverse disorders characterized by lower extremity spasticity and weakness
   b. Progressive spasticity of the lower extremities that may be accompanied by a mild decrease in proprioception and urinary sphincter dysfunction
   c. Leg stiffness, weakness in the hip flexors, and impaired foot dorsiflexion in the second through fourth decades
   d. Extensor plantar response
   e. Tendon reflexes are pathologically increased
   f. Complicated HSP indicates spasticity with additional neurological impairment, such as optic neuropathy, retinopathy, extrapyramidal disturbance, dementia, ataxia, ichthyosis, mental retardation, and deafness.
10. Cauda equina syndrome
   a. LMN weakness of lower limbs
   b. Painful onset—pain is radicular

c. Later on, it is followed by hypoesthesia or anesthesia in the dermatome supplied by the affected root.
N.B.: Motor and sensory manifestations are usually unilateral; if bilateral, it is mostly found to be asymmetrical
d. Bladder is involved usually later on unless the lesion is bilateral (sensory atonic bladder/motor atonic bladder/autonomic bladder).

11. Lathyrism
    a. It is due to *khesari dal* (lathyrus sativus)
    b. May involve families in locality
    c. The causative factor is BOAA (Beta N Oxalyl Aminoalanine), α-neurotoxin.

Paraplegia with loss of deep tendon jerks
1. In paraplegia the tendon jerks are brisk. They can only become absent when patient is either in spinal shock or there is involvement of afferent or efferent side of reflex
2. Neural shock (spinal)
3. Hematomyelia/Myelomalacia
4. Radiculitis—the jerk whose root is involved will be absent
5. Peripheral neuropathy—bilateral ankle jerks may be absent
6. Reflex activity may be absent in presence of severe infection due to suppression.

Causes of paraplegia with optic atrophy
1. Friedreich's ataxia
2. Multiple sclerosis
3. Infections like TB, syphilis
4. Subacute combined degeneration
5. Subacute myelo-optic neuropathy.

Causes of pure motor paraplegia
1. Hereditary spastic paraplegia
2. Lathyrism
3. GB syndrome
4. Amyotrophic lateral sclerosis
5. Erb's spastic paraplegia (syphilitic)-rare
6. Fluorosis.

Causes of cord compression at multiple levels
1. Neurofibromatosis
2. Arachnoiditis
3. IVDP
4. AV malformations
5. Secondary deposits.

Compressive versus noncompressive paraplegia

Features	Compressive	Noncompressive
Bony deformity	Present	Not seen
Bony tenderness	Present	Not seen
Girdle-like sensation	Present	Not seen
Upper level of sensory loss	Present	Not seen
Zone of hyperesthesia	Present	Not seen
Root pain	Present	Not seen
Onset and progress	Gradual	May be acute
Symmetry	Asymmetrical	Majority symmetrical
Flexor spasm	Common	Usually absent
Pattern of neurodeficit	U-shaped	Bilaterally symmetrical
Bowel and bladder involvement	Early	Late (early in acute transverse myelitis)
Classical example	Caries spine	MND

Difference between extramedullary and intramedullary paraplegia

Features	Extramedullary	Intramedullary
Root pains	Common	Rare
Dissociated anesthesia	Rare	Common
Brown-Séquard syndrome	May occur	Does not occur
Wasting	Minimal	Marked
Pyramidal signs	Marked	Not so marked
Sphincter disturbances	Occur late	Early involvement
Trophic changes	Minimal	Marked
Tenderness over spine	May be present	Usually absent
CSF proteins	Raised	Normal
Common tumors	Meningioma	Glioma
	Neurofibroma	Ependymoma
	Chordoma	
	Lipoma	

Differences between cauda equina and conus medullaris

Features	Conus medullaris syndrome	Cauda equina syndrome
Presentation	Sudden and bilateral	Gradual and unilateral
Reflexes	Knee jerk preserved but ankle jerk affected	Both ankle and knee jerk affected
Radicular pain	Less severe	More severe
Low back pain	More	Less
Sensory symptoms and signs	Numbness is symmetrical and bilateral; sensory dissociation occurs	Numbness is asymetrical, may be unilateral; no sensory dissociation
Motor strength	Typically symmetric, hyper-reflexic distal paresis of lower limbs	Asymmetric areflexic paraplegia
Impotence	Frequent	Less frequent
Sphincter dysfunction	Overflow urinary incontinence and fecal in continence; tend to present early in the course of disease	Urinary retention; tends to present late in the course of disease

Differences between Frederick's ataxia, Tabes dorsalis, subacute combined degeneration of cord

Features	Frederick's ataxia	Tabes dorsalis	Subacute combined degeneration of cord
Tracts involved	Classically and long tracts degenerate Pyramidal, Dorsal, Spinocerebellar	Chronic progressive Demyelination Post column of spinal cord, Dorsal root ganglia, Nerve roots	Post column, Pyramidal tract Peripheral nerves Usually present can be lost in late stages under reflexes
Reflexes	Areflexia in lower limbs	Absent at patella and Achilles	
Babinski's sign	Positive	Absent	Positive

Contd...

Contd...

Joint position and vibration sense	Lost	Lost	Lost
Pain and temp	Intact	Intact	Intact
Other nervous system abnormality	Wide based ataxia nystagmus, dysarthria dysmetria	Anisocoria, Argyll Robertson pupil, Lightening pain in legs	Progressive spastic and ataxic weakness
Associated anomalies	Cardiomyopathy Skeletal abnormality Optic atrophy Increased incidence of diabetes mellitus	Bladder disturbance	Low serum B_{12} Megaloblastic anemia Pernicious anemia

Cardinal features of Parkinsonism

1. Bradykinesia or akinesia
2. Rigidity
3. Parkinson's tremor (tremor at rest)
4. Postural instability.

Differentiating features of supranuclear palsy from Parkinson's disease

1. Early falling
2. Rarity of tremor
3. Axial rigidity (cervical dystonia)
4. Lack of response to l dopa.

Triad of Huntington's Disease

1. Autosomal dominant inheritance
2. Choreoathetosis
3. Dementia.

Brain tumors

1. MC intracranial tumor—glioma
2. Most common Glial tumor—glioblastoma multiforme
3. Second most common Glial tumor—astrocytoma
4. Most common posterior fossa tumor in childhood—cerebellar astrocytoma
5. Second most common posterior fossa tumor in childhood—medulloblastoma
6. Most common tumor of childhood—astrocytoma
7. Most common astrocytoma of childhood—juvenile pilocytic astrocytoma
8. Most common malignant tumor of childhood—medulloblastoma.

Causes of Bacterial Meningitis

1. *Neonates*: *E. coli* (most common); Streptococcus B (2nd most common); listeria
2. *Infants*: *H. influenzae*
3. Children and young adults—Neisseria Meningitis
4. Adult and older people—*Streptococcus pneumoniae*
5. Overall most common cause of acute meningitis is *Streptococcus pneumoniae* (50%).

Differences between bilateral UMN and LMN facial palsy

Features	Bilateral UMN	Bilateral LMN
Bell's phenomenon	Absent	Present
Emotional fibers	Spared	Affected
Long tract signs	Present	Absent
Jaw jerk	Exaggerated	Normal
Corneal reflex	Present	Absent

Components of Reflex ARC

1. Sensory receptor
2. Afferent pathway
3. Center
4. Efferent pathway
5. Effector organ.

Definitions

1. *Acalculia*: A leashing or speech disorder characterized by the inability to perform arithmetic calculations
2. *Adie pupil*: Characterized by absent or delayed (pupillary) constriction to light or to accommodation or convergence
3. *Ageusia*: Loss/absence of sense of taste
4. *Agraphia*: Loss of the ability to write
5. *Agnosia*: Defined as loss of ability to comprehend the meaning or recognize stimulation
6. *Alexia*: Loss of the power to grasp the meaning of written or printed words and sentences
7. *Anorexia nervosa*: Weight loss of 25% or more of original body weight in the absence of organic disease
8. *Anosmia*: Absence of the ability to smell
9. *Aphasia*: Disturbance in the structure and organization of language
10. *Apraxia*: It is a defect in the ability to carry out known acts in the absence of motor weakness, sensory loss or ataxia
11. *Athetosis*: A complex writhing involuntary movement usually more pronounced in distal than in proximal
12. *Bell's phenomenon*: A patient with peripheral facial paralysis cannot close the eyelids on the affected side without at the same time moving the eyeball upward and outward
13. *Brown-Séquard syndrome*: Hemiparaplegia and hyperesthesia but with loss of joint and muscle sense on the side of the lesion and hemianesthesia of the opposite side
14. *Capgras syndrome*: Illusion of doubles; failure to recognize a familiar person and instead believing him to be double
15. *Chorea*: A disorder usually of childhood, characterized by irregular, spasmodic, involuntary movements of the limbs or facial muscles
16. *Charcot's joint*: Diabetic osteoarthropathy; enlargement with osteoarthritis due to trophic disturbances in patients with tabes dorsalis
17. *Coma*: A state of unconsciousness in which the patient does not respond to any type of external stimuli or inner need
18. *Depression*: Dejection; a sinking of spirits so as to constitute a clinically discernible condition
19. *Dementia*: It is a syndrome of acquired global or multifocal impairment of cognitive function involving decline in intellect, memory or personality in the presence of normal consciousness
20. *Delusion*: These are false beliefs which continue to be held despite evidence to contrary
21. *Dysarthria*: The defects of articulation and enunciation of speech
22. *Epilepsy*: It is a tendency to have recurrent seizures
23. *Fasciculation*: It is applied to an irregular, nonrhythmic contraction of muscle fascicules
24. *Hallucination*: These are false impressions referred to the organs of special senses in the absence of a stimulus
25. *Illusion*: These are misinterpretations of stimuli
26. *Internuclear ophthalmoplegia*: It is a result of lesions in the medial longitudinal fasciculus and is characterized clinically by the failure of adduction of the eye on the side of lesion of MLF and a mild weakness of abduction with nystagmus on the contralateral side
27. *Nystagmus*: It is a disturbance of ocular movement characterized by involuntary, conjugate often rhythmical oscillations of the eye
28. *Obsession*: These are recurrent and persistent thoughts, which intrudes into the patient's mind despite best efforts to get rid of them
29. *Papilloedema*: Edema of the optic disc may be due to raised intracranial pressure or part of a diffuse retinal edema as in malignant hypertension
30. *Prosopagnosia*: It is inability to identify a familiar face including sometimes the reflection of his or her own face in the mirror
31. *Reflex*: It is a consistent involuntary adaptive response to the stimulation of sense organ
32. *Status epilepticus*: It is defined as a state in which the patient suffers a series of seizures without fully recovering consciousness between these seizures
33. *Strabismus or squint*: It is an abnormality of ocular movement in which the visual axis do not meet at the point of fixation
34. *Stupor*: It is a state of disturbed consciousness from which only vigorous external stimuli can cause arousal
35. *Tremor*: It is defined as a rhythmical and oscillatory movement of a body part caused by regular, rhythmical contractions of the agonist and antagonist muscles
36. *Vertigo*: It is a hallucination of movement of either the body or part of it or the surroundings
37. *Young stroke*: Refers to stroke occurring in persons below 40 years of age.

RENAL SYSTEM

Oliguria: It is the passage of < 500 mL urine per day.
Urgency: It is the loss of the normal ability to postpone micturition beyond the time when the desire to pass urine is initially perceived.
Hesitancy: It is difficulty in initiating the process of micturition.
Nephritic syndrome: It is defined as the presence of heavy proteinuria (> 3 g/day compared with normal of < 150 mg/day), hypoalbuminemia, hypercholesterolemia and edema.

Effects of Renal Failure on Other Organ Systems

Cardiovascular system
1. Cardiac failure or angina associated with fluid overload, hypertension, anemia and impaired ventricular function (uremic cardiomyopathy)
2. Precordial chest pain due to pericarditis
3. Cardiac arrhythmias associated with hyperkalemia/hypokalemia.

Respiratory system
1. Breathlessness and hemoptysis from fluid overload
2. Chest pain due to pleurisy.

Nervous system
1. Hypertensive stroke and encephalopathy
2. Clouding of consciousness, fits and coma in advanced renal failure
3. Impaired sensation or paresthesia in the feet due to peripheral neuropathy in long standing uremia
4. Impaired higher mental or intellectual function.

Hematological system
1. Lethargy and breathlessness associated with anemia due to impaired production of erythropoietin by the kidneys
2. Defective coagulation and excessive bruising (advanced renal failure)
3. Hemorrhage from gastrointestinal tract or lungs.

Water and electrolyte balance
1. Breathlessness due to salt and water overload
2. Deep sighing breathing (Kussmaul respiration) due to acidosis
3. Weakness and postural fainting due to hypotension caused by salt and water depletion
4. Lethargy and weakness due to hypokalemia.

Musculoskeletal system
1. Muscular weakness and bone pain due to impairment of vitamin D activation and to excessive parathyroid gland activity
2. Acute pain due to gout.

Urine diagnostic indices in differentiation of prerenal vs intrinsic renal failure

Diagnostic index	Prerenal ARF	Intrinsic renal ARF
Fractional excretion of Na	< 1	> 1
Urine sodium concentration (mmol/L)	< 10	> 20
Urine creatinine to plasma creatinine ratio	> 40	< 20
Urine osmolality (mosmol/kg H_2O)	> 500	~300
Renal failure index	< 1	> 1
Urine urea nitrogen to plasma urea nitrogen	> 8	< 3
Plasma BUN/creatinine ratio	> 20	< 10–15
Urinary sediment	Hyaline casts	Muddy brown granular casts
Urine specific gravity	> 1.020	~1.010

Pathogenesis of renal conditions

1. **Minimal change disease**
   Light microscopy: No abnormality
   Electron microscopy: Fusion of foot processes
   Immunofluorescence: Absence of immunoglobulin or complement.
2. **Membranous glomerulonephritis**
   Light microscopy: Diffuse thickening of basement membrane which is most apparent on staining with PAS
   Electron microscopy: Demonstrates that the diffuse thickening are caused by irregular dense deposits between the basement membrane and the overlying epithelial cells (subepithelial deposits)
   Immunofluorescence: Demonstrates that these granular deposits contain immunoglobulins and various amount of complement (IgG and C3).
3. **Acute poststreptococcal glomerulonephritis—immune complex formation**
   Light microscopy: Diffuse proliferation and leukocyte infiltration
   Electron microscopy: Subepithelial deposits
   Fluorescence microscopy: Granular IgG and C3 in GBM and mesangium.
4. **IgA nephropathy—unknown**
   Light microscopy: Mesangial proliferation and widening; focal proliferative glomerulonephritis
   Electron microscopy: Mesangial and paramesangial dense deposits
   Fluorescence microscopy: IgA +/- IgG, IgM and C3 in mesangium.

Differentiating features between IgA nephropathy and poststreptococcal glomerulonephritis

IgA nephropathy	Poststreptococcal glomerulonephritis
Onset of hematuria 2–4 days after URTI	Onset of hematuria 7–21 days following URTI and skin infection
Serum complement C3 level normal	Serum compliment C3 level decreased
Recurrence common	Recurrence rare, one attack confers life long immunity
No elevation of antibody titer	Elevation of antistreptococcal antibody titer

Histological varients of renal cell carcinoma

1. Clear cell carcinoma—(nonpapillary)
   a. Most common type (70–80%)
   b. Cells have clear or granular cytoplasm and are nonpapillary
   c. Defect lies in chromosome 3.
2. Papillary carcinoma
   a. Second most common type (10–15%)
   b. Papillary growth pattern is characteristic (clear cells not seen)
   c. Psammoma bodies may be present
   d. Most common cytogenetic abnormality are trisomy of chromosome 7, 16 and 17 and loss of Y in male patients in sporadic form; trisomy 7 in familial form
   e. Striking characteristic of tumor is tendency to invade the renal vein and grow as a solid column of cells within the vessels; extension may produce a continuous cord of tumor in IVC and even in the right side of heart.
3. Chromophobe renal carcinoma
   a. Least common
   b. Pale eosinophilic cytoplasm
   c. Multiple chromosomal losses and extreme haploploidy.

Indications for dialysis in acute renal failure

1. Severe hyperkalemia (serum potassium > 6.5 mEq/L)
2. Dysnatremia (serum sodium < 130 or > 150 mEq/L)
3. Severe acidosis (pH < 7.2, TCO_2 < 12 mEq/L)
4. Uremic encephalopathy
5. Pulmonary edema; congestive heart failure.

Renal Tubular Acidosis

Systemic hyperchloremic acidosis, resulting from impaired urinary acidification

1. Type 1 or distal RTA
   a. Defective H ion secretion by DCT
   b. 5–15% of filtered HCO_3 lost in the urine
   c. Urine pH cannot be reduced to < 5.5
   d. Hypokalemia
   e. Hyperchloremia
   f. Hypercalciuria-nephrocalcinosis.
   Causes: obstructive/sickle cell/transplant rejection/lupus/ amphotericin B/Li
2. Type 2 or proximal RTA
   a. Defective reabsorption of HCO_3 by PCT—85%
   b. Severe hypokalemia (in exchange for Na)
   c. Hyperchloremia (decreased ECF volume)
   d. Urine acidifiable to pH < 5.5.
3. Type 3
   a. Decreased production or responsiveness to aldosterone
   b. Hyperkalemia
   c. Urine pH < 5.5.

OBJECTIVE STRUCTURED CLINICAL EXAMINATION (MEDICINE)

General Examination

1. **Patient with Pallor-Examine eyes, hands and oral cavity. Describe findings. Give 4 causes. Most important investigations to find out diagnosis. Explain abnormalities in the investigations**

   Eyes – look in lower palpebral conjunctiva. Always in daylight. Compare.
   Hands – look for nail beds, palm, palmar creases. Not seen if Hb below 7, Platonychia, Koilonychia, Ridging of nails-Iron deficiency anemia
   Oral cavity – tongue, hard palate

   The most common cause in India is hookworm infestation.
   Nutritional: Iron deficiency anemia, megaloblastic anemia
   Increased blood loss: GI malignancies, menorrhagia
   Marrow failure: Hematological malignancies, aplastic anemia
   Increased destruction: Hereditary spherocytosis
   Nonanemic causes of pallor: Myxedema, nephritic syndrome, vasovagal attack, peripheral circulatory failure
   Investigations:
   Hb Low
   MCV High - RDW low—Aplastic anemia
   - RDW high—Megaloblastic anemia
   MCV Low - RDW low—Thalassemia
   - RDW high—Iron deficiency anemia

   a. *Peripheral smear*: Normocytic normochromic-posthemorrhagic, anemia of chronic disease. Microcytic hypochromic-Fe deficiency anemia, thalassemia, sideroblastic anemia
   b. *Serum ferritin*: Low in iron deficiency anemia (first change in iron deficiency is associated with a decrease in levels of serum ferritin only. Other indices will be WNL)
   c. *Serum iron*: Low in iron deficiency
   d. *TIBC*: High in iron deficiency.

   Features of hemolytic anemia
   a. Hb low
   b. Increased unconjugated bilirubin
   c. High LDH
   d. High AST
   e. Low haptoglobin
   f. Increased urobilinogen in urine
   g. Increased stercobilinogen in urine
   h. Increased reticulocytosis
   i. Increased MCV/MCH
   j. Macrocytes, polychromasia and nucleated red cells
   k. Erythroid hyperplasia in marrow.

   Proteins defective in hereditary spherocytosis
   a. Ankyrin
   b. Protein 3 (anion transport channel)
   c. Spectrin
   d. Palladin.

High reticulocyte count: Hemolysis, blood loss
Low reticulocyte count: Aplastic anemia, nutritional deficiency anemia
Mycoplasma pneumonia can cause cold antibody hemolytic anemia.

2. Patient with jaundice, subconjunctival hemorrhage—Examine the eyes. Conditions causing jaundice—sites-upper bulbar conjunctiva (area where bilirubin is not photo oxidized) soft palate, palms, skin.
Conditions:

Jaundice with subconjunctival hemorrhage

a. Chronic liver disease
b. Infections—Leptospirosis, Dengue fever.

Jaundice

a. Viral hepatitis
b. Hemolysis.

Subconjunctival hemorrhage

a. Acute leukemia
b. Aplastic anemia.

Tests to identify the cause of LFT abnormality

Diagnosis	Clinical clue	Initial test	Additional tests
Alcoholic liver disease	AST > ALT; high MCV		Random blood alcohol
Non-alcoholic fatty liver disease (NAFLD)	Metabolic syndrome (central obesity, diabetes, hypertension)		
Chronic hepatitis B	Injection drug use, blood transfusion	HBsAg	HBeAg, HBeAb HBV-DNA
Chronic hepatitis C		HCV antibody	HCV-RNA
Primary biliary cirrhosis	Raised alkaline phosphatase	AMA	
Primary sclerosing cholangitis	Inflammatory bowel disease	MRCP	ANCA antibody
Autoimmune hepatitis	Other autoimmune diseases	ASMA, ANA, LKM, immunoglobulin	
Hemochromatosis	Diabetes/joint pain	Transferrin saturation, ferritin	HFE gene test
Wilson's disease	Neurological signs	Ceruloplasmin	24-hour urinary copper
α1-antitrypsin	Lung disease	α1-antitrypsin level	α1-antitrypsin phenotype
Drug-induced liver disease	Drug/herbal remedy history		
Celiac disease	Malabsorption	Endomysial antibody	

3. Patient with pedal edema, ichthyosis, clubbing. Examine feet. Give two causes for each.

Causes of edema

Low plasma oncotic pressure

a. Low serum albumin due to
b. Increased loss—nephrotic syndrome
c. Decreased synthesis—liver failure
d. Malnutrition/malabsorption.

Increased capillary permeability

a. Leakage of proteins into the interstitium, reducing the osmotic pressure gradient which draws fluid into the lymphatics and blood
b. Local-infection/inflammation
c. Systemic-severe sepsis
d. Drug-related, e.g. calcium channel blockers.

Increased hydrostatic pressure high venous pressure/obstruction

a. Deep venous thrombosis or venous insufficiency—local edema
b. Pregnancy
c. Pelvic tumor
d. Congestive heart failure
e. Intravascular volume expansion (iatrogenic, renal failure, Conn's syndrome).

Lymphatic obstruction

a. Infection-filariasis, lymphogranuloma venereum
b. Malignancy
c. Radiation injury
d. Congenital abnormality.

Causes of ichthyosis

a. Dehydration
b. Chronic liver disease
c. Paraneoplastic syndrome
d. Familial
e. Congenital.

Causes of clubbing

a. CVS—cyanotic heart diseases, infective endocarditis
b. Respiratory—lung abscess, bronchogenic carcinoma
c. GIT—cirrhosis, celiac disease
d. Others—genetic, normal in some people.

4. **Patient with clubbing. Examine hands and feet. Finding. Causes.**
   a. Examine the finger nails tangentially or do Shamroth's sign
   b. Palpate the nailbed for fluctuation
   c. Look for widening and tenderness of end of long bones—hypertrophic osteoarthropathy.

   Grading of clubbing

   Grade 1: Obliteration of the angle between nail and nailbed and positive fluctuation test
   Grade 2: Parrot beak appearance
   Grade 3: Drumstick appearance
   Grade 4: Hypertrophic osteoarthropathy

   Types of clubbing

   a. *Drum stick*: Congenital cyanotic heart disease and bronchiectasis
   b. *Parrot beak*: Bronchogenic carcinoma
   c. *Painful clubbing*: Bronchogenic carcinoma and SBE
   d. *Unilateral*: Presubclavian coarctation of aorta, bronchogenic carcinoma, cervical rib, aneurysm of subclavian artery, erythromelalgia, arteriovenous fistula of branchial vessels
   e. *Unidigital*: Hereditary, local trauma, sarcoidosis, rarely from median nerve injury or deposition of tophi
   f. *Pseudoclubbing*: Scleroderma, acromegaly, hyperthyroidism and leprosy.

   Causes of clubbing

   a. Cardiac causes
      i. Congenital cyanotic heart disease like Fallot's tetralogy
      ii. SBE
      iii. Rarely in cardiac tumors (e.g. in atrial myxoma)
      iv. Eisenmenger's syndrome, primary pulmonary hypertension.
   b. Lung and pleural causes (ABCDEF)
      i. Abscess (lung)
      ii. Bronchiectasis (including CF)
      iii. Cancer (lung)
      iv. Decreased oxygen (hypoxia)
      v. Empyema
      vi. Fibrosing alveolitis.
   c. Ulcerative colitis—GIT
      Biliary cirrhosis, sometimes in hepatocellular failure
      Intestinal causes
      i. Malabsorption syndrome
      ii. Crohn's disease
      iii. Polyposis coli
      iv. Celiac disease.
   d. Normal—found normally in some people
   e. Genetic—may be a familial condition.

5. **Patient with edema. Give physiological, cardiovascular, respiratory, gastrointestinal, renal, infective and drug induced causes of edma.**

   Physiological - pregnancy
   Cardiovascular - CCF
   Respiratory - Cor pulmonale
   GIT - Hepatic failure

Renal - Nephrotic syndrome, renal failure
Infective - Filariasis, lymphogranuloma venereum
Drug - Calcium channel blockers.

6. **General examination. What will you look for in eyes, oral cavity, axillae, arms, palms, nails, chest and abdomen? Importance of examination of supraclavicular fossa.**

Eyes

a. Icterus - Upper bulbar conjunctiva
b. Pallor - Lower palpebral conjunctiva
c. Subconjunctival hemorrhage
d. Bitot spots - Vitamin A deficiency
e. KF ring - Wilson's disease
f. Sunflower cataract - Wilson's disease.

Oral cavity and tongue

a. Ask the patient to show you their teeth then open wide and look carefully at the state of the teeth, the tongue and the inner surface of the cheeks. You should also subtly attempt to smell the patient's breath
b. *Angular stomatitis*: A reddening and inflammation at the corners of the mouth. A sign of thiamine, vitamin B_{12}, and iron deficiencies
c. *Circumoral pigmentation*: Hyperpigmented areas surrounding the mouth. Seen in Peutz-Jeghers syndrome
d. *Telangiectasia*: Dilatation of the small vessels on the gums and buccal mucosa. Seen in Osler-Weber-Rendu syndrome
e. *Gums*: Look especially for ulcers (causes include celiac disease, inflammatory bowel disease, Behcet's disease and Reiter's syndrome) and hypertrophy (caused by pregnancy, phenytoin use, leukemia, scurvy [vitamin C deficiency] or inflammation [gingivitis])
f. *Breath*: Smell especially for:
   i. Fetor hepaticus a sweet-smelling breath.
   ii. *Ketosis*: Sickly sweet pear-drop smelling breath
   iii. *Uremia*: a fishy smell.
g. *Tongue*: Look especially for:
   i. *Glossitis*: Smooth, erythematous swelling of the tongue. Causes include deficiencies of iron, vitamin B_{12}, and folate deficiencies
   ii. *Macroglossia*: Enlarged tongue. Causes include amyloidosis, hypothyroidism, acromegaly, Down's syndrome, and neoplasia
   iii. *Leukoplakia*: A white-colored thickening of the tongue and oral mucus membranes. A premalignant condition caused by smoking, poor dental hygiene, alcohol, sepsis and syphilis
   iv. *Geographical tongue*: Painless red rings and lines on the surface of the tongue looking rather like a map. Can be caused by vitamin B_2 (riboflavin) deficiency or may be a normal variant
   v. *Candidiasis*: Thrush. A fungal infection of the oral membranes seen as creamy white curd-like patches which can be scraped off revealing erythematous mucosa below. Causes include immunosuppression, antibiotic use, poor oral hygiene, iron deficiency and diabetes.

Axillae

a. Lymphadenopathy
b. Acanthosis nigricans (a thickened, blackening of the skin. Velvety in appearance. May be associated with intra-abdominal malignancy).

Arms

a. *Bruising*: May be a sign of:
   i. Hepatocellular damage and the resulting coagulation disorder
   ii. Thrombocytopenia due to hypersplenism
   iii. Marrow suppression with alcohol.
b. *Petechiae*: Pin-prick bleeds which do not blanche with pressure. Possibly a sign of thrombocytopenia
c. *Muscle wasting*: Seen as in muscle mass, possibly with overlying skin hanging loosely. A late manifestation of malnutrition and often seen in patients with chronic alcoholic liver disease
d. *Scratch marks (excoriations)*: Suggests itch (pruritus) is present and may be the only visible feature of early cholestasis.

Palms

a. Palmar erythema
b. Dupuytren's contracture
c. Flapping tremor (asterixis)
d. Small muscle wasting
e. Pallor.

Nails

a. *Leukonychia*: Whitening of the nail bed due to hypoalbuminemia (e.g. malnutrition, malabsorption, hepatic disease, nephritic syndrome)
b. *Platynychia and Koilonychia*: Flattening and spooning of the nails making a concave shape instead of the normal convexity. Causes include congenital and chronic iron deficiency
c. *Muehrcke's lines*: These are transverse white lines. Seen in hypoalbuminemic states including severe liver cirrhosis
d. *Clubbing*: Abdominal causes are cirrhosis, inflammatory bowel disease and celiac disease
e. *Blue lunulae*: A bluish discoloration of the normal lanulae seen in Wilson's disease.

Chest

a. *Spider nevi*: Telangiectatic capillary lesions
   i. A central red area with engorged capillaries spreading out from it in a spidery manner
   ii. Caused by engorgement of capillaries from a central feeder vessel
   iii. If the lesion is truly a spider nevus, it will be completely eliminated by pressure at the center using a pen-point or similar and will fill outwards when the pressure is released
   iv. Can range in size from those that are only just visible up to 5 or 6 mm in diameter
   v. Found in the distribution of the superior vena cava
   vi. A normal adult is allowed up to 5 spider nevi
   vii. Causes include chronic liver disease and estrogen excess.
b. *Gynecomastia*: The excessive development of male mammary glands due to ductal proliferation such that they resemble post-pubertal female breasts
   i. This is often embarrassing for the patient so be sensitive
   ii. Caused by alcoholic liver disease, congenital adrenal hyperplasia and several commonly used drugs including spironolactone, digoxin, and cimetidine
   iii. Can also be seen during puberty in the normal male.

Abdomen

a. Hepatomegaly
b. Splenomegaly-cardinal feature in portal hypertension
c. Ascites
d. Dilated veins-caput medusa
e. Umbilicus—smiling umbilicus in ascites.

Supraclavicular fossa

Troisier's sign—Virchow's node seen in malignancy of GIT, lung, testes and ovaries

Hepatic flap (asterixis)

a. This is identical to the flap seen in hypercapnic states
b. Ask the patient to stretch out their hands in front of them with the hands dorsiflexed at the wrists and fingers outstretched and separated
c. The patient should hold that position for at least 15 seconds. If flap is present, the patient's hands will move in jerky, irregular flexion/extension at the wrist and MCP joints. The flap is nearly always bilateral. May be subtle and intermittent
d. This is characteristic of encephalopathy due to liver failure
e. If a sign of hepatic encephalopathy in a patient with previously compensated liver disease, it may have been precipitated by infection, diuretic medication, electrolyte imbalance, diarrhea or constipation, vomiting, centrally acting drugs, upper GI bleeding, abdominal paracentesis, or surgery.

7. **Patient with lymphadenopathy. What are the findings? Give causes.**

Causes of lymphadenopathy

Infectious diseases

a. *Viral*: Infectious mononucleosis syndromes (EBV, CMV), infectious hepatitis, herpes simplex, herpes virus-6, varicella-zoster virus, rubella, measles, adenovirus, HIV, epidemic keratoconjunctivitis, vaccinia, herpes virus-8
b. *Bacterial*: Streptococci, staphylococci, cat-scratch disease, brucellosis, tularemia, plague, chancroid, melioidosis, glanders, tuberculosis, atypical mycobacterial infection, primary and secondary syphilis, diphtheria, leprosy
c. *Fungal*: Histoplasmosis, coccidioidomycosis, paracoccidioidomycosis
d. *Chlamydial*: Lymphogranuloma venereum, trachoma
e. *Parasitic*: Toxoplasmosis, leishmaniasis, trypanosomiasis, filariasis
f. *Rickettsial*: Scrub typhus, rickettsialpox, Q fever.

Immunologic diseases

a. Rheumatoid arthritis
b. Juvenile rheumatoid arthritis
c. Mixed connective tissue disease
d. Systemic lupus erythematosus
e. Dermatomyositis
f. Sjögren's syndrome
g. Serum sickness
h. Drug hypersensitivity—diphenylhydantoin, hydralazine, carbamazepine
i. Angioimmunoblastic lymphadenopathy
j. Primary biliary cirrhosis
k. Graft vs. host disease
l. Silicone-associated
m. Autoimmune lymphoproliferative syndrome.

Malignant diseases

a. *Hematologic*: Hodgkin's disease, non-Hodgkin's lymphomas, acute or chronic lymphocytic leukemia, hairy cell leukemia, malignant histiocytosis, amyloidosis
b. *Metastatic*: From numerous primary sites.

Lipid storage diseases: Gaucher's, Niemann-Pick, Fabry, Tangier

Endocrine diseases: Hyperthyroidism

Other disorders

a. Castleman's disease (giant lymph node hyperplasia)
b. Sarcoidosis
c. Dermatopathic lymphadenitis
d. Lymphomatoid granulomatosis
e. Histiocytic necrotizing lymphadenitis (Kikuchi's disease)
f. Sinus histiocytosis with massive lymphadenopathy (Rosai-Dorfman disease)
g. Mucocutaneous lymph node syndrome (Kawasaki's disease)
h. Histiocytosis X
i. Familial mediterranean fever
j. Severe hypertriglyceridemia
k. Vascular transformation of sinuses
l. Inflammatory pseudotumor of lymph node
m. Congestive heart failure.

8. Patient with pallor, petechia, LNE and subconjunctival hemorrhage. Do general examination. Describe findings. Diagnosis. Investigations.

Diagnosis: Hematological malignancies

Investigations: Total count, differential count, platelets, Hb, HCT, peripheral smear, bone marrow aspiration, trephine biopsy.

9. Patient with small muscle wasting. Inspect hand. Give causes.

Leprosy
Carpal tunnel syndrome
Cervical spondylosis

10. Patient with glossitis. Inspect tongue. Give findings and causes for each.

Glossitis : Smooth, erythematous swelling of the tongue. Causes include deficiencies of iron, vitamin B_{12}, and folate deficiencies.

Macroglossia : Enlarged tongue. Causes include amyloidosis, hypothroidism, acromegaly, Down's syndrome, and neoplasia.

Leukoplakia : A white-colored thickening of the tongue and oral mucus membranes. A premalignant condition caused by smoking, poor dental hygiene, alcohol, sepsis and syphilis.

Geographical tongue : Painless red rings and lines on the surface of the tongue looking rather like a map. Can be caused by vitamin B_2 (riboflavin) deficiency or may be a normal variant.

Beefy tongue : B_{12} deficiency.

Strawberry tongue : Scarlet fever, Kawasaki disease.

11. Patient with thyroid swelling, cervical lymphadenopathy. Examine neck of the patient. Findings. Investigations.

Most probably carcinoma thyroid. Papillary carcinoma most common. Investigations-TFT, FNAC, biopsy.

12. Patient with unilateral pitting edema. Do general examination. Finding. Complications.

Unilateral pitting edema causes—Cellulitis, DVT, Filariasis, Femoral venous obstruction
Complication—pulmonary embolism

13. Patient with swan neck deformity, pitting nails, psoriatic plaques and small muscle wasting. Examine hand. Findings. Diagnosis. Management.

Diagnosis—Psoriasis

Management

a. Easily applied topical agents such as emollients, corticosteroids, vitamin D agonists, or 'weak' tar or dithranol preparations
b. Ultraviolet therapies such as PUVA and UVB
c. Systemic agents such as retinoids or immunosuppressives such as ciclosporin, or one of a range of new biological therapies ('biologics')
d. Intensive inpatient or day-patient care with topical agents and UVR under medical supervision.

Deformities of finger joint

a. *Swan neck*: Fixed flexion at the DIP and extension at the PIP joints associated with rheumatoid arthritis
b. *Boutonniere*: Fixed extension at the DIP and flexion at the PIP joints associated with rheumatoid arthritis
c. *Z-shaped thumb*: Flexion at the MCP joint of the thumb with hyperextension at the interphalangeal joint associated with rheumatoid arthritis
d. *Ulnar deviation*: A feature of rheumatoid arthritis and other conditions, the fingers are deviated medially (toward the ulnar aspect of the forearm) at the MCP joints
e. *Wrist subluxation*: Deviation (either ulnar or radial) at the wrist
f. *Heberden's nodes*: Swelling (due to osteophytes) at the DIP joints a feature of osteoarthritis
g. *Bouchard's nodes*: Similar to Heberden's nodes but at the PIP joints a feature of osteoarthritis.

Nail changes

a. *Leukonychia*: Whitening of the nail bed due to hypoalbuminemia (e.g. malnutrition, malabsorption, hepatic disease, nephritic syndrome)
b. *Koilonychia*: Spooning of the nails making a concave shape instead of the normal convexity. Causes include congenital and chronic iron deficiency
c. *Muehrcke's lines*: These are transverse white lines. Seen in hypoalbuminemic states including severe liver cirrhosis
d. *Clubbing*: Causes are cyanotic HD, bronchiectasis, lung abscess, endocarditis, cirrhosis, inflammatory bowel disease and celiac disease
e. *Blue lunulae*: A bluish discoloration of the normal lanulae seen in Wilson's disease
f. *Splinter hemorrhages*: Tiny, longitudinal streak hemorrhages under the nails caused by micro-emboli or trauma (small streak-like bleeds in the nail bed) seen especially in bacterial endocarditis but may also be a sign of rheumatoid arthritis, vasculitis, trauma, or sepsis from any source. Can be a normal finding in manual workers
g. *Pitting*: Tiny indentations in the surface of the nail. A feature of psoriasis and less commonly eczema, lichen planus and alopecia areata
h. *Onycholysis*: Premature lifting of the nail
i. *Beau's lines*: Transverse depressions in the nail. Coincide with arrested nail growth during a period of acute severe illness
j. *Paronychia*: Infection of the skin adjacent to the nail causing pain, swelling, redness, and tenderness
k. *Onychomycosis*: Fungal nail infection causing the nail to become thickened, opaque, crumbly and yellow. Often with onycholysis and may be indistinguishable from psoriatic nail changes.

14. Patient with cyanosis. Examine oral cavity. Difference between central and peripheral cyanosis.

a. Ensure adequate lighting
b. Examine over tongue, oral mucosa, lips
c. Other areas—cheeks, ear lobes, tip of nose, hands, nailbeds.

Sites in peripheral cyanosis

a. Tip of the nose
b. Ear lobules
c. Outer aspect of lips, chin and cheek
d. Tip of the fingers and toes
e. Palms and soles
f. Tongue remains unaffected.

Sites to be looked for in central cyanosis

a. Tongue (mainly the margin as well as the undersurface)
b. Inner aspect of lips
c. Mucous membrane of gum, soft palate, cheeks.
d. Lower palpebral conjunctiva.
e. Plus, the sites mentioned in the peripheral cyanosis.

Central cyanosis	Peripheral cyanosis
Tongue and periphery cyanosed	Not on tongue
Limb warm	Limb cool
Clubbing may be ++	Usually not present
On warming cyanosis remains	Cyanosis disappears
On breathing 100% O_2 cyanosis	Cyanosis persists
Disappears in upper column	

Cardiovascular System

15. Auscultate aortic area and describe findings.

Auscultatory areas

a. Mitral - 5th light ICS 1 cm medial to MCL
b. Tricuspid - Lower part of sternum
c. Aortic - 2nd right ICS at the sternal margin
d. Pulmonary - 2nd light ICS at the sternal margin
e. Neoaortic area - 3rd light ICS at the sternal margin
f. Apex (if cardiomegaly+).

Auscultation

a. Expose the patient adequately
b. Ask the patient to lie supine
c. Ensure adequate lighting
d. Always time with carotid pulse to avoid confusion between systolic and diastolic events
e. Look for the following in all the auscultatory areas
f. First and second HS
g. Additional sounds (IIIrd and IVth HS)
h. Any murmurs
i. Adventitious sounds (click, rub)
j. Pericardial rub if present.

Murmur 10 points

a. Site
b. Pitch
c. Timing
d. Grade
e. Character
f. Radiation
g. Positional variation
h. Variation with respiration
i. Best heard with bell/diaphragm
j. Variation with exercise/exertion.

Murmurs

Mitral stenosis

- Low pitched rough rumbling mid-diastolic murmur with pre-systolic accentuation of grade III intensity heard best in the mitral area without any radiation with the bell of the stethoscope with the patient lying in the left lateral position and the breath held in expiration.
- Intensity of the murmur increases with mild exercise.

Mitral regurgitation: High pitched soft blowing pansystolic murmur of grade IV intensity heard best in the mitral area radiating to the left axilla and inferior angle of scapula heard best with the diaphragm of the stethoscope with the patient lying in the left lateral position and the breath held in expiration.

Aortic stenosis: Low pitched harsh ejection systolic murmur of grade V intensity heard best in the aortic area radiating to the carotids best heard with the diaphragm of the stethoscope with the patient sitting up and leaning forward with the breath held in expiration.

Aortic regurgitation: High pitched soft blowing. Early diastolic murmur of grade III intensity heard best in the neoaortic area with the diaphragm of the stethoscope with the patient sitting up and leaning forward with the breath held in expiration.

16. **Patient with irregular pulse. Examine pulse. Describe causes.**
Pulse-rate, rhythm, character, volume, condition of vessel wall, radiofemoral delay, radioradial delay, peripheral pulses
Rate rhythm-radial pulse
Character, volume-carotid pulse
Causes of irregular pulse
a. Atrial fibrillation
b. Ventricular extrasystoles.

17. **Patient with CCF. Examine wrist, ankle, neck, back and abdomen. Findings.**
Wrist : Resting tachycardia, hypokinetic pulse
Ankle : Edema
Neck : JVP
Back : Presacral edema
Abdomen : Tender hepatomegaly

18. **Patient with MS. Auscultate mitral area. DDs of MDM. Complications and prophylaxis.**
DDs MDM : MS, TS, AF, severe AR, Severe MR, Carey comb murmur (rheumatic valvulitis). In MS presystolic accentuation, loud S1, Opening snap present
Complications : Portal hypertension, atrial fibrillation, embolic phenomenon
Prophylaxis : Infective endocarditis, anticoagulants

19. **Patient with bradycardia. Examine pulse in detail. Causes.**
Pulse—Rate, rhythm, volume, character, condition of vessel wall, brachiofemoral delay, no radioradial delay. Peripheral pulses both sides.
a. *Radial pulse*: Semipronated forearm; flex the wrist feel the pulse near the wrist and examine it for a minute
b. *Carotid pulse*: Ask the patient to look straight ahead use your thumb and press it backwards at the level of medial border of sternomastoid muscle and lateral to thyroid cartilage. Character of the pulse is best felt
c. *Popliteal pulse*: Ask the patient to lie supine make knee partially flexed feel pulse with fingers encircling and supporting the knee from both sides
d. *Posterior tibial pulse*: Ask the patient to lie supine and feel the pulse in the groove midway between medial malleolus and the heel (tendo-Achilles)
e. *Dorsalis pedis pulse*: Feel the pulse lateral to the extensor hallucis longus tendon and proximal to first metatarsal space. Examine both sides simultaneously except carotid pulse.

Bradycardia—causes
Physiological: Athelets, sleep, elderly
Drugs: Beta blockers
Pathological: Hypothyroidism, IWMI, sick sinus syndrome, raised ICT (Cushing reflex)

20. **Palpate apex beat. Describe.**
Heaving apex : Aortic stenosis
Hyperdynamic apex : Aortic regurgitation and mitral regurgitation
Tapping apex : Mitral stenosis

21. **Patient with cardiomegaly. Palpate precordium and describe findings. What are the causes?**
Causes of cardiomegaly.

Respiratory System

22. **Patient with accessory muscles of respiration+, pursed lip breathing, plethoric facies. Examine the patient. Describe findings. Give your diagnosis. Explain the complications.**
Accessory muscles of respiration
a. Pectoralis major
b. Alae nasae
c. Sternomastoid
d. Scalene
e. Serratus anterior
f. Abdominal muscles
g. Latissimus dorsi
h. Trapezius.

Pursed lip breathing-prevent alveolar collapse
a. Plethoric facies
   - Cor pulmonale-pulsatile JVP
     - COPD
b. SVC obstruction-nonpulsatile JVP
   - Pancoast syndrome, thymoma, retrosternal thyroid, mediastinal fibrosis

Diagnosis

COPD: COPD is a heterogeneous condition embracing several overlapping pathological processes including chronic bronchitis, chronic bronchiolitis (small airway disease) and emphysema

Complications: Exacerbation of COPD, Cor-pulmonale, Spontaneous pneumothorax

23. Patient with bronchial breath sounds. Auscultate chest. Types of breath sounds.

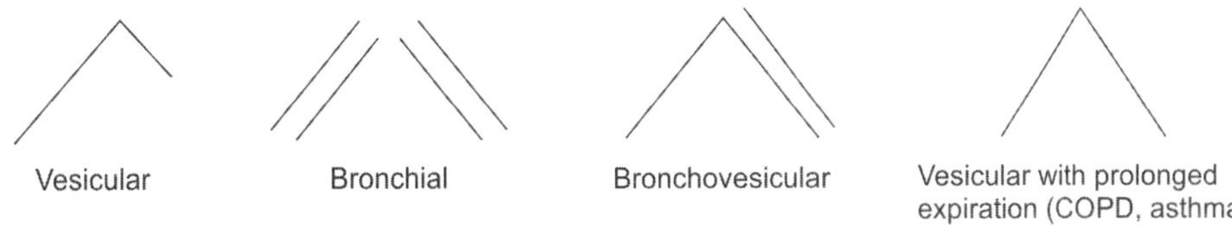

Breath sounds

Normal vesicular: Produced by airflow in the large airways and larynx and altered by passage through the small airways before reaching the stethoscope. Often described as rustling. Heard especially well in inspiration and early expiration.

Reduced sound: If local = effusion, tumor, pneumothorax, pneumonia or lung collapse. If global=COPD or asthma (the silent chest is a sign of a life threatening asthma-attack).

Bronchial breathing: It is caused by density of matter in the peripheral lung allowing sound from the larynx to the stethoscope unchanged. Has a hollow, blowing quality, heard equally in inspiration and expiration, often with a brief pause between. Heard over consolidation, lung abscess at the chest wall and dense fibrosis. Also heard at the upper border of a pleural effusion.

Types

Tubular: High pitched. Consolidation, partial collapse and above the level of pleural effusion

Cavernous: Low pitched. Cavity.

Amphoric: Low pitched with high pitched overtone. Thin walled cavity, tension pneumothorax

Added sounds

Wheeze (rhonchi): Musical whistling sounds caused by narrowed airways. Heard easier in expiration. Different caliber airways = different pitch note as asthma and COPD can cause a chorus of notes termed polyphonic wheeze.

Monophonic wheeze indicates a single airway is narrowed, usually by a foreign body or carcinoma.

Crackles (crepitations, rales): It is caused by air entering collapsed airways and alveoli producing an opening snap. Heard in inspiration.

Coarse crackles made by larger airways opening and sound like the snap and pop of a certain breakfast cereal. *Causes*: fluid or infection.

Fine crackles occur later in inspiration. The sounds can be reproduced by rolling the hair at your temples between the thumb and forefinger.

Causes: Fluid, infection or fibrosis (particularly at lung bases).

Crackles are often a normal finding at the lung bases. If so, they will clear after asking the patient to cough.

Rub: Creaking sound likened to the bending of new leather. Heard at the height of inspiration. Caused by inflamed pleural surfaces rubbing against each other.

Causes: pneumonia, pulmonary embolism with infarction.

Differences between pleural rub and crepitation

Pleural rub	Crepitation
Continuous	Interrupted
Do not disappear with cough	May disappear with cough
Superficial	Deep
Scratchy leathery char	Bubbling character
Through out cycle	During inspiration mainly
Localized	Not localized
Associated with pain	Not usually associated with pain

24. Patient with barrel shaped chest. Inspect chest. Auscultate lung bases. Describe the findings.
Barrel shaped chest—COPD

25. Patient with succession splash.
Gastrointestinal system

26. Palpate abdomen. Give two bedside investigations to confirm.
Inspection
Abdominal palpation
a. Right side of patient
b. Consent
c. Expose area
d. Flex hip and knee to relax fascia
e. Tilt head to left side
f. Warm your hands
g. Always palpate from nontender to tender area
h. Palpate all areas. Start from left iliac fossa in anticlock wise direction
i. Comment on:
   i. Temperature
   ii. Tenderness
   iii. Any mass
   iv. Pulsations
   v. Direction of flow of engorged veins
   vi. Liver and gallbladder
   vii. Spleen
   viii. Kidney (renal angle tenderness)
   ix. Hernial orifice and external genitalia.

Percussion and auscultation
Bedside invesigations: Complete blood count, peripheral smear

27. Patient with hepatomegaly, splenomegaly and axillary LN. Examine abdomen and axilla. What are the differential diagnosis.
Abdomen—HSM
Axillary LN
DDs-IMN, TB, lymphoma, ALL, AML

28. How to look for minimal hepatomegaly and minimal splenomegaly.
Minimal hepatomegaly—Tidal percussion
Minimal splenomegaly—Dullness in Traube's space
(Traube's space—6th rib, midaxillary line, left coastal margin)

29. Patient with ascites. What are investigations? Drug of choice.
Investigations
a. Diagnostic paracentesis
b. LFT-A/G reversal
c. USG-portal venous system
d. OGD scopy.
Drug of choice in management of ascites—spironolactone-aldosterone antagonist.

30. Demonstrate shifting dullness.
Patient in supine position:
a. Percuss over the midline downwards till the bladder dullness is reached (keep your finger horizontally)
b. Keep fingers vertically, percuss from midline laterally till dullness is reached, continue percussing till it is completely dull and percuss back to the point where the dullness started
c. Now ask the patient to lie in the opposite lateral position, wait for 2 minutes and percuss from resonant to dull area.

Fluid required:

Shifting dullness	500–1000 mL
Fluid thrill	2000 mL
Puddle sign	120 mL

Causes of ascites
Common causes
Malignant disease
a. Hepatic
b. Peritoneal.

Cardiac failure
Hepatic cirrhosis
Other causes
Hypoproteinemia
a. Nephrotic syndrome
b. Protein-losing enteropathy
c. Malnutrition.
Hepatic venous occlusion
a. Budd-Chiari syndrome
b. Veno-occlusive disease.
Pancreatitis
Lymphatic obstruction
Infection
a. Tuberculosis
b. Spontaneous bacterial peritonitis.
Rare
a. Meigs' syndrome
b. Vasculitis
c. Hypothyroidism
d. Renal dialysis.

Management of ascites
a. Dietary sodium restriction
b. Diuretic therapy—spironolactone drug of choice
c. Large volume paracentesis
d. Correction of hypoprotenemia
e. Shunts.

31. Locate renal angle.
Space between angle formed by 12th rib with lateral vertebral border.

32. Ryle's tube. Identify. Give two uses and complications.
Nasogastric tube : Long tubes with 3 lead balls at one end. Its position is confirmed by pushing 5-10 mL of air and auscultating in the epigastrium or by aspirating the gastric juice.
Uses : Life saving use is in acute gastric dilatation, used to aspirate in intestinal obstruction or pyloric stenosis, used in the diagnosis of GI hemorrhage, used to feed coma or tetanus patients, Nasogastric feeding, aspiration of gastric contents in poisoning. Complications-perforation, aspiration pneumonia

33. Examination of dilated veins of abdomen. Relevance of lower limb examination in this patient.
Can be examined in standing/sitting position.
Direction of flow is found by using two index fingers.
In lower limb there can be—Varicosity, DVT, edema.

34. How do you find out borders of liver and spleen?
Liver
Upper border—heavy percussion
Lower border—palpation and light percussion
Spleen
Traube's space boundaries—6th rib, left coastal margin and mid axillary line.

Nervous System

35. Demonstrate signs of meningeal irritation. Name the organisms producing meningitis.
Signs of meningeal irritation
Neck stiffness
Patient actively flexes his neck as fully as he can and then relaxes then passively flex the neck (normally the chin should touch the chest without causing pain).
Kernig's sign
The patient is made to lie supine. The opposite leg is fully extended Flex the hip to 90 degrees on the same side passively extend the patient's knee.
Brudzinski's sign
Head sign-
Leg sign-
Flex the head the thighs and knees also flex. Flex one thigh fully. The opposite thigh also flexes.

Causes of meningitis

Infective

Bacteria

a. Gram-negative bacilli (*Escherichia coli, Proteus,* etc.)—neonate
b. Group B streptococci—neonate
c. *Haemophilus influenzae*—preschool child
d. *Neisseria meningitidis*—older child and adult
e. *Streptococcus pneumoniae*—older child and adult
f. Brucella.

Viruses

a. Enteroviruses (echo, Coxsackie, polio)
b. Mumps
c. Influenza
d. Herpes simplex
e. Varicella zoster
f. Epstein-Barr
g. HIV
h. Lymphocytic choriomeningitis
i. Mollaret's meningitis (HSV type 2).

Protozoa and parasites

a. Toxoplasma
b. Ameba
c. Cysticercus.

Fungi

a. *Cryptococcus neoformans*
b. *Candida*
c. *Histoplasma*
d. *Blastomyces*
e. *Coccidioides*
f. *Sporothrix.*

Noninfective (sterile) malignant disease

a. Breast cancer
b. Bronchial cancer
c. Leukemia
d. Lymphoma.

Inflammatory disease (may be recurrent)

a. Sarcoidosis
b. SLE
c. Behçet's disease.

36. Demonstrate ankle and patellar clonus.

Seen in hyper reflexia and hypertonia.

Knee clonus

With the patient relaxed and the knee extended and the skin over knee stretched, sharply push with your thumb and forefinger above the patella towards the foot, sustaining the pressure for few seconds.

Ankle clonus

Support the patient's leg with both the knee and ankle resting in 90 degree flexion. Briskly dorsiflex and partially evert the foot and sustain the pressure.

37. Patient with dilated pupil-examine eyes. Write findings. Give four causes.

Dilated pupil (mydriasis) causes

Physiological : (children, anxiety)
Pathological : (3rd nerve palsy)
Drugs : (atropine, tropicamide)

38. Look for plantar reflex. What is the response? What is the root value?

Plantar reflex

a. Look for weakness of extensor hallucis longus
b. Expose upto midthigh to see tensor fascia lata
c. Assess mobility of Bigtoe, sole thickness
d. Stroke up to 3rd toe within 3–5 seconds and do 3–5 times only.

Response

a. Flexor
b. Extensor
c. Minimal plantar response—Contraction of tensor fascia lata only
d. Equivocal
e. No response.

Root value

Afferent : S1
Efferent : Flexor - S1
: Extensor - L5 (EHL-L5)

Plantar extensor

a. Physiological—children, deep sleep
b. Pathological—hemiplegia.

39. Patient with Parkinsonism. Comment on face of patient. Describe tone in upper limb. Elicit palmomental reflex and glabellar tap.
Face: Mask like facies
Resting tremor
Tone in upperlimb: Cogwheel type
Plastic (leadpipe) type, mostly legs
Palmomental reflex and glabellar tap: Degenerative conditions

40. Muscles supplied by median nerve LOAF.
Lumbricals
Opponens pollicis ion
Abductor pollicis brevis
Flexor pollicis brevis

41. Foley catheter. Identify. Give two uses and complications.
Long latex rubber tube with silicon coating. There is a bulb and before inflating make sure that the catheter is in the urinary bladder and not in urethra.
Uses: Urinary retention, BPH, to drain peritoneal fluid as in biliary peritonitis. Inflated bulb compresses the prostatic bed and controls the bleeding after prostatectomy.
Complications: UTI, Urethral rupture.

42. Patient with Pes cavus. Inspect feet of the patient. Finding. Causes.
Causes of pes cavus
a. Friedreich's ataxia
b. Spina bifida
c. Peripheral neuropathy
d. Syringomyelia

43. Patient with Inverted supinator jerk.
44. Patient with Internuclear ophthalmoplegia.
45. Patient with facial palsy-LMN.
46. Patient with Horners syndrome.

CHARTS

Urine Examination Findings

Examination	AGN	Nephrotic syndrome
Quantity	350 mL/24 hours	1500 mL/24 hours
Color	Smoky	Clear
Specific gravity	1.028	1.016
Chemical		
pH	6.6	6.4
Albumin	++	+++
Blood	++	Nil
Sugar	Nil	Nil
Ketone bodies	Nil	Nil
Bile	Nil	Nil
Microscopic		
RBC	Plenty	Nil
WBC/ PUS cells	2/HPF	1/HPF
Hyaline cast	+	+
RBC cast	++	Absent

Contd...

Contd...

Epithelial cast	+	–
Fatty cast	–	++
Bacteria	Nil	Nil
Crystals	Nil	Nil
Interpretation	Oliguria, smoky urine RBC and RBC cast moderate albuminuria	Macroscopically normal urine massive albuminuria Fatty cast

Jaundice

	Normal	Hemolytic	Hepatocellular	Obstructive
S. Bilirubin (mg%)	0.3–1.3	10	10	10
Conjugated (mg%)	0.1–0.4	0.5	5.5	8.5
Unconjugated (mg%)	0.2–0.9	9.5	4.5	1.5
S. ALP (IU/L)	33–96			
ALT (SGPT) (IU/L)	7–41	26	260	80
AST (SGOT) (IU/L)	12–38	30	290	90
Urine				
Bile salts	–ve	–ve	++	++

(Modified Fouchets Test-$FeCl_3$ in Trichloroacetic Acid)

Bile pigments (Hay's test)	–ve	–ve	+	++
Urobilinogen	+	+++	+	–ve

(**Ehrlich's Test**—Para-aminobenzaldehyde in Conc. HCl)

Feces				
Stercobilinogen	+	+++	normal color	clay color
Examples		Hereditary spherocytosis (hs) Sickle cell Thalassemia Gilbert's syndrome Chemicals, drugs burns, lead	Viral hepatitis Alcohol abuse C/c liver disease	Cholangiocarcinoma Stricture of biliary tree, Carcinoma head of pancreas, Carcinoma gallbladder

Examination of CSF

Examination	Normal	A/C pyogenic	Tuberculous	A/C viral
Pressure		++	++	++
Appearance		Turbid/cloudy	Clear	Clear
On standing		No coagulum	Cobweb coagulum	No coagulum
Chemical				
Protein (mg%)	15–50	180	600	150
Sugar (mg%)	40–70	12	30	65
Chloride (mEq/L)	116–122	675	580	730

Contd...

Contd...

Microscopic				
Total cells (per microL)	0–5	4000	450	140
Polymorphs	None	92	8	10
Lymphocytes (%)	60–70	8	92	90
Microscopic		Gram +ve cocci	Sterile	Sterile

CSF Normal Values

Electrolytes:
Na 137–145 mEq/L
K 2.7–3.9 mEq/L
Chloride 116–122 mEq/L
PCO_2 45–49 mm Hg
pH 7.31–7.34

Total protein: 15–50 mg/dL
Albumin 6.6–44.2 mg/dL
Glucose 40–70 mg/dL
Leukocytes
Total: 0–5 per microL
Lym 60–70% *Mono* 30–50% *Neut*-none

DRUGS

Cholinergic Agonists

1. Choline esters : Acetylcholine, Methacholine, Carbachol, Bethanechol.
2. Alkaloids : Muscarine, Pilocarpine, Arecoline.

Anticholinesterases

1. Reversible
   a. Carbamates : Physostigmine, neostigmine, edrophonium
   b. Acridine : Tacrine.
2. Irreversible
   a. Organophosphates : Diazinon, parathion, malathion, tabun, sarin, soman
   b. Carbamates : Carbaryl, propoxur.

Adrenergic Drugs

1. Pressor agents : Noradrenaline, Dopamine
2. Cardiac stimulants : Adrenaline, Isoprenaline, Dobutamine
3. Bronchodilators : Salbutamol, Terbutaline, Salmeterol
4. Nasal decongestants : Phenylephrine, Oxymetazoline
5. CNS stimulants : Amphetamine, Dexamphetamine
6. Anorectics : Fenfluramine
7. Uterine relaxants : Ritodrine, Isoxsuprine, Terbutaline.

α adrenergic blocking agents

1. Nonequilibrium type
2. Equilibrium type
   a. Nonselective
      i. Ergot alkaloids : Ergotamine
      ii. Hydrogenated ergot alkaloids : Dihydroergotamine
      iii. Imidazolines : Phentolamine
      iv. Miscellaneous : Ketanserin
      v. α1 selective : Prazosin
      vi. α2 selective : Yohimbine

α adrenergic blocking agents

1. Nonselective
   a. Without intrinsic sympathomimetic activity : Propranolol, Timolol, Sotalol
   b. With intrinsic sympathomimetic activity : Pindolol
   c. With additional α blocking property : Labetalol, Carvedilol
2. Cardioselective α1 : Metoprolol, atenolol, esmolol
3. Selective α2 : Butoxamine.

Antihistaminics

1. Highly sedative : Diphenhydramine, Promethazine
2. Moderately sedative : Pheniramine, Cyproheptadine, Cinnarizine, Meclizine
3. Mild sedative : Chlorpheniramine, Mepyramine, Cyclizine, Clemastine
4. Second generation antihistaminics : Loratadine, Cetirizine, Azelastine.

NSAIDs

Nonselective COX inhibitors

1. Salicylates : Aspirin
2. Propionic acid derivatives : Ibuprofen, Naproxen
3. Anthranilic acid derivatives : Mefenamic Acid
4. Aryl acetic acid derivatives : Diclofenac
5. Oxicam derivatives : Piroxicam, Tenoxicam
6. Pyrrolo-pyrrole derivatives : Ketorolac

Preferential COX 2 inhibitors : Nimesulide, Nabumetone
Selective COX 2 inhibitors : Celecoxib, Rofecoxib, Valdecoxib
Aspirin-adverse effects : Gastric mucosal damage and peptic ulceration.
Uses: Acute rheumatic fever, rheumatoid arthritis, postmyocardial and poststroke patients.

DMARDs (Disease modifying antirheumatic drugs)

1. Gold
2. D-penicillamine
3. Chloroquine or hydroxyl chloroquine
4. Sulfasalazine
5. Leflunomide
6. Immunosuppressants—methotrexate, azathioprine, cyclosporine.

Gout

1. Acute gout : NSAIDs, Corticosteroids, Colchicine
2. Chronic gout/hyperuricemia
   a. Uricosurics : Probenecid, Sulfinpyrazone
   b. Synthesis inhibitor : Allopurinol.

Bronchial Asthma

Bronchodilators

Sympathomimetics : Salbutamol, Terbutaline
Methylxanthines : Theophylline, Aminophylline
Anticholinergics : Ipratropium, tiotropium (more useful in COPD)
Leukotriene antagonists : Montelukast, Zafirlukast
Mast cell stabilizers : Sodium cromoglycate, Nedocromil.

Corticosteroids

Systemic : Hydrocortisone, prednisolone
Inhalational : Beclomethasone dipropionate, budesonide, fluticasone.

Antithyroid

Inhibit hormone synthesis (antithyroid drugs) : Carbimazole, Propylthiouracil
Inhibit iodide trapping (ionic inhibitors) : Thiocyanates, Perchlorates
Inhibit hormone release : Iodine, Iodides of Na and K, Organic iodide
Destroy the thyroid tissue : Radioactive I131, I125, I123.

Newer Insulin Delivery Devises

1. Insulin syringes
2. Pen devices
3. Jet injectors
4. Insulin pumps
5. Implantable pumps
6. External artificial pancreas.

Other routes: Intraperitoneum, rectal, oral, intranasal.

Oral hypoglycemic agents

1. Sulphonyl ureas
   - *1st generation* : Tolbutamide, Chlorpropamide
   - *2nd generation* : Glibenclamide, Glimepiride, Glipizide, Gliclazide
2. Biguanides : Metformin, Phenformin
3. Meglitinide analogs : Repaglinide, Nateglinide
4. Thiazolidinediones : Rosiglitazone, Pioglitazone
5. Alpha glucosidase inhibitors : Acarbose, Miglitol.

Selective estrogen receptor modulators

1. Tamoxifen citrate
2. Raloxifene
3. Ormeloxifene.

Newer antiepileptics

Vigabatrin, topiramate, tiagabine, levetiracetam.

Antihypertensive drugs

ACE inhibitors : Enalapril, Ramipril, Lisinopril, Captopril
Angiotensin antagonist : Losartan, Candesartan, Irbesartan, Telmisartan, Olmesartan
Calcium channel blockers : Nifedipine, Amlodipine, Verapamil, Diltiazem.

Diuretics

Beta adrenergic blockers : Propranolol, Atenolol, Metoprolol
Beta+alpha adrenergic blockers : Labetalol, Carvedilol
Alpha adrenergic blockers : Prazosin, Phentolamine
Central sympatholytics : Clonidine, Methyldopa
Vasodilators-arteriolar : Hydralazine, Minoxidil, Diazoxide
Arteriolar + venous : Sodium Nitroprusside.

Diuretics

Loop diuretics : Frusemide, Torsemide (longest acting), Bumetanide (most potent), Ethacrynic acid, Azosemide
Thiazides : Hydrochlorothiazide, Chlorothiazide, Methyclothiazide
Thiazide like : Chlorthalidone, Indapamide, Metolazone
Carbonic anhydrase inhibitors : Acetazolamide, Dichlorphenamide, Methazolamide
Osmotic diuretics : Mannitol, Glycerol, Urea, Isosorbide
Potassium sparing : Spironolactone, Amiloride, Triamterene.

Antiarrhythmic Drugs—Vaughan William's

All are blockers

I-Na II-Beta III-K IV-Ca V-miscellaneous

Class I
a : Quinidine, procainamide, disopyramide
b : Lignocaine, mexiletine, phenytoin, tocainide
c : Propafenone, encainide, flecainide, moricizine
Class II : Propranolol, esmolol, metoprolol
Class III : Amiodarone, Bretyllium, Ibutilide, Dofetilide, Sotalol
Class IV : Verapamil, Diltiazem
Class V : Adenosine, Digoxin, Magnesium, Atropine, Potassium.

Hypolipedimic Drugs

HMG COA reductase inhibitors-(Statins) : Atorvastatin, Lovastatin, Simvastatin, Pravastatin
BILE acid sequestrants (Resins) : Cholestyramine, Colestipol.

Activate Lipoprotein Lipase

(Fibric acid derivatives) : Clofibrate, Gemfibrozil
Inhibit Pg synthesis and lipolysis : Nicotinic acid
Others : Probucol, Gugulipid.

Treatment for Peptic Ulcer

Reduction of Gastric Acid Secretion

H_2 antihistaminics : Ranitidine, Cimetidine, Famotidine, Roxatidine, Nizatidine
Proton pump inhibitors : Omeprazole, Pantoprazole, Rabeprazole, Esomeprazole, Lansoprazole
Anticholinergics : Pirenzepine, Telenzepine, Propantheline, Oxyphenonium
PG analogs : Misoprostol, Enprostil, Rioprostil.

Neutralization of Gastric Acid (Antacids)

Systemic : Sodium Bicarbonate, Sodium Citrate
Nonsystemic : Magnesium hydroxide, Aluminum hydroxide gel
Ulcer protectives : Sucralfate, Colloidal Bismuth Subcitrate (CBS)
Ulcer healing drugs : Carbenoxolone sodium
Anti H pylori drugs : Amoxicillin, Clarithromycin, Metronidazole, Tinidazole and Tetracycline.

Antimicrobials Based on Mechanism of Action

1. *Inhibit cell wall synthesis*: Penicillins, Cephalosporins, Cycloserine, Vancomycin, Bacitracin. Echinocandins (antifungals-micafungin, Caspofungin, Anidulafungin)
2. *Cause leakage from cell membranes*: Polypeptides (Polymyxins, Colistin, Bacitracin) and Polyenes (Amphotericin B, Nystatin, Hamycin)
3. *Inhibit protein synthesis*: Tetracyclines, Chloramphenicol, Erythromycin, Clindamycin, Linezolid
4. *Cause misreading of mRNA code and affect permeability*: Aminoglycosides, e.g. Streptomycin, Gentamicin
5. *Inhibit DNA gyrase*: Fluoroquinolones, e.g. Ciprofloxacin
6. *Interfere with DNA function*: Rifampin, Metronidazole
7. *Interfere with DNA synthesis*: Idoxuridine, Acyclovir, Zidovudine
8. *Interfere with intermediary metabolism*: Sulphonamides, Sulfones, PAS, Trimethoprim, Trimethylamine, Ethambutol.

Beta-lactam Antibiotics (Penicillins, Cephalosporins, Monobactams, Carbapenems) Penicillins

Penicillin G : Procaine and Benzathine (longest acting penicillin)
Aminopenicillins : Ampicillin, Amoxicillin
Carboxypenicillins : Carbenicillin, Ticarcillin
Ureidopenicillins : Mezlocillin, Azlocillin, Piperacillin
Orally active penicillins : Penicillin V, Oxacillin, Dicloxacillin, Cloxacillin, Amoxicillin and Ampicillin
Penicillinase resistant penicillin : Cloxacillin, Oxacillin, Nafcillin, Dicloxacillin, Methicillin.

Cephalosporins

First generation

Parenteral : Cephalothin, Cefazolin
Oral : Cephalexin, Cephradine, Cefadroxil.

Second generation

Parenteral : Cefuroxime, Cefoxitin
Oral : Cefaclor, Cefuroxime axetil.

Third generation
Parenteral : Cefotaxime, Ceftizoxime, Ceftriaxone, Ceftazidime, Cefoperazone
Oral : Cefixime, Cefpodoxime Proxetil, Cefdinir, Ceftibuten.
Fourth generation
Parenteral : Cefepime, Cefpirome, Ceftazidime.

Fifth generation
Ceftaroline
Ceftobiprole-effective against MRSA and pseudomonas
Monobactams : Aztreonam
Carbapenems : Imipenem, Doripenem, Meropenem, Ertapenem
Beta lactamase inhibitors : Clavulanic acid, Sulbactam, Tazobactam.

Fluoroquinolones

First generation : Norfloxacin, Lomefloxacin
Second generation : Ofloxacin, Ciprofloxacin
Third generation : Levofloxacin, Sparfloxacin, Gatifloxacin, Pefloxacin
Fourth generation : Moxifloxacin, Fleroxacin, Garenoxacin, Gemifloxacin, Trovafloxacin.

Tetracyclines

Group 1 : Tetracycline, Chlortetracycline, Oxytetracycline
Group 2 : Demeclocycline, Lymecycline
Group 3 : Doxycycline, Minocycline
Glycylcyclines-mechanism similar to tetracyclines, e.g. Tigecycline
Macrolides : Erythromycin, Azithromycin, Roxithromycin and Clarithromycin
Ketolides : Telithromycin
Lincosamides : Clindamycin, Lincomycin
Streptogramins : Quinupristin, Dalfopristin
Oxazolidinones : Linezolid
Aminoglycosides : Streptomycin, Gentamicin, Kanamycin, Tobramycin, Amikacin, Sisomicin, Netilmicin, Neomycin, Framycetin
Pleuromutilins : Retapamulin.

Antitubercular Drugs

First line drugs
Isoniazid, Rifampin, Pyrazinamide, Ethambutol, Streptomycin.

Second line drugs
Thiacetazone, PAS, Ethionamide, Cycloserine, Kanamycin, Amikacin, Capreomycin,
Newer drugs—ciprofloxacin, ofloxacin, clarithromycin, azithromycin, rifabutin.

Antileprotic Drugs

Sulfones : Dapsone
Phenazine derivative : Clofazimine
Antitubercular drug : Rifampin and Ethionamide
Other antibiotics : Ofloxacin, Minocycline and Clarithromycin.

Antifungal Drugs

1. Antibiotics
   a. *Polyenes*: Amphotericin B, nystatin, hamycin, natamycin
   b. *Heterocycline benzofuran*: Griseofulvin.
2. *Antimetabolite*: Flucytosine

3. Azoles
   a. *Imidazoles*: Topical (Clotrimazole, Miconazole, Econazole) Systemic (Ketoconazole)
   b. *Triazoles*: Systemic (Fluconazole and Itraconazole).
4. *Allylamine*: Terbinafine
5. *Other topical agents*: Tolnaftate, Undecylenic acid, Benzoic acid, Quiniodochlor, Ciclopirox Olamine, Sodium Thiosulphate
6. Echinocandins-Micafungin, Caspofungin, Anidulafungin.

Antiviral drugs

Antiherpes virus : Acyclovir, Idoxuridine, Famciclovir.
Anti-influenza virus : Amantadine, Rimantadine
Non selective antiviral drugs : Ribavirin, Lamivudine and Interferon alpha

Antiretroviral drugs

Nucleoside reverse transcriptase inhibitor: Zidovudine, Stavudine, Lamivudine, Zalcitabine, Didanosine, Aba**cavir**, Emtricitabine.
Non-nucleoside reverse transcriptase inhibitors: Efavirenz, Nevirapine, Delavirdine, Etravirine.
Protease inhibitors: Saqui**navir**, Rito**navir**, Indi**navir**, Nelfi**navir**, Ampre**navir**, Fosampre**navir**, Lopi**navir**, Ataza**navir**, Daru**navir**, Tipra**navir.**
Nucleotide reverse transcriptase inhibitor : Tenofovir
Entry inhibitor : Enfuvirtide, Maraviroc
Integrase inhibitor :Ralte**gra**vir, Elvite**gra**vir

Antihelminthic drugs

Drugs inhibiting polymerization of beta tubulin: Albendazole, Mebendazole, Thiabendazole, Triclabendazole.
Drugs causing spastic paralysis (Novel nicotinic receptor agonist): Pyrantel pamoate, Levamisole
Drugs causing flaccid paralysis (GABA A agonist): Piperazine, Ivermectin
Drugs altering microfilarial membrane and increasing phagocytosis: Diethylcarbamazine (DEC)
Drugs causing uncoupling of oxidative phosphorylation: Bithional, Niclosamide
Drugs causing influx of calcium: Praziquantel

DRUGS OF CHOICE FOR MICROBIAL PATHOGENS

INFECTIVE ORGANISM	DRUGS OF CHOICE
Gram-positive cocci	
Staphylococcal infections	
Sensitive to penicillin	Penicillin
Sensitive to methicillin	Naficillin or oxacillin
Resistant to methicillin	Vancomycin
Resistant to methicillin with Intermediate or complete Resistance to vancomycin	Linezolid
Streptococcal infections	
Group A	
Pharyngitis	Benzathine penicillin G
Impetigo	Benzathine penicillin G
Erysipelas/cellulitis severe	Penicillin G
Mild to moderate	Procaine penicillin G
Necrotizing fascitis/myositis	Surgical debridement +Penicillin G + clindamycin
Pneumonia/empyema	Penicillin G + drainage of empyema
Streptococcal TSS	Penicillin G + clindamycin + IV Ig
Group B	Penicillin
Group D	
Enterococci and nonenterococcal	
(Enterococci are resistant to all cephalosporins)	

Combination therapy	Penicillin or ampicillin + gentamycin
If penicillin is allergic	Vancomycin in combination with gentamycin
Viridans streptococci	Penicillin
Streptococcus pneumoniae	
For otitis media	Amoxicillin
For pneumococcal pneumonia	Oral therapy-amoxicillin quinolone Parenteral therapy-penicillin, Ampicillin, ceftriaxone, cefotaxime, Quinolone
Streptococcus meningitis	
Antibiotic susceptibility unknown	Ceftriaxone + vancomycin
Susceptibility report available	Susceptible-ceftriaxone Resistant-ceftriaxone+vancomycin
Life threatening penicillin allergy	Imipenem
Gram negative cocci	
Meningococcus (Neisseria meningitidis)	Penicillin for confirmed invasive meningococcal disease
Moraxella catarrhalis	Penicillin/clavulanic acid
Gonococcal infection	
Cx, urethra, pharynx, rectum	Ceftriaxone, ciprofloxacin, Ofloxacin
Gonococcal conjunctivitis	ceftriaxone
Ophthalmia neonatarum	ceftriaxone
Disseminated gonococcal infection	
Patient tolerant to β lactam drugs	Ceftriaxone, cefotaxime, ceftizoxime
Patient allergic to β lactam drugs	Ciprofloxacin, ofloxacin, spectinomycin
Gonorrhea epididymitis	Ceftriaxone followed by doxycycline
Gonococcal urethritis	Cefopodoxime or ceftriaxone or flouro quinolones
PID	Oral Regimen A—ofloxacin or levofloxacin + metronidazole Regimen B—ceftriaxone + doxycycline + metronidazole Parenteral Regimen A—cefotetan or cefoxitin + gentamicin Regimen B—clindamycin + gentamicin
Gram-positive bacilli	
Bacillus anthrax	Ciprofloxacin or doxycycline+ Rifampicin, penicillin or chloramphenicol
Clostridium	
Gas gangrene	Penicillin (IV) + clindamycin
Clostridial sepsis	Penicillin (IV) + clindamycin
Suppurative deep tissue infections	Penicillin (IV) + gentamicin or 3rd gen cephalosporin
Clostridium difficile (diarrhea)	Metronidazole and vancomycin
Clostridium tetani	IV penicillin
Diphtheria (respiratory)	Erythromycin/procaine penicillin
Listeria monocytogenes	IV ampicillin/penicillin
Enteric gram-negative bacilli	
E. coli	
Sepsis	Cefotaxime, ceftizoxime,ceftriaxone
Urinary infection	Fluoroquinolones, nitrofurantoin
Klebsiella infections	Carbapenems imipenem is most active drug against *Klebsiella*
Salmonella	Ciprofloxacin, ceftriaxone
Shigella	Nalidixic acid, ampicillin
Campylobacter	Erythromycin
Yersinia pestis	Streptomycin
Other gram-negative bacilli	
Haemophilus ***infections***	
H. influenzae b	Ceftriaxone or cefotaxime
H. ducreyi	Azithromycin (single 1 g oral dose)

Pertussis	Macrolides-erythromycin, Clarithromycin, azithromycin
Legionella	Newer macrolides—Clarithromycin, Azithromycin, Respiratory Quinolones-Levofloxacin
Donovanosis	Azithromycin, erythromycin, Tetracycline, doxycycline
Brucella	Monotherapy-streptomycin Dual therapy-streptomycin and tetracycline
Tularemia	Streptomycin (IM)
Gardnerella vaginalis	Metronidazole
Chlamydia	
Chlamydia trachomatis	Azithromycin
Chlamydia psittaci	Tetracycline
Chlamydia pneumoniae	Erythromycin, Tetracycline, Azithromycin
Chlamydia urethritis	Azithromycin/doxycycline
Rickettsial infections	
Rocky mountain spotted fever	Doxycycline
Rickettsial pox	Doxycycline/ciprofloxacin
Endemic typhus	Doxycycline/chloramphenicol
Epidemic typhus	Doxycycline
Scrub typhus	Doxycycline/chloramphenicol
Spirochaetes	
Syphilis	
Primary, secondary or early latent	Penicillin G benzathine
Late latent cardiovascular or benign tertiary	Normal CSF-penicillin benzathine Abnormal CSF- Rx as neurosyphilis
Neurosyphilis	Aq. penicillin G or Aq. Penicillin G procaine
Leptospirosis	Mild-doxycycline, Ampicillin or Amoxicillin Moderate/severe-penicillin G, Ampicillin, Amoxicillin, Erythromycin
Borrelia	
Relapsing fever	Doxycycline (tetracyclines), Erythromycin, Chloramphenicol
Lyme disease	Oral-adult-doxycycline < 9 years-amoxicillin IV-ceftriaxone
Mycoplasma	Erythromycin or doxycycline
Actinomycetes	
Actinomycosis	Penicillin
Nocardia	Sulphonamides, minocycline
Helminthic infections	
Cestodes	
Hymenolepis nana	Praziquantel
Taenia saginata	Praziquantel
Taenia solium	Praziquantel
Trematodes	
Schistosomiasis	Praziquantel
Liver flukes	Praziquantel
Lung flukes	Praziquantel
Nematodes-*Trichinella* (tissue)	Enteric stage-mebendazole and albendazole
Intestinal nematodes	
Ascariasis	Albendazole, mebendazole, pyrantel pamoate
Hookworm	Albendazole, mebendazole, pyrantel pamoate
Strongyloidiasis	Ivermectin
Trichuriasis (whipworm)	Albendazole or mebendazole
Enterobiasis (pinworm)	Albendazole, mebendazole, pyrantel pamoate

Extraintestinal nematodes	
Filarial (filariasis, tropical pulmonary eosinophilia)	Diethylcarbamazine
Onchocerciasis	Ivermectin
Dracunculiasis	Metronidazole
Protozoal infections	
Ameba	
Asymptomatic carrier	Iodoquinol paramomycin
Acute colitis	Metronidazole + luminal agent
Amoebic liver abscess	Metronidazole
Trichomoniasis	Metronidazole
Giardiasis	Metronidazole
Toxoplasma infection	
Congenital infection	Oral pyrimethamine and sulphadiazine
Immunocompetent patients	Usually do not require Rx
Immunocompromised patients	Trimethoprim sulphamethoxazole.

Antiviral

Influenza A and B	
Prophylaxis	Amantadine or rimantadine amantadine for influenza A only
Treatment	Oseltamivir, zanamivir, amantadine
RSV infection	Ribavirin
CMV-retinitis	Ganciclovir
Varicella	Acyclovir
Herpes simplex	
Encephalitis	Acyclovir
Neonatal	Acyclovir
Genital	Acyclovir
Keratitis	Trifluridine
Herpes zoster	
Immunocompromised	Acyclovir
Immunocompetent	Valacyclovir
Herpes zoster ophthalmicus	Cyclovir
Condyloma acuminatum	IFN-α 2bm, IFN-α n3
Chronic hepatitis B	IFN-α 2b, lamivudine, adefovir, dipivoxil.

Antifungal

Histoplasmosis	
Acute pulmonary	IV amphotericin B
C/c pulmonary	None (alternative Amphotericin B)
Disseminated immunocompetent	Itraconazole
Rapid progressive,CNS involvement	Itraconazole
HIV infection	Amphotericin B
Coccidioidomycosis	
No risk factors	Itraconazole or fluconazole
Risk factors	Amphotericin B Switch to itraconazole/Fluconazole
Chronic dissemination	Itraconazole or fluconazole
Meningitis	Fluconazole/Intrathecal amphotericin B
Blastomycosis	
Rapidly progressing/severe	Amphotericin B Switch to itraconazole
CNS disease	Amphotericin B for 10–12 weeks Switch to fluconazole
Indolent infection	Itraconazole

Cryptococcosis	
Disease in AIDS patients	Amphotericin B
Non-AIDS patients	Meningitis-amphotericin B Switch to fluconazole
Candidiasis	
Cutaneous	Topical azole
Vulvovaginal	Azole cream/Suppository/Oral fluconazole
Oropharyngeal	Clotrimazole or fluconazole
Esophageal	Fluconazole tab
Deeply invasive	Non-neutropenic-fluconazole/Amphotericin, Caspofungin Neutropenic-amphotericin B
Aspergillosis	
Fungus base of lung	Surgical resection
ABPA	Short course of glucocorticoids Itraconazole-Prophylaxis
Invasive aspergillosis	Vorticonazole liposomal/ Conventional amphotericin B
Mucormycosis	IV amphotericin B
Pityriasis versicolor	Azole creams, Application of selenium itraconazole
Sporotrichosis	Itraconazole
Mycetoma	
Actinomycetoma	Streptomycin, dapsone and cotrimoxazole
Eumycetoma	Rarely responds to chemotherapy
Pneumocystosis	
Pneumocystis jiroveci	Trimethoprim sulfamethoxazole.

DRUGS OF CHOICE

Absence seizure	Ethosuximide/valproate
Acetaminophen (poisoning)	N-Acetyl cysteine
Acute bronchial asthma	Salbutamol
Acute gout	NSAIDs except aspirin do not use allopurinol
Acute hyperkalemia	Calcium gluconate
Acute severe migraine	Sumatriptan
Alzheimer's disease	Donepezil/rivastigmine/galantamine
Anaphylactic shock	Adrenaline
Antithyroid in pregnancy	Propylthiouracil
Atonic seizures	Valproate
Atropine poisoning	Physostigmine
Atypical pneumonia	Erythromycin/tetracycline
Benzodiazepine poisoning	Flumazenil
Beta blocker poisoning	Glucagon
Bipolar disorder	Lithium
Carbamate poisoning	Atropine
Chemotherapy induced vomiting	Ondansetron
CLL	Fludarabine+Rituximab
Clonidine withdrawal	Phentolamine
Cyanide toxicity	Amyl nitrate/hydroxocobalamin
Depression	Fluoxetine
DKA	Regular insulin
Drug induced Parkinsonism	Benzhexol
SMR for ET intubation	Succinylcholine
Epilepsy in pregnancy	Phenobarbitone
Ethylene glycol poisoning	Fomepizole
Febrile seizures	Diazepam
Grand mal epilepsy	Valproate

Hairy cell leukemia	Cladribine
Heparin overdose	Protamine
Hypertension in pregnancy	Alpha methyldopa
Hypertension wtih BHP	Prazosin
Hypertensive emergencies in pregnancy	Labetalol/hydralazine
Hypertensive emergencies	Nitroprusside
Hypothyroidism	Levothyroxine
Infantile spasms	Vigabatrin
Iron toxicity	Desferrioxamine
Malignant hyperthermia	Dantrolene
Methanol poisoning	Fomepizole
Mydriatic in adults	Tropicamide
Mydriatic in children	Atropine
Myoclonic seizures	Valproate
Neuroleptanesthesia	Fentanyl+Droperidol+Nitrous oxide
Neuroleptanalgesia	Fentanyl+droperidol
Neuroleptic malignant syndrome	Dantrolene
OCD	Fluoxetine
Opioid poisoning	Naloxone
Organophosphate poisoning	Atropine
Prevention of RF	Benzathine penicillin
Panic disorder	Fluoxetine
Partial seizures	Carbamazepine
Peptic ulcer	PPI
Performance anxiety	Propranolol
PTSD	Fluoxetine
Prevention of MI	Aspirin
Prevention of DVT	Warfarin
Secondary shock	Alpha blockers
Shock with oliguria	Dopamine
SMR in asthma	Vecuronium
SMR in kidney/hepatic failure	Cysatracurium
Status epilepticus	Lorazepam IV
Surgical prophylaxis	Cefazolin
Termination of acute angina	Sl nitroglycerine
Termination of PSVT	Adenosine
PPH	Oxytocin
Trigeminal neuralgia	Oxcarbazepine/Carbamazepine
Ulcerative colitis	Sulfasalazine
Warfarin overdose	Vitamin K
Wegener's granulomatosis	Cyclophosphamide.

MNEMONICS

Appearance of rash in a febrile patient—(Very sick people must take double tea)

1. 1st day—**V**aricella (mainly in trunk; all forms seen at a time; no umbilication of the vesicle)
2. 2nd day—**S**carlet fever (over chest, neck, scapula; mainly macular)
3. 3rd day—Small**p**ox (peripheral distribution; rashes come in a sequence; umbilication of the vesicle)
4. 4th day—**M**easles (maculopapular; over forehead, hairline near ears, face and trunk)
5. 5th day—**T**yphus (macular over shoulders, chest extremities, palms and soles)
6. 6th day—**D**engue (morbilliform; over dorsum of hands and feet, trunk)
7. 7th day—**T**yphoid (rose spots over abdomen, flanks and back; pale-pink fades on pressure).

Common Causes of Travelers Diarrhea (SEC. SNAP)

1. *Shigella* spp
2. ETEC
3. Campylobacter jejuni
4. *Salmonella* spp
5. Noncholera vibrio spp
6. *Aeromonas* spp
7. *Plesiomonas shigelloides.*

Complications of *Falciparum* Malaria (CHAR BACHA HSP)

1. **C**oma
2. **H**yperpyrexia
3. **A**nemia (severe)
4. **R**enal failure (acute)
5. **B**leeding (spontaneous) and coagulopathy
6. **A**cidosis (metabolic)
7. **C**onvulsions
8. **H**ypoglycemia
9. **A**spiration pneumonia
10. **H**yperparasitemia
11. **S**hock
12. **P**ulmonary edema (acute).

Investigations of Typhoid Fever (BASU)

1st week : **B**lood culture
2nd week : **A**gglutination test
3rd week : **S**tool culture
4th week : **U**rine culture.

Complications of Typhoid Fever (SBT)

Septicemic foci-bone and joint infection, meningitis, cholecystitis
Bowel—hemorrhage and perforation
Toxic phenomena—myocarditis and nephritis.

Cardinal Features of Leprosy (SAT)

Skin lesion—typical anesthetic at the tubercular end of spectrum
Acid fast bacilli on skin smear or biopsy
Thickened peripheral nodes.

Oral Lesions of HIV (POSH COLASH)

1. **P**eriodontitis
2. **O**ral hairy leukoplakia
3. **S**yphilis
4. **H**erpes simplex and zoster
5. **C**MV
6. **O**ropharyngeal candidiasis
7. **L**ymphoma
8. **S**arcoma-Kaposi's
9. **H**uman papilloma virus.

Risk Factors for Suicide after Deliberate Self-harm (PALM CURD HSV)

1. **P**sychiatric illness
2. **A**ge over 45
3. **L**iving alone
4. **M**ale sex
5. **C**hronic physical ill health
6. **U**nemployed
7. **R**ecently bereaved
8. **D**rug or alcohol misuse
9. **H**istory of previous attempt
10. **S**uicide note written
11. **V**iolent method used.

Diagnostic Criteria of Anorexia Nervosa (WADA)

1. **W**eight loss of at least 25% of body weight
2. **A**voidance of high calorie food
3. **D**istortion of body image
4. **A**menorrhea for at least 3 months.

Medical Complications of Weight Gain (GOD's SHARP WISH)

1. **G**all stones
2. **O**bstructive sleep apnea
3. **D**iabetes mellitus type 2
4. **S**troke
5. **S**tress incontinence
6. **H**ypertension
7. **A**rthritis
8. **R**espiratory disease
9. **P**regnancy complications
10. **W**eight related musculoskeletal disorders
11. **I**ncreased risk of certain cancers
12. **S**ulphonyl ureas and sodium valprovate (drugs)
13. **H**yperlipidemia.

Causes of Aortic Regurgitation (AIR AIR)

1. **A**ortic dissection
2. **I**nfective endocarditis
3. **R**heumatic disease (common)
4. **A**ortic dilatation
5. **I**njury (trauma)
6. **R**uptured sinus of Valsalva.

Radiological Features of Heart Failure (Small PEG)

1. **S**eptal or kerly B Lines
2. **P**rominence of upper lobe blood vessels
3. **E**nlarged—hilar vessels and cardiac silhouette
4. **G**round glass appearance of alveolar edema.

Complications of Heart Failure (UTI AH3)

1. **U**remia
2. **T**hromboembolism
3. **I**mpaired liver function
4. **A**rrhythmia
5. **H**ypokalemia
6. **H**yponatremia
7. **H**yperkalemia.

Jones Criteria for Acute Rheumatic Fever

Major (CANCHE)

1. **C**arditis
2. **A**rthritis
3. **N**odules (subcutaneous)
4. **C**horea
5. **E**rythema marginatum.

Minor

Clinical (FAP)

1. **F**ever
2. **A**rthralgia
3. **P**revious history of rheumatic fever or heart disease.

Laboratory (CEL.PR)

1. **C** reactive protein ++
2. **E**levated ESR
3. **L**eukocytosis
4. **P**rolonged **PR** interval.

Essential Criteria (SAT)

Scarlet fever recent
Antistreptolysin O titer increased
Throat culture +.

Symptoms and Signs of Acute Limb Ischemia (6 Ps)

1. **P**ain
2. **P**allor
3. **P**ulselessness
4. **P**erishing cold
5. **P**arasthesia
6. **P**aralysis.

Tetralogy of Fallot (VARP)

1. **V**entricular septal defect
2. Overriding of ventricular septal defect by **A**orta
3. **R**ight ventricular hypertrophy
4. **P**ulmonary stenosis.

Clinical Features of Constrictive Pericarditis (HALF PERK)

1. **H**epatomegaly
2. **A**scites
3. **L**oud early third heart sound
4. **F**atigue
5. **P**ulses paradoxus and peripheral edema
6. **E**levated jugular venous pressure
7. **R**apid low volume pulse
8. **K**ussmaul's sign.

Complications of Pneumonia (PAS DEEP ITIS)

1. **P**arapneumonic effusion
2. **A**RDS
3. **S**uppurative pneumonia
4. **D**evelopment of thromboembolic disease
5. **E**ctopic abscess formation (*Staphylococcus aureus*)
6. **E**mpyema
7. **P**neumothorax
8. **H**epa**titis**
9. **P**ericar**ditis**
10. **M**yocar**ditis**
11. **M**eningoencepha**litis**.

Clinical Features of Diabetic Ketoacidosis

Symptoms (PAWN LBW)

1. **P**olyuria
2. **A**bdominal pain
3. **W**eight loss
4. **N**ausea, Vomiting
5. **L**eg cramps
6. **B**lurred vision
7. **W**eakness.

Signs (CHATS DDC)

1. **C**onfusion
2. **H**ypotension, hypothermia
3. **A**ir hunger (Kussmaul's breathing)
4. **T**achycardia
5. **S**mell of acetone
6. **D**ehydration
7. **D**rowsiness
8. **C**oma.

Dermatological Manifestations of Hyperthyroidism (Digital VIP SOAP3)

1. **Digital** clubbing
2. **V**itiligo
3. **I**ncreased sweating
4. **P**almar erythema
5. **S**pider nevi
6. **O**nycholysis
7. **A**lopecia
8. **P**igmentation
9. **P**ruritus
10. **P**retibial myxedema.

Features of Insulin Resistance (Metabolic X Syndrome) (CHIL TIME)

1. **C**entral obesity
2. **H**yperinsulinemia, hypertension
3. **I**ncreased fibrinogen
4. **L**ow HDL
5. **T**ype 2 diabetes
6. **I**ncreased Plasminogen activated inhibitor 1
7. **M**icroalbuminuria
8. **E**levated plasma uric acid.

Complications of Portal Hypertension (VH CHAR)

1. **V**ariceal bleeding
2. **H**ypersplenism
3. **C**ongestive gastropathy
4. **H**epatic encephalopathy
5. **A**scites
6. **R**enal failure.

Extraintestinal Manifestations of Familial Adenomatous Polyposis (BDS LDC)

1. **B**enign osteomas
2. **D**esmoid tumors
3. **S**ubcutaneous epidermal cysts
4. **L**ipomas
5. **D**ental abnormalities
6. **C**ongenital hypertrophy of the retinal pigment epithelium.

Causes of Cirrhosis (WASH PAPA)

1. **W**ilson's disease
2. **A**lcohol
3. **S**econdary biliary cirrhosis (stones, stricture)
4. **H**emochromatosis
5. **P**rimary biliary cirrhosis
6. **A**ny cause of chronic hepatitis
7. **P**rimary sclerosing cholangitis
8. α antitrypsin deficiency.

Complications of Acute Hepatic Failure (PHIR BHI CRIME)

1. **P**ancreatitis
2. **H**ypotension
3. **R**espiratory failure
4. **B**leeding
5. **H**ypothermia
6. **C**erebral edema
7. **R**enal failure
8. **I**nfection
9. **M**etabolic (hypoglycemia, hypokalemia, hypocalcemia, hypomagnesemia)
10. **E**ncephalopathy.

Sites of Hemorrhage (PTCP)

1. **P**utamen
2. **T**halamus
3. **C**erebellum
4. **P**ons.

Factors Precipitating Hepatic Encephalopathy (ABCDEFGHI)

1. **A**lcohol, **A**spiration pneumonia
2. **B**leeding
3. **C**onstipation
4. **D**rugs, **D**ehydration, **D**iuretics
5. **E**xcessive protein
6. **F**luid paracentesis
7. Sur**G**ery
8. **H**ypokalemia
9. **I**nfection.

Common Red Cell Appearance and their Causes

Microcytosis

1. Iron deficiency
2. Sideroblastic anemia
3. Thalassemia.

Macrocytosis

1. Vitamin B_{12} or folate deficiency
2. Hypothyroidism and liver disease.

Target Cells

1. Liver disease
2. Postsplenectomy
3. Thalassemia
4. HbC disease.

Spherocytes

1. Autoimmune hemolysis
2. Postsplenectomy
3. DIC
4. Hereditary spherocytosis.

Howell Jolly Bodies

1. Hyposplenism
2. Dyshemopoisis
3. Postsplenectomy.

Basophyllic Stippling

1. Dyshematopoiesis
2. Lead poisoning.

Criteria for Diagnosis of Rheumatoid Arthritis (MADR3AS)

1. **M**orning stiffness (> 1 hour)
2. **A**rthritis of three or more joints
3. **D**uration of 6 weeks or more
4. **R**heumatoid nodules
5. **R**heumatoid factor
6. **R**adiological changes
7. **A**rthritis of hand joints
8. **S**ymmetrical arthritis.

(Diagnosis of rheumatoid arthritis is made with 4 or more criteria.)

Criteria for SLE (Aim on Sharp Disk)

1. **A**rthritis
2. **I**mmunological disorders
3. **M**alar rash
4. **O**ral ulcers
5. **N**eurological disorders
6. **S**erositis
7. **H**ematological disorders
8. **A**ntinuclear antibody disorder
9. **R**enal disorders
10. **P**hotosensitivity
11. **D**iscoid rash.

(Diagnosis of SLE is made when 4 out of 11 are present serially or simultaneously.)

Narcolepsy Tetrad (Chess)

1. Cataplexy
2. Hypnagogic hallucinations
3. Sleep paralysis
4. Sleep attacks.

Abdominal Pain: Medical Causes [ABDOMENAL PANE (Abdominal Pain)]

1. **A**cute rheumatic fever
2. **B**lood (Purpura, a/c hemolytic crisis)
3. **D**KA
4. c**O**llagen vascular disease
5. **M**igraine (abdominal migraine)
6. **E**pilepsy (abdominal epilepsy)
7. **N**ephron (uremia)
8. **A**bdominal angina
9. **L**ead
10. **P**orphyria
11. **A**rsenic
12. **N**SAID's
13. **E**nteric fever.

Anion Gap Metabolic Acidosis: Causes (AIM CAT PUDLE)

1. **A**lcohol
2. **I**ron/Isoniazid
3. **M**ethanol
4. **C**arbamazepine
5. **A**spirin
6. **T**oluene
7. **P**araldehyde
8. **U**remia
9. **D**iabetic ketoacidosis
10. **L**actic acidosis
11. **E**thylene glycol.

Metabolic Acidosis: Causes (USED CAR)

1. **U**reteroenterostomy
2. **S**aline hydration
3. **E**ndocrinopathies (hyperparathyroid, hyperthyroid, Addison's)
4. **D**iarrhea/**D**KA/**D**rugs
5. **C**arbonic anhydrase inhibitors
6. **A**mmonium chloride
7. **R**enal tubular acidosis.

Alternatively: **USED CARP,** to include **P**arenteral nutrition/**P**ancreatic fistula.

Toxicity/Sepsis: Signs (6 T's)

1. Tachycardia
2. Tachypnea
3. Tremors
4. Toxic look
5. Tiredness
6. Temperature (fever).

Gynecomastia

1. **G**enetic **G**ender disorder (Klinefelter)
2. **Y**oung boy (pubertal)*
3. **N**eonate*
4. **E**strogen
5. **C**irrhosis/**C**imetidine/**C**a Channel blockers
6. **O**ld age*
7. **M**arijuana
8. **A**lcoholism
9. **S**pironolactone
10. **T**umors (Testicular and adrenal)
11. **I**soniazid/**I**nhibition of testosterone
12. **A**ntineoplastics (Alkylating Agents)/**A**ntifungal (Ketoconazole).

* Asterisk indicates physiologic cause.

Hypernatremia: Causes (6 D's)

1. **D**iuretics
2. **D**ehydration
3. **D**iabetes insipidus
4. **D**ocs (iatrogenic)
5. **D**iarrhea
6. **D**isease: kidney, sickle cell, etc.

SIADH

1. **S**pasms
2. **I**s not any pitting edema (key DDx)
3. **A**norexia
4. **D**isorientation (and other psychoses)
5. **H**yponatremia.

Horner's Syndrome: Components (SAMPLE)

1. **S**ympathetic chain injury
2. **A**nhidrosis
3. **M**iosis
4. **P**tosis
5. **L**oss of ciliospinal reflex
6. **E**nophthalmos.

Causes of Clubbing

1. Cardiac causes
   a. Congenital cyanotic heart disease like Fallot's tetralogy
   b. SBE
   c. Rarely in cardiac tumors (e.g. in atrial myxoma)
   d. Eisenmenger's syndrome, primary pulmonary hypertension.
2. Lung and pleural causes (ABCDEF)
   a. **A**bscess (lung)
   b. **B**ronchiectasis (including CF)
   c. **C**ancer (lung)
   d. **D**ecreased oxygen (hypoxia)
   e. **E**mpyema
   f. **F**ibrosing alveolitis.
3. **U**lcerative colitis
4. **B**iliary cirrhosis, sometimes in hepatocellular failure

5. Intestinal causes
   a. Malabsorption syndrome
   b. Crohn's disease
   c. Polyposis coli
   d. Celiac disease.
6. Normal—found normally in some people
7. Genetic—may be a familial condition.

CHOREA: Common Causes (St VITUS'S DANCE)

1. **S**ydenhams
2. **V**ascular
3. **I**ncreased RBCs (polycythemia)
4. **T**oxins: CO, Mg, Hg
5. **U**remia
6. **S**LE
7. **S**enile chorea
8. **D**rugs
9. **A**PLA syndrome
10. **N**eurodegenerative conditions: HD, neuroacanthocytosis, DRPLA
11. **C**onception related: pregnancy, OCPs
12. **E**ndocrine: hyperthyroidism, hypo-, hyperglycemi
13. Cranial nerves which one is sensory and which is motor can be learned by
    "Some Says Money Matters But My Brother Says Big Books Matter More". Here, S = Sensory; M = Motor and B = Both.

Guillain-Barré Syndrome: Features (4 A's)

1. Acute inflammatory demyelinating polyneuropathy
2. Ascending paralysis
3. Autonomic neuropathy
4. Arrythmias.

Raised JVP: Causes (PQRST)

1. **P**ericardial effusion, **P**ulmonary embolism, **P**ulmonary hypertension (chronic)
2. **Q**uantity of fluid is more (fluid overload)
3. **R**ight heart failure
4. **S**uperior venacaval obstruction (distended veins without pulsation)
5. **T**ricuspid regurgitation, **T**ricuspid stenosis, **T**amponade (cardiac).

Atrial Fibrillation: Causes (PIRATES)

1. **P**ulmonary: Pulmonary embolism, COPD
2. **I**atrogenic
3. **R**heumatic heart disease
4. **A**therosclerotic heart disease
5. **T**hyrotoxicosis
6. **E**ndocarditis
7. **S**ick sinus syndrome.

Heart Murmur: Characteristics (SCRIPT)

1. **S**ite
2. **C**haracter
3. **R**adiation, **R**espiratory variation
4. **I**ntensity (grade)
5. **P**itch, **P**ositional variation
6. **T**iming.

Thrombocytosis: Causes (MAKE MAPS)

1. **M**yeloproliferative disorders (CML or PRV)
2. **A**cute hemorrhage
3. **K**awasaki syndrome
4. **E**ssential thrombocytosis
5. **M**alignancy
6. **A**cute/chronic inflammation
7. **P**ostoperative
8. **S**plenectomy.

Sarcomas with Lymph Node Metstatis (SCARE)

1. **S**ynovial sarcoma
2. **C**lear cell sarcoma
3. **A**ngiosarcoma
4. **R**habdomyosarcoma
5. **E**pitheliod sarcoma.

2
CHAPTER
Surgery

SWELLING OR LUMP

History of Present Illness

1. *Duration*: Shorter—benign; Longer—malignant
2. *Mode of onset*: Sudden or gradual
3. Associated symptoms
4. *Pain*: Nature, site, time of onset, radiation, difficulty in respiration/swallowing
5. Fever
6. Impairment of function
7. *Progress of swelling*: Stationary or continued
8. History of trauma
9. *Secondary changes*: Softening, ulceration, fungation, inflammatory changes
10. *History of recurrence*: Malignant—recurs after removal
11. *Cystic swelling*: If cyst wall not completely removed
12. History of loss of appetite and weight loss.

History of Past Illness

Similar illness, TB, syphilis.

Personal History

Betel chewing (Nut, slaked lime, tobacco) responsible for growth in cheek, tongue, mouth, lip.

Family History

Similar illness; TB; von Recklinghausen's disease.

General Examination

1. PICCLE (**P**allor, **I**cterus, **C**yanosis, **C**lubbing, **L**ymph node enlargement, **E**dema).
2. Vitals
3. Local examination (L/E).

Inspection

1. Site
2. Shape
3. Size
4. Surface—cauliflower (Squamous cell carcinoma) irregular numerous branched (Papilloma).

5. Extent
6. Color—blue (Ranula); black (Nevus, melanoma); red (Hemangioma)
7. Margin—well defined, poorly defined
8. Number
9. Pulsation
10. Impulse on cough—meningocele, hernia
11. Skin over swelling
12. Any sinuses, scar, prominent veins.

Palpation

1. Local rise of temperature and tenderness
2. Site, size, shape, number, extent, surface, margin
3. Consistency
4. Fluctuation
5. Transillumination
6. Impulse on cough
7. Pulsatility—transmitted (swelling superficial to artery); expansile (originates from arterial wall)
8. Reducibility
9. Compressibility
10. Fixity to overlying skin—papilloma, epithelioma, sebaceous cyst
11. Skin over the swelling—pinchable (if not fixed to skin)
12. Relation to superficial and deep part—skin, subcutaneous (s/c) tissue, muscle, tendon, bone, joint, vessels.

Examination of Regional Lymph Node

Percussion

Auscultation
Bruit-aneurysm.

Measurements
Compare with opposite side in case of wasting.

Movements
Examine the movement of nearby joints.

Examination of Pressure Effects

1. Arterial pulse—weak distal to swelling
2. Nerve—wasting, paresis, paralysis
3. Vein—distal edema, venous engorgement.

Diagnosis

1. Anatomical location
2. Pathological nature
3. Complication.

Anatomical	Pathological
Skin, subcutaneous (s/c) tissue, muscle, tendon, bones, joints	Congenital, traumatic, inflammatory-acute and chronic
Vessels, arteries	Neoplasm—benign and malignant

Example: Lipoma—this person having benign subcutaneous tissue swelling probably lipoma without any features of complication.

Investigations

1. Routine (R/E) investigations of blood and urine
2. X-ray of swelling—to find out bony erosion
3. X-ray chest—to rule out pulmonary metastasis
4. Fine needle aspiration cytology (FNAC)

5. Aspiration—for cystic swelling
6. Angiography—for aneurysms
7. Biopsy
8. USG, CT, MRI (only for special situations).

Discussion

Common Swellings of Soft Tissue

Lipoma

Clinical features
1. Ubiquitous
2. Pseudofluctuant
3. Free from skin and deeper tissue
4. Commonly subcutaneous lipoma
5. Slipping edge.

Complications
1. Myxomatous degeneration
2. Infection
3. Saponification
4. Malignant change to liposarcoma
5. Ulceration due to repeated trauma.

Management

Investigation + treatment (Rx)—excision.

Sebaceous Cyst

Commonly on scalp and scrotum, has connection with a hair follicle in majority of cases. Adherent to skin at punctum and is fluctuant.

Complications

1. Infection
2. Calcification
3. Rupture and sinus formation
4. Carcinomatous changes
5. Cock's peculiar tumor
6. Sebaceous horn.

Management

Investigation + treatment (Rx)—incision and avulsion of cyst with wall.

Classification of Tumors

1. **Congenital**
   a. Dermoid cyst
   b. *Hemangioma*:
      i. Capillary
      ii. Cavernous
      iii. Plexiform
      iv. Congenital AV fistula
      v. Glomangioma.
2. **Traumatic**
   a. Hematoma
   b. Implantation dermoid.
3. **Inflammatory**
   a. Erysipelas—spreading cuticular lymphangitis
   b. Cellulitis—spreading of inflammation of subcutaneous and facial tissues leading to suppuration, sloughing or even gangrene
   c. Abscess-pyogenic, pyemic and cold
   d. Boil furuncle
   e. Carbuncle.
4. **Neoplastic**

I. **Benign neoplasms**
   1. *Papilloma*: Overgrowth of all layers of skin.
   2. *Fibroma*: Tumors of fibrous tissue.
   3. *Lipoma*: Encapsulated subcutaneous lipoma, diffuse variety, multiple lipoma.
   4. *Neurofibroma*: This tumor contains both neural (abdermal) and fibrous (mesodermal elements)
      a. Local neurofibroma
      b. Generalized neurofibromatosis—von Recklinghausen's disease, congenital autosomal dominant, associated with light brown pigmentation, acoustic neuroma, pheochromocytoma
      c. Plexiform neurofibromatosis-branches of fifth cranial nerve
      d. Elephantiasis neurofibromatosis
      e. Pachydermatocele.
   5. *Schwannoma (neurilemmoma)*: Schwann cell neurilemma, benign well encapsulated tumor.
   6. *Lymphangioma*:
      a. Simple/capillary lymphangioma b. Cavernous lymphangioma c. Cystic hygroma.
   7. *Moles (pigmented nevus, freckles, benign melanoma)*:
      a. Hairy mole
      b. Nonhairy or smooth moles
      c. Blue nevus
      d. Junctional nevus
      e. Compound nevus
      f. Juvenile mole
      g. Hutchisons freckle (lentigo).

II. **Malignant**
   1. Basal cell carcinoma
   2. Squamous cell carcinoma
   3. Malignant melanoma
   4. Sarcoma
   5. Synovial sarcoma.

   Other swellings
   a. Sebaccous cyst
   b. Condyloma
   c. Warts
   d. Keloid and hypertrophic scar
   e. Callosity and corn
   f. Keratoacanthoma
   g. Seborrheic wart
   h. Solar keratosis
   i. Bowen's disease.

THYROID SWELLING

History

1. Age
   a. *Teenage girls*: Simple goiter
   b. *Women of 20 to 30*: MNG and SNT
   c. *Young girls*: Papillary CA, primary toxic goiter
   d. *Middle aged women*: Hashimoto's disease, follicular CA
   e. *Old age*: Anaplastic CA.
2. Sex
   a. *Female*: Male—3:1
   b. History of swelling—onset, duration, rate of growth.
   c. Associated with pain—inflammatory conditions are painful—goiter and CA are painless
   d. *History of pressure effect*:
      i. Dyspnea
      ii. Dysphagia
      iii. Hoarseness of voice
      iv. Stridor
   e. History of precipitating emotional or psychic trauma
   f. Physiological stress—puberty, pregnancy, lactation, menopause
   g. History of endemicity.

Symptoms of Primary Thyrotoxicosis

1. Loss of weight in spite of good appetite
2. Excessive sweating
3. Insomnia
4. Protruding eyes (exophthalmos)

5. Intolerance to heat
6. Smooth and moist skin—irritability
7. Tremor of hands
8. Diplopia (ophthalmoplegia).

Symptoms of Secondary Thyrotoxicosis (Cardiovascular)

1. Palpitation
2. Dyspnea on exertion
3. Swelling of ankles
4. Chest pain.

Symptoms of Hypothyroidism (Myxedema)

1. Increase of weight in spite of poor appetite
2. Dry skin
3. Loss of memory
4. Loss of hair and eyebrows (lateral 1/3rd)
5. Constipation
6. Intolerance to cold
7. Dull expression
8. Puffiness of face
9. Fatigability
10. Lethargy.

Past History

1. *History of radiation*: Papillary CA
2. *History of HTN + thyroid swelling*: Sipple's syndrome
3. *History of similar illness*: Recurrence
4. History of intake of drugs.

Personal History

1. Sleep decreased—hyperthyroidism
2. Menstrual history in females
3. Diet—excessive use of cabbage—goitrogens (brassica family).

Family History

Medullary CA, papillary CA, MNG run in family.

General Examination

Body built and nourishment
1. *Thin and underweight*: Thyrotoxicosis
2. *Obese and overweight*: Hypothyroidism.

Facies

1. *Thyrotoxicosis*: Facial expressions of excitement, tension, nervousness, agitations with exophthalmos
2. *Hypothyroidism*: Puffy face without expression.

Skin

1. *Thyrotoxicosis*: Hot and moist palm
2. *Myxedema*: Dry and inelastic skin.

Local Examination

Inspection

1. *Pizzillo's method*: Hands are placed behind the head, push the head against resistance
2. Shape, size
3. Extent
   a. Vertically—from lower part of thyroid cartilage to 1 cm above suprasternal notch
   b. Horizontally—from anterior border of sternocleidomastoid (SCM) on both side.

4. Moving with deglutition
5. Lower border visible or not
6. Plane of swelling—deep to deep fascia
7. Skin over the swelling—dilated veins, sinus, scar, fistula, visible pulsations
8. Pemberton's sign—ask patient to lift the hands so that hand touches the ear lobes.

Dilated vein (obstruction of superior vena cava)—Retrosternal goiter.

Sipple's syndrome (Men Type 2)
- Hyperparathyroidism
- Pheochromocytoma
- Medullary carcinoma thyroid.

Pendred's syndrome (Peroxidase enzyme deficiency)
- Congenital deafness
- Goiter
- Hypothyroidism.

Palpation

Three Berry's in Thyroid

Berry's sign: Absent carotid pulsations (anaplastic carcinoma).

1. Palpated with neck slightly flexed
2. Palpation of each lobe
   a. *Lahey's method*: In front of the patient
   b. *Crile's method*: Thumb on thyroid gland on swallow
   c. *Naffziger's method*: Stand behind the patient
3. Local rise of temperature or tenderness
4. Site, size, shape, extent, consistency, margin
5. Surface
   a. *Smooth*: Primary thyrotoxicosis
   b. *Bosselated*: Multinodular goiter (MNG)
6. Mobility
7. Get above the swelling
8. Plane of the swelling—deep to deep fascia
9. *Kocher's test (Test for large swelling)*: Push the thyroid swelling laterally—stridor.

Vitals

1. *Pulse rate*: Rapid and irregular—secondary thyrotoxicosis
2. *Sleeping pulse rate*: Access the degree of toxicity
   a. *Mild*: < 90/min
   b. *Moderate*: 90 to 110/min
   c. *Severe*: 110/min.

Signs of Toxicity

I. *Eye Signs*

1. *Lid retraction*: Over activity of involuntary part of muscle—Smooth part of levator palpebrae superioris and Mullers muscles supplied by cervical sympathetic plexus
2. *Exophthalmos*: Due to infiltration of retrobulbar connective tissue with mucopolysaccharide, immunoglobulins, fluid occurs probably due to lymphatic/venous obstruction
   a. *von Graefe's sign (lid lag)*
   b. *Joffroy's sign (wringling of forehead absent)*
   c. *Stellwag's sign (infrequent blinking of eyes)*: Due to toxic contraction of striated fibers of levator palpebrae superioris
   d. *Möbius sign (inability to converge the eyeball)*
   e. *Dalrymple's sign (upper sclera visible)*: Due to retraction of upper eyelid

3. *Ophthalmoplegia*: Weakness of ocular muscles
   Muscles affected—superior and lateral rectus, inferior oblique.
4. *Chemosis (edema of conjunctiva)*:

II. *Delayed Ankle Jerk (Hypothyroidism)*

III. *Tachycardia*

IV. *Tremor*

V. *Moist Skin*

VI. *Thyroid Bruit*

Cardiovascular System Changes

Inc heart rate (HR) → ectopics → AF → VT → VF.

Mechanism of Eye Signs

1. **Lid lag and lid spasm** are due to hyperthyroidism and are also seen in secondary hyperthyroidism and disappears on correcting hyperthyroidism.
2. **Diplopia** develops in Grave's disease due to weakness of elevators especially internal oblique.
3. **Edema** of the eye lid conjunctival congestion and chemosis are due to compression of ophthalmic vein.
   Thyroidectomy or radio iodine therapy are contraindicated in proptosis of recent onset as it may produce malignant **exophthalmos.**

Percussion

1. Normally resonant over manubrium sterni
2. Dull in retrosternal goiter.

Auscultation

1. Lateral aspect of upper lobe
2. Bruit due to increased vascularity.

Skull and Spine

Cardiovascular System (CVS)

Gastrointestinal System (GIT)

Respiratory

Position of trachea.

Diagnosis

Treated multinodular thyroid without any features of thyrotoxicosis or malignancy.

Investigations

1. Blood and urine R/E
2. Thyroid function test
3. X-ray neck—retrosternal thyroid
4. Indirect laryngoscopy

5. FNAC—cannot distinguish between follicular adenoma and CA
6. Isotope scan I-123
7. Bone scan
8. Thyroid antibodies
9. Trucut biopsy
10. Serum cholesterol increased in hypothyroidism
11. Serum calcitonin increased in medullary CA (normal < 0.08 mg/L)
12. USG, CT, MRI.

Thyroid Function Test

1. T4 (10–30) nmol/L
2. T3 (3.5–7.5) micromol/L
3. TSH (0.3–3.3) milliunit/L.

Treatment

Medical

Hyperthyroidism

1. Thyroid inhibitors (Inhibiting thyroid hormone synthesis) methimazole, carbimazole, propylthiouracil
2. *Inhibit iodide trapping*: Thiocyanates, perchlorates, nitrates
3. *Destroy thyroid tissue*: Radioactive iodine I-131, I-125, I-123
4. *β blockers (Prevent T4 → T3)*: Propranolol.

Hypothyroidism

Thyroxine doses OD.

Surgical

Preoperative Preparations

1. Carbimazole 30–40 mg/day for 8 to 12 weeks after 12 weeks reduce the dose to 5 mg 8th hourly
2. Last dose given on evening before surgery
3. Thyroxine added to maintain the euthyroid state
4. Lugol's iodine (5–10 drops) orally with milk (to decrease vascularity and size of tumor)
5. Potassium iodide (KI)/Sodium iodide (NaI) (60 mg tid) alternative to Lugol's iodine—10 days before operation
6. Propranolol (40 mg TDS) or nadolol (160 mg once daily)—inhibit the conversion of T4 → T3
7. Indirect laryngoscopy (ENT consultation) medicolegal purposes
8. Three drug regime—Antithyroid + Lugol's iodine + β blocker.

Block and Replacement Surgeries

T3 (20 mg up to 4 times daily) or T4 (0.1 mg/day) + antithyroid drugs → Less danger of producing thyroid insufficiency and increase in size of goiter.

Thyroxine Doses

1. Supplementary 0.1 mg
2. Replacement 0.2 mg
3. Suppressive 0.3 mg.

Thyroid Surgeries

1. Isthumusectomy
2. *Lobectomy*: Total lobectomy + isthumusectomy
3. *Subtotal thyroidectomy*: Total lobectomy + total lobectomy+ isthumusectomy
4. *Near total thyroidectomy*: Total lobectomy + isthumusectomy + subtotal lobectomy.

Strap Muscles of Neck

1. *Superficial*: Sternohyoid, omohyoid
2. *Deep*: Thyrohyoid, sternothyroid.

Postoperative assessments

1. Indirect laryngoscopy
2. Serum Ca after surgery
3. Withhold the thyroxine until HPR results are available and proceed accordingly
4. Life long follow-up for thyrotoxicosis
5. Propranolol should be continued for 7 days postoperative as it does not inhibit thyroxin synthesis but acts on the end organs.

Postoperative Complications

Immediate

1. *Hemorrhage*: Tension hematoma; subcutaneous hematoma.
2. *Respiratory obstruction*: Collapse of trachea; laryngeal edema; tension hematoma.
   Rx: Release tension hematoma; endotracheal tube (ET) intubation; steroids reduce edema tracheostomy (rarely); needle tracheostomy (temporary measure).
3. *RLN paralysis*
   a. Unilateral/bilateral
   b. Transient/permanent—recovers in 3 weeks to 3 months.
4. *Thyroid crisis or thyroid storm*
   a. Acute exacerbation of hyperthyroidism
   b. Occurs in a thyrotoxic patient inadequately prepared for thyroidectomy.

Management of thyroid crisis

General

1. IV fluids
2. Cooling the patient with ice packs
3. Oxygen administration
4. Diuretics for cardiac failure
5. Digoxin for uncontrolled AF
6. Sedation
7. Hydrocortisone IV.

Specific

1. Carbimazole 10–20 mg 6th hourly
2. Lugol's iodine 10 drops 6th hourly orally or NaI IV
3. Propranolol 40 mg 6th hourly orally.

Late Complications

Hypoparathyroidism (hypocalcemia)

1. Due to removal of parathyroid gland or damage to parathyroid end artery
2. Occurs at the end of 2nd day (half-life of parathyroid is 2 to 5 days).

Symptoms

1. Perioral numbness
2. Carpal spasm
3. Tingling sensation of fingers
4. Tetany
5. Severe painful cramps
6. Laryngeal spasm.

Management: 10% calcium gluconate IV 10 mL slowly for 10 minutes.

1. *Thyroid insufficiency*: Occurs within 2 years
2. Wound infection
3. *Hypertrophic/keloid scar Rx*: Intradermal injection of corticosteroid
4. Stitch granuloma
5. Laryngeal paralysis.

Berry's Ligament

Berry picking: Removal of lymph nodes.

Stages of development of thyrotoxic arrhythmias.

1. Multiple extrasystole
2. Paroxysmal atrial tachycardia
3. Paroxysmal atrial fibrillation
4. Persistent atrial fibrillation not responding to digoxin.

Sites of Aberant Thyroid Tissue

1. Lingual
2. Cervical
3. Intrathoracic.

Neuberg's artery: Thyroid ima artery
Koker's vein: Vein between middle and inferior thyroid vein draining into internal jugular vein (IJV).
Nerve of galagussi: External laryngeal nerve—supplying cricothyroid.

Multiple Endocrine Neoplasia

MEN 1 or Wermer Syndrome

1. Pituitary adenoma or hyperplasia
2. Parathyroid adenoma or hyperplasia
3. Pancreatic islet cell hyperplasia, adenoma or carcinoma
4. Less common manifestations—foregut carcinoids; pheochromocytoma; subcutaneous or visceral lipomas.

MEN 2A or Sipple Syndrome

1. Medullary carcinoma of thyroid
2. Pheochromocytoma
3. Parathyroid adenoma or hyperplasia
4. Hirschsprung's disease
5. Cutaneous lichen amyloidosis.

MEN 2B

1. Medullary carcinoma of thyroid
2. Pheochromocytoma
3. Marfanoid features
4. Mucocutaneous and gastrointestinal neuromas.

Multinodular Goiter—Stages

Stage 1: Diffuse hypertrophy and hyperplasia of gland
Stage 2: Fluctuating levels of thyroid stimulating hormone (TSH)
Stage 3: Active lobules undergo central necrosis leads to nodular formation.

Complications of Multinodular Goiter

1. Acute respiratory obstruction due to hemorrhage
2. Secondary thyrotoxicosis
3. Calcification
4. Carcinomatous changes.

Treatment

1. *If asymptomatic*: No surgery
2. *If symptomatic*: Subtotal thyroidectomy after toxic symptoms are decreased—postoperative thyrotoxins.

Indications for Operation

1. Malignancy
2. Toxic adenoma
3. Pressure symptoms
4. Cosmetic
5. Patient wishes.

Wayne's Clinical Diagnostic Index

Score

1. < 11 Hypothyroidism
2. 11–13 Euthyroid
3. > 13 Hyperthyroidism
4. > 19 Toxic.

Eye Manifestations in Toxic Goiter (No Specs Criteria)

Grade 0 : No signs
Grade 1 : Only signs
Grade 2 : Symptoms present—diplopia, periorbital edema
Grade 3 : Proptosis > 1.5 cm
Grade 4 : Extraocular manifestations
Grade 5 : Corneal ulcer
Grade 6 : Sight loss.

Clinical Features of Hyperthyroidism

1. Weight loss
2. Tachycardia
3. Atrial fibrillation/heart failure
4. Eye signs—lid lag, lid retraction, exophthalmos (Grave's disease)
5. Sweating
6. Thyroid gland enlargement and bruit (Grave's disease)
7. Fine distal tremor
8. Thinning of hair
9. Proximal weakness; cannot rise from squat
10. Chorea.

Clinical Features of Hypothyroidism

1. Weight gain
2. Shallow complexion and dry skin
3. Thinning of scalp and lateral eyebrow hair
4. Cold intolerance
5. Deepened gruff voice
6. Slow physical and mental activity
7. Unsteadiness and slightly slurred speech
8. Tingling in toes and fingers
9. Aching muscles with cramp
10. Mild proximal weakness
11. Slow pulse and shortness of breath.

Causes for Hypothyroidism (GET AIDS)

1. Goitrogens
2. Endemic
3. Thyroid agenesis
4. Autoimmune—Chronic lymphoma, Hashimoto's disease
5. Iatrogenic
6. Dyshormonogenesis
7. Secondary to pituitary or hypothalamic disease.

Myxedema Coma

Clinical Features

1. Altered mental state
2. Hypothermia
3. Precipitating cardiac failure
4. Infection.

Management

1. Slow warming of body
2. Broad spectrum antibiotics IV
3. Injection hydrocortisone divided dose
4. 500 ng T4 /10 mg T3 IV/orally every 4 to 6th hourly.

Thyroiditis

Autoimmune Thyroiditis

Clinical features

Bosselated goiter (hyperthyroidism)—initially and later hypothyroidism due to fibrosis sudden and painful, common after menopause associated with papillary CA, malignant lymphoma.

Diagnosis

1. Raised thyroid antibody titer
2. Thyroid function test (TFT) gives hypothyroid status
3. FNAC.

Treatment

1. Replacement dose 0.2 mg TID
2. Steroid—if goiter increases in size or no response to thyroxin
3. Thyroidectomy—if goiter is large and causes discomfort.

Granulomatous Thyroiditis

Granulomatous thyroiditis (Subacute thyroiditis, De Quervain's thyroiditis)—due to viral infection.

Clinical features

Pain in neck, fever, malaise, firm irregular enlargement of one/two lobes.

Diagnosis

1. Raised ESR
2. Thyroid antibodies absent
3. Serum T4 level high normal or slightly raised
4. I-131 reuptake decreased.

Treatment

Subsides spontaneously within few months.
Prednisolone 10 to 20 mg once daily (OD) for 7 days (dose is gradually reduced over next month).

Riedel's Thyroiditis

1. Thyroid tissue is replaced by cellular fibrous tissue which infiltrates—muscles, adjacent structures, parathyroid, recurrent nerves, carotid sheath
2. Goiter may be U/L or B/L
3. Very hard and fixed-hypothyroidism.

Diagnosis

Wedge biopsy.

Treatment

High dose steroid.
Thyroxine replacement dose.
Isthmusectomy—reduction in size of goiter.

Risk of Malignancy in Thyroid Swelling

Rule of Twelve

Isolated thyroid swelling		Dominant thyroid swelling	
Solid 24%	Cystic 12%	Solid 12%	Cystic 6%
Male 48%	Female 12%	Male 24%	Female 6%
Male 24%	Female 6%	Male 12%	Female 3%
Generalized thyroid swelling 3%			

Neck Dissection

Levels of Lymph Nodes of Neck

Level 1: 1a–Submental LN 1b–Submandibular LN

Level 2: (Upper jugular LN) upper 1/3rd of jugular vein (i.e. between the base of skull and level of hyoid bone up to bifurcation of carotid artery)

Level 3: (Middle jugular LN)
1. Above → hyoid bone; 2. Below → cricoid cartilage

Level 4: (Lower jugular LN)-Upper border of cricoid cartilage to clavicle

Level 5: (Postcervical group)-LN of spinal accessory chain; supraclavicular LN; transverse cervical LN

Level 6: (Anterior compartment nodes)
1. Laterally → medial borders of SCM
2. Above → hyoid bone
3. Below → suprasternal notch (prelaryngeal LNs; pretracheal LNs; paratracheal LNs)

Level 7: (Nodes of upper mediastinum); below → suprasternal notch.

Neoplasms of Thyroid Gland

Important points about thyroid carcinoma

1. *Most malignant*: Anaplastic carcinoma
2. *Least malignant*: Papillary carcinoma
3. *MC type of thyroid carcinoma after radiation*: Papillary carcinoma
4. *Thyroid carcinoma associated with dystrophic calcification*: Papillary carcinoma
5. *Psammoma bodies are seen in*: Papillary carcinoma
6. *Orphan Annie Eyed nuclei are seen in*: Papillary carcinoma
7. *Thyroid carcinoma occurring in long standing multinodular goiter*: Follicular carcinoma
8. *Carcinoma derived from C cells of thyroid*: Medullary carcinoma
9. *Thyroid carcinoma associated with MEN*: Medullary carcinoma
10. *Thyroid carcinoma associated with amyloidosis*: Medullary carcinoma.

Carcinoma	Papillary (80%)	Follicular (11%)	Anaplastic (2%)	Medullary (4%)
Etiology	Irradiation	Endemic goiter	Unknown	Sporadic/familial (MEN2 syndrome)
Age	20–40	30–50	50 and above	Middle age
Diagnosis	Thyroid swelling with LN	Thyroid swelling metastasis—bone	Thyroid swelling	Difficulty to diagnose clinically
Microscopy	Orphan Annie eyed nucleus psammoma bodies	Angioinvasion, capsular invasion	Poorly differentiated cell	Amyloid stoma like carcinoid
Spread	Lymphatic	Blood	Local infiltration	Lymphatic + blood
Investigations	FNAC	Frozen section	FNAC, biopsy	FNAC, calcitonin
Rx of primary	Near total thyroidectomy	Near total thyroidectomy	Isthmusectomy external RT	Total thyroidectomy
Rx of metastasis	Functional block dissection	Radio I131 or external RT	Palliative external RT	Radical block dissection
Prognosis	Excellent	Good	Worst	Bad

List of Important Tumor Markers

Tumor site	Tumor markers
Medullary carcinoma of thyroid	Calcitonin
Papillary carcinoma of thyroid	Thyroglobulin

Contd...

Contd...

Prostate	Prostate specific antigen; prostate acid phosphatase
Liver	Alpha feto protein (AFP); carcinoembryonic antigen
Ovary	CA125; Placental alkaline phosphatase; b hCG
Breast	CEA (Carcinoembryonic antigen)
Testicle	AFP; b hCG; lactate dehydrogenase (LDH)
Lung (small cell carcinoma)	Neuron specific enolase; creatinine kinase brain isoenzyme
Carcinoid	5 HIAA
Neuroblastoma	Neuron specific enolase
Pancreas	Insulin
Stomach	Gastrin
Pituitary	Adrenocorticotropic hormone (ACTH)
Bone	Alkaline phosphatase
Multiple myeloma	Bence-Jones proteins

Types of Neck Dissection

1. **Classical radical ND**—Entire removal of:
   a. Submandibular gland
   b. Sternomastoid muscle
   c. Internal jugular vein
   d. Cervical lymphatics and LNs
   e. Submandibular lymph node
   f. Lower deep cervical LN
   g. Fat and fascia from midline to anterior border of trapezius from lower border of mandible
   h. Accessory nerve
   i. Submental
   j. Upper deep cervical LN.
2. Extended radical neck dissection
3. Modified radical neck dissection
   a. Preservation of nerve
   b. Preservation of nerve and muscle
   c. Preservation of nerve, muscle and vein.

Selective Neck Dissection

1. *Supraomohyoid neck dissection* in primary tumor of oral cavity
2. *Jugular neck dissection* in primary tumor of hypopharynx and larynx
3. *Central compartment neck dissection*—in thyroid carcinoma (CA) and medullary CA
4. *Posterolateral neck dissection* in melanoma; squamous cell CA of posterior scalp.

Pendred Syndrome (Dyshormonogenesis)

1. Congenital deafness associated with goiter and hypothyroidism
2. Absence of enzyme peroxidase
3. Goiter + sensorineural hearing impairment and abnormality of bony labyrinth
4. Diagnosed by CT scan of temporal bone.

Retrosternal Goiter

Etiology—strong pretracheal muscles; short neck; obesity
Clinical features—dyspnea at night; cough; stridor; dysphagia
***On examination (O/E)*—Pemberton's sign** positive; lower border not palpable.

Diagnosis

1. X-ray chest—shadow in superior mediastinum with calcification
2. Venogram—obstruction of superior vena cava (SVC); flow volume
3. Loop pulmonary function test.

Types

1. Substernal—lower border below sternum
2. Intrathoracic—no thyroid seen in neck, diagnosed by radioisotope scan
3. Plunging—intrathoracic pressure increases (cough) thyroid plunges out lower border of gland is seen in neck.

Treatment

1. Resection of thyroid gland from neck and midline followed by sternotomy
2. Retrosternal goiter delivered by traction and finger mobilization
3. 90% cases do not need sternotomy
4. Sternotomy needed in carcinoma.

CARCINOMA BREAST

History

Age

1. Fibroadenoma—below 35 years
2. Breast abscess—lactating young women
3. Fibroadenosis—at any age
4. CA breast—above 40 years.

Presenting Complaints

Complaints of Lump

1. Following trauma, hematoma or fat necrosis
2. Long history and slow growth—benign
3. Short history and fast growth—malignant (except atrophic scirrhous CA).

Complaints of Pain

1. Painless and accidently felt—carcinoma (CA)
2. Pain main complaint—acute mastitis
3. Throbbing pain—pus is formed
4. Cyclical breast pain aggravated during menstruation—fibroadenosis
5. Pain at the back hip or shoulder—long standing CA—bony metastasis.

Complaints of Discharge

1. Fresh blood or altered blood in duct papilloma or CA
2. Pus in mammary abscess
3. Milk in lactation or galactocele
4. Serous or greenish discharge in fibroadenosis and mammary duct ectasia.

Complaints of Retraction of Nipple

1. Since puberty—developmental
2. Recent retraction—CA.

Complaints of Loss of Weight–TB and Carcinoma

Past history

1. TB
2. Recurrence of symptoms
3. Fibroadenosis
4. Previous biopsy
5. Breast surgery
6. Chemo/radiation to chest
7. Surgery on opposite side.

Menstrual history

1. History of cyclical dysmenorrhea
2. Early menarche
3. Late menopause.

Personal history

1. Fibroadenosis and CA in unmarried or nulliparous
2. Suppurative mastitis in first lactational period.

Family history

1. Carcinoma recur in family
2. History of CA in its degree relatives
3. Use of oral contraceptive pills (OCP).

Hereditary Syndrome Associated with Breast Cancer

Hereditary syndrome	Gene defect
Li-Fraumeni	p^{53}
Cowden's	PTEN
Peutz-Jeghers	*LKB1*
Hereditary nonpolyposis colorectal cancer	*MSH 2 MLH 1*

General Examination

Pallor; LNs; alopecia.

Examination of Breast

1. Sitting posture—level of nipples, axillary LN
2. Semirecumbant position
3. Recumbent position
4. Bending forward position—retraction of nipple.

Inspection

1. Arms by the side of the body
2. Arms raised—lump is more marked
3. Hands on her hips pressing and relaxing—exaggeration of skin dimples
4. Patient bending forwards—abnormal fibrosis.
5. *Breasts*:
   a. Position
   b. Any puckering or dimpling
   c. Size and shape
   d. Any visible swelling or ulcer.
6. Skin over the breast—color and texture acute mastitis—skin is red warm and edematous
7. Engorged veins—large fibroadenoma, rapidly growing sarcoma
8. Dimple, retraction, or puckering—scirrhous CA
9. Peau d'orange appearance—CA
10. Nodules; ulceration and fungation **cancer en cuirasse** (Armour plate)
11. *Nipple*:
    a. Presence
    b. Position, comparing both sides
    c. Number—accessory nipples present or not
    d. Size and shape—prominent flattened or retracted
    e. Paget's disease—nipple is completely destroyed
    f. Fissures and ulcers; discharge.

12. *Areola*:
    a. Color
    b. Size—larger in case of large fibroadenoma
    c. Ulceration
    d. Destruction
    e. Paget's disease
13. *Arm and thorax*: Cancer en cuirasse and edematous arm
14. Axilla and supraclavicular fossa.

Palpation (Sitting, Recumbent, Semirecumbent, Arms Above Her Head)

1. Palpate normal breast first
2. Palpate with palmar surface of fingers
3. Four quadrants are palpated.

Palpation of a Lump

1. Local rise of temperature and tenderness
2. Situation
    a. Fibroadenosis in upper and outer quadrant
    b. Fibroadenoma in lower half
    c. Carcinoma anywhere and common in upper and outer.
3. Number—fibroadenosis—multiple
4. Size and shape
5. Surface
6. Margin
7. Consistency
8. Fluctuation
9. Transillumination test
    a. Fat is transilluminant
    b. Solid tumor is opaque.
10. Fixity to skin
    a. Dimpling or tethering
    b. Sliding of skin
    c. Pinching of skin.
11. Fixity to breast tissue — **fibroadenoma**—not fixed-breast mouse
12. Fixity to underlying fascia and muscles—feel the anterior fold of axilla by pressing the hand on the hip
13. Fixity to the chest wall—tumor fixed irrespective of muscle contraction
14. Palpation of nipple—nipple retraction or discharge.

Examination of Lymph Nodes

1. Palpation of axillary lymph nodes—pectoral; branchial; subscapular; central; apical
2. Palpation of cervical lymph nodes—supra- and infraclavicular LN.

Examination of Abdomen

1. Hepatomegaly
2. Peritoneal deposits
3. Ascites
4. Jaundice (secondaries).

Examination of Chest

Hemoptysis (secondaries).

Examination of Skull and Spine

Per Rectal Examination

Deposits in pouch of Douglas.

Per Vaginal Examination

Krukenberg tumor.

Provisional Diagnosis

Carcinoma of breast stage tumor node metastasis (TNM)
Side (Right/left), whether postchemo/RT.

Eczema	Paget's disease
Lactating women	Elderly women
Bilateral	Unilateral
Itching present	Absent
Responds to antibiotics	Does not respond

Investigations

1. Routine
2. Specific.

1. *Mammography*: Views—craniocaudal and oblique/mediolateral
2. *Chest X-ray*: Pleural effusion
   Metastasis: Cannon ball appearance
3. *Ultrasound abdomen*: Liver
4. *Biopsy*: Trucut and excision
   First investigation: FNAC
   Definitive investigation: Open biopsy
5. Bone scan and bone X-ray for metastasis
6. CT scan/MRI.

BIRADS (Breast imaging reporting and data system)—grades 0-6
Grade 0: Incomplete assessment
Grade 1: Negative
Grade 2: Benign
Grade 3: Probably benign
Grade 4: Suspicious
Grade 5: Malignant
Grade 6: Biopsy proven malignant.

Grading of FNAC

C0—No epithelial cells present; C1—Scanty benign cells; C2—Benign cells; C3—Probably benign; C4—Probably malignant; C5—Malignant.

Order of Metastasis

Lumbar vertebrae > femur > thoracic vertebrae > ribs.

Grading of CA Breast by Modified Bloom Richardson Grading

(Nottingham Combined Histological Grading System)
1. Tubule formation
2. Nuclear pleomorphism
3. Mitotic count.

Mammographic Signs of Malignancy

1. *Spiculation*: Mass with irregular edges
2. *Tentaculation*: Long tentacles
3. *Microcalcification*: Fine scatter calcification
4. Distortion of **architectural pattern** of breast.

Distinguishing Features between Benign and Malignant Breast Disease by Mammography

Feature	Benign	Malignant
Opacity	Smooth margin Low density Homogeneous Thin halo	Ill-defined margin, irregular stellate spiculated margins High density Inhomogeneous Wide halo
Calcification	Macrocalcification	Microcalcification
Breast parenchyma	Normal	Architectural distortion
Nipple/areola	May be retracted/not	May be retracted/not
Skin	Normal	Thickened
Cooper ligaments	Normal	Thickened
Ducts	Normal	Focal dilatation
Subcutaneous retromammary space	Normal	Obliterated

T—Primary Tumor

Tx—primary tumour cannot be assessed
T0: No evidence of primary tumor
Tis: CA *in situ*
Tis (DCIS)—ductal carcinoma *in situ*
Tis (LCIS)—lobular carcinoma *in situ*
T1: Tumor < 2 cm in greatest dimension
T1mic: Microinvasion < 0.1 cm
T1a: 0.1 to 0.5 cm
T1b: 0.5 to 1 cm
T1c: 1 to 2 cm
T2: Tumor 2 to 5 cm in greatest dimension
T3: Tumor > 5 cm in greatest dimension
T4: Any tumor size with direct extension to chest wall or skin or both
T4a: Chest wall
T4b: Edema/ulceration of skin or satellite nodules confined to breast (Peau d'orange)
T4c: T4a + T4b
T4d: Inflammatory CA breast.

Note: Chest wall includes ribs, intercostal muscles, and serratus anterior muscle but not pectoral muscles.

N—Nodes Status

Nx—Regional lymph nodes cannot be assessed
N0: No regional LN present
N1: Mobile ipsilateral axillary nodes
N2: N2a + N2b
N2a: Ipsilateral axillary nodes fixed/matted
N2b: Ipsilateral internal mammary nodes in the abscence of axillary metastasis
N3: N3a + N3b + N3c
N3a: Ipsilateral infraclavicular LN
N3b: Ipsilateral internal mammary LN and axillary LN
N3c: Ipsilateral supraclavicular LN.

Distant Metastasis

M—Distant metastasis
Mx: Distant Metastasis cannot be assessed
M0: No distant metastasis
M1: Distant metastasis.

Tumor Node Metastasis Classification

Stage	Tumor	Node	Metastasis
0	Tis	N0	M0
IA	T1	N0	M0
IB	T0	N1mi	M0
	T1	N1mi	M0
IIA	T0	N1	M0
	T1	N1	M0
	T2	N0	M0
IIB	T2	N1	M0
	T3	N0	M0
IIIA	up to T3	Up to N2	M0
IIIB	any T4	N0/N1/N2	M0
IIIC	any T	N3	M0
IV	any T	Any N	M1

Treatment

1. **General management**
   a. Confirm the disease (histological)
   b. Stage the disease (histological)
   c. Chart out prognostic factors.
2. *Early carcinoma (Stage 1 and 2)*: Breast conservative surgery/Simple mastectomy with axillary dissection
3. **Other procedures**
   a. Radical mastectomy
   b. Modified radical mastectomy
   c. Quart.
4. **Advanced carcinoma (Stage 3 and 4)**
   a. Downstage by chemotherapy or radiotherapy
   b. Reassess if surgery possible do modified radical mastectomy and axillary dissection
   c. Continue chemotherapy and radiotherapy
   d. If not resectable/fungating—toilet mastectomy.

Operative Procedures

1. *Lumpectomy*: Removal of lump with 1 cm margin
2. *Quadrantectomy*: Removal of lump with 3 cm margin
3. *Radical mastectomy*: (Halsted)-breast + pectoralis major + minor + regional lymph nodes up to costoclavicular ligament
4. **Modified radical mastectomy**
   a. *Patey's*: Pectoralis minor is **removed** + level 1, 2, 3
   b. *Scanlon*: Pectoralis minor is **divided** + level 1, 2, 3
   c. *Auchincloss*: Pectoralis minor **retained** + level 1, 2
5. *Simple mastectomy*: Skin, areola, all of breast + axillary tail + axillary sampling of lymph nodes
6. **QUART** by Umberto Veronesi from Milan – quadrantectomy + axillary dissection + radiotherapy to breast and axilla.
7. *Breast reconstructive procedures*
   a. Silicon gel implant under pectoralis major—subcutaneous tissue and under muscle
   b. Pedicled flap—TRAM—Transverse rectus abdominis myocutaneous flap
   c. Latissimus dorsi (LD) flap—latissimus dorsi myocutaneous

d. Nipple reconstruction—labia skin, tattooing, prosthetic
e. Reduction/Augmentation mammoplasty/mammopexy—to achieve symmetry
f. External breast prosthesis.

Haagensen's Criteria of Inoperability

1. Extensive edema of the breast
2. Satellite nodules of carcinoma
3. Inflammatory carcinoma
4. A parasternal tumor, indicating spread to the internal mammary nodes
5. Supraclavicular metastasis
6. Edema of the arm
7. Distant metastasis.

Complications of Mastectomy

1. Psychological trauma to the patient
2. Bleeding
3. Infection
4. Flap necrosis
5. Edema of arm
6. Hematoma
7. Injury to axillary vein
8. Injury to thoracodorsal nerve
9. Injury to long thoracic nerve (winging of scapula)
10. Seroma (fluid collection)
11. Lymphangiosarcoma (Stewart-Treves syndrome)
12. Recurrence.

Triple Assessment of Breast Symptoms

1. Confident diagnosis in 99% cases
2. Triple assessment—Clinical, imaging and pathology
   i. Clinical—Age, examination
   ii. Imaging—USS, mammography
   iii. Pathology—FNAC, corecut.

Cancer Risks Associated with Benign Breast Diseases

Abnormality	Relative risk
Nonproliferative lesions	No increased risk
Sclerosing adenosis	No increased risk
Intraductal papilloma	No increased risk
Florid epithelial hyperplasia	1.5 to 2 fold
Atypical lobular hyperplasia	4 fold
Atypical ductal hyperplasia	4 fold
Ductal involvement by cells of atypical ductal hyperplasia	7 fold

Nottingham Prognostic Index (NPI)

I - (.2 × size) + grade + node size in cm; grade 1 to 3; nodes 1 to 3

Based on index—excellent moderate poor-prognostic group.

1. *Stage 1*: NPI—84%
2. *Stage 2*: NPI—71%
3. *Stage 3*: NPI—45%
4. *Stage 4*: NPI—26%.

Levels of Axillary Lymph Nodes

1. *Level 1*: Axillary tail to lateral border of pectoralis minor
2. *Level 2*: Lateral border to medial border (Rotor's nodes/interpectoral node)
3. *Level 3*: Up to apex of axilla.

Sentinel lymph nodes: First lymph nodes draining the tumor bearing areas of breast.

Biopsy: Inject a patent blue dye (Sulfur colloid) or radioisolabeled albumin in peritumor area and follow-up with gamma camera and do frozen section of the drained lymph nodes for histopathological analysis.

Indications for Adjuvant Chemotherapy (Cyclophosphamide, Methotrexate and 5-Fluorouracil/ Cyclophosphamide, Adriamycin and 5-Fluorouracil/Taxanes)

1. All node positive cancers
2. Node negative > 1 cm
3. Node negative > 0.5 cm with adverse prognostic factors (blood vessel/lymphatic invasion, high nuclear/histological grade, HER2/neu overexpression, negative hormone receptor status)
   Neoadjuvant chemotherapy—chemo given before surgery/radiation to downstage the disease.
   Adjuvant hormone therapy with tamoxifen if ER/PR positive cases.

C - Cyclophosphamide	**M** - Methotrexate
F - 5 Fluorouracil	**A** - Adriamycin

TAC regime

Docetaxel	Doxorubicin	Cyclophosphamide.

Hormone therapy
1. Tamoxifen-antiestrogen LHRH agonist—buseriline
2. Oral aromatase inhibitor anastrozole, letrozole goserelin
3. Medical adrenalectomy naphazoline
4. Progestrogens
5. Pure anti-estrogen—Fulvestrant.

Prognostic Factors of CA Breast

1. Node metastasis
2. Tumor size
3. Histological grade
4. Age at presentation (young age bad prognosis)
5. Lymphovascular invasion
   a. Grade 1—no nodes
   b. Grade 2—(1-3) nodes
   c. Grade 3 to 4 or more nodes.

Breast Conservative Surgery

Ductal carcinoma *in situ* (DCIS)/stage I and II breast disease.

Contraindications

1. More than 1 macroscopic carcinoma in more than 1 quadrant
2. Diffuse microcalcifications on mammography
3. Multicentricity
4. Persistent positive margins
5. Centrally located tumor
6. Contraindicated for radiation
7. Fixity to chest wall/overlying skin
8. Where regular follow-up is not feasible.

Differential Diagnosis

1. Chronic breast abscess
2. Traumatic fat necrosis
3. Giant fibroadenoma
4. Hematoma
5. Antibioma.

Risk Factors of Carcinoma

1. Age—incidence increases with increasing age
2. Gender—more in females
3. Common in western countries
4. Family history
5. Genetic factors—BRCA1(17q), BRCA2(13q) tumor suppressor genes
6. Past history of ovarian/endometrial/contralateral breast carcinoma
7. Hormonal factors—increased exposure to estrogen—early menarche, late menopause, nulliparity, obesity
8. Diet—alcohol and high fatty food increases the risk
9. Previous benign breast disease
10. High socioeconomic status
11. Irradiation
12. Hormone replacement therapy
    a. OCP—do not appear to increase the risk
    b. Smoking is not a risk factor
    c. Longer durations of breast feeding has protective effect.

CARCINOMA STOMACH

History of Present Illness

Clinical picture can be:

1. *Insidious type*: Indigestion, vague discomfort, fullness in upper abdomen after meals, loss of appetite, weight loss, pain is seen in late stage.
2. *Obstructive type*: Carcinoma at the pyloric end present with features of GOO (Gastric outlet obstruction) with nonbilious vomiting and rolling sensation in the upper abdomen after food intake.
3. *Lump*: Patient may present with an epigastric lump.
4. *Peptic ulcer type*: Malignancy is suspected if there is:
    a. Loss of periodicity
    b. Sharp pain replaced by dull aching pain
    c. Loss of appetite
    d. Loss of weight.

The most common symptom is **recent onset dyspepsia**.

History of Past Illness

1. History of acid peptic disease or dyspepsia
2. History of surgery (Partial gastrectomy or gastrojejunostomy).

Personal History

Bowel movements altered; micturition difficulties; alcoholism; cigarette smoking.

Family History

History of malignancy or acid peptic disease.

General Examination

Pallor; lymph nodes; built and nourishment are important.

Abdominal Examination

Inspection

1. Any visible mass; engorged veins or pulsations
2. Any visible peristalsis; umbilical nodule.

Palpation

1. Local rise of temperature and tenderness
2. Features of palpable mass—well defined margin; irregular borders with mass in the epigastrium; hard in consistency; non-pulsatile; upper border palpable; moving with respiration
3. Hepatosplenomegaly
4. Renal angle tender or nontender.

Percussion

1. Shifting dullness or fluid thrill
2. Resonant note.

Auscultation

1. Bowel sounds; succussion splash

Examination of external genitalia

Examination of left supraclavicular lymph nodes (Virchow's nodes)

Per rectal examination—metastatic deposits

Skull and spine.

Differential Diagnosis

1. *Tumors of epigastrium*: Left lobe of liver
2. Lymphoma
3. Intestinal obstruction
4. Gallbladder disease
5. Tuberculosis (ulcerative and hyperplastic lesion)
6. Ca hepatic flexure of colon.

Investigations

1. Complete blood picture—anemia, iron deficiency
2. Liver function test (LFT) (differentiate between hepatocellular from obstructive jaundice)
3. Stool and blood examination
4. Barium meal—persistent filling defect (Decreased capacity of stomach in linitis plastica)
5. USG; X-ray; FNAC
6. Endoscopy is the diagnostic modality of choice. Endoscopic USG gives better assessment of TNM staging of the tumor
7. CT abdomen gives better delineation about invasion of surrounding organs.

Discussion

Risk Factors of Carcinoma Stomach

1. Diet—long-term ingestion of dried, smoked and salted food, gastric bacteria converting nitrate to nitrite which is a carcinogen.
   Diet low in animal fat and animal proteins, high in complex carbohydrates, salt, low in fresh fruits and vegetable.
2. Smoking—increases the risk
3. *H. pylori*
4. Previous gastric surgery

5. Ménétrier's disease
6. Family history
7. Genetic factors
8. Hereditary nonpolyposis colorectal cancer (HNPCC)
9. Premalignant conditions—strophic gastritis, gastric polyps, intestinal metaplasia and dysplasia.

Clinical Signs of Inoperability

1. Mass per abdomen
2. Ascites
3. Liver nodules
4. Left supraclavicular nodes
5. Left axillary nodes (**Irish's node**)
6. Umbilical nodes (**Sister Mary Joseph's nodes**)
7. Rectal shelf (**Blumer's shelf**)
8. Migratory thrombophlebitis
9. Krukenberg's tumor.

Spread of Carcinoma of Stomach

1. Direct spread
2. Lymphatic spread
3. Blood borne metastasis
4. Transperitoneal spread—common mode of spread:
   a. Rectal shelf
   b. Krukenberg's tumor
   c. Sister Mary Joseph's nodes.

Precancerous Conditions

1. Atrophic gastritis
2. Pernicious anemia
3. Adenomatous polyps
4. Ménétrier's disease
5. *H. pylori* infection
6. Gastric ulcer
7. Type A and B gastritis
8. Previous gastric resection.

Tnm Staging of Carcinoma Stomach

T: Primary tumor
Tx: primary cannot be assessed
T0: No evidence of primary tumor
Tis: Carcinoma *in situ*
T1: *T1a* + *T1b*
T1a: Invasion of lamina propria or muscularis mucosa
T1*b*: Invades submucosa
T2: Invasion of muscularis propria
T3: Penetration of serosa without invasion of visceral peritoneum or adjacent structures
T4: T4a + T4b
T4a: Invasion of serosa
T4*b*: Invasion of adjacent structures
N: Lymph nodes
Nx: regional nodes cannot be assessed
N0: No regional lymph nodes
N1: 1–2 lymph nodes metastasis
N2: 3–6 lymph nodes metastasis
N3: More than 7 lymph nodes metastasis
N3*a*: 7–15 regional lymph nodes
N3*b*: metastasis in 16 or more lymph nodes
M: Distant Metastasis
M0: No distant metastasis
M1: Distant metastasis

Tumor Node Metastasis Classification

Stage	0	Tis N0 M0
Stage	IA	T1 N0 M0
Stage	IB	T1 N1 M0/ T2 N0 M0
Stage	IIA	T3 N0 M0/ T2 N1 M0/ T1 N2 M0
Stage	IIB	T4A N0 M0/ T3 N1 M0/ T2 N2 M0
Stage	IIIA	T4A N1 M0/ T3 N2 M0/ T2 N3 M0
Stage	IIIB	T4B N0 M0/ T4B N1 M0/ T4A N2 M0/ T3 N3 M0
Stage	IIIC	T4B N2 M0/ T4B N3 M0/ T4A N3 M0
Stage	IVC	Any T, Any N, M1

LN stations

1–6: N1 nodes (perigastric nodes)
7–11: N2 nodes (along the named vessels)
12–14: N3 nodes (intra peritoneal nodes)
15–16: N4 nodes.

1. Right cardia
2. Left cardia
3. Lesser curvature
4. Greater curvature
5. Suprapyloric
6. Infrapyloric
7. Left gastric artery
8. Common hepatic ART
9. Celiac artery
10. Splenic hilum
11. Splenic artery
12. Hepatoduodenal
13. Retropancreatic
14. Superior mesenteric artery
15. Middle colic artery
16. Para-aortic nodes.

R Classification of Completeness of Resection

R0: No gross or microscopic residual disease
R1: Microscopic residual disease
R2: Gross residual disease.

Types of dissection

D1 Dissection—removal of perigastric lymph nodes LN 1-6
D2 Dissection—also removes LN 7–12 (requires distal pancreatectomy and splenectomy)
D3 Dissection—also removes para-aortic nodes in addition to 1–12
Billroth I: End to end gastroduodenostomy
Billroth II: Duodenal stump closure + side to side gastrojejunostomy.

Japanese Classification of Early Gastric Carcinoma

Early gastric carcinoma involves the mucosa and submucosa with or without LN involvement
1: Protruding type
2a: Superficial elevated
2b: Flat type
2c: Superficial depressed type
3: Excavated type
15% of early gastric carcinoma have lymph nodes deposits.

Classification of Gastric Cancer

Gross types

1. Cauliflower type
2. Infiltrative type
3. Ulcerative type
4. Colloid carcinoma.

Borrmann's Classification

(Classification of advanced gastric carcinoma tumor invading the muscularis propria)
Type 1: Polypoid/fungating carcinoma
Type 2: Ulcerating lesion surrounded by elevated borders
Type 3: Ulcerating lesion infiltrating the gastric wall
Type 4: Diffuse infiltrating type (linitis plastica)
Type 5: Unclassified CA.

Ming Classification

1. Expansive form (good prognosis)
2. Infiltrating form (poor prognosis).

Treatment of Carcinoma Stomach

Curative resection
Carcinoma of pyloric antrum and body of stomach.
Radical subtotal gastrectomy with gastrojejunal anastomosis (Removes 70–80% of stomach).

Carcinoma of the fundus
Esophagogastrectomy with esophagogastric anastomosis or esophagojejunal anastomosis.

Diffuse growth (linitis plastica)
1. Radical total gastrectomy with esophagojejunostomy
2. Early gastric carcinoma (confined to mucosa, < 2 cm size with no nodal involvement)
3. Endoscopic mucosal resection.

Palliative Surgery

Carcinoma pyloric antrum
1. Anterior gastrojejunostomy (GJ) done
2. Palliative gastrectomy.

Chemotherapy for Carcinoma Stomach

1. *FAM*: 5 fluorouracil, adriamycin, mitomycin C
2. *ECF*: epirubicin, cisplatin and 5 fluorouracil

Mitomycin C impregnated charcoal given intraperitoneally.

Newer Treatment

Hematoporphyrin derivatives injected and is concentrated into the malignancy followed by resection or laser.

Comparison of Intestinal and Diffuse Type of Adenocarcinoma

Features	Intestinal	Diffuse
Histogenesis	Areas of intestinal Metaplasia	Normal gastric Mucosa
Early CA type	Protruding type 1 and 2a	Flat, depressed and excavated 2b, 2c and 3
Infiltration	Localized	Diffuse
Peritoneal metastasis	Infrequent	Frequent
Hepatic metastasis	Nodular	Diffuse
Sex	M > F	F > M

Contd...

Contd...

Age	Elderly	Young
Prognosis	Better	Worse
Association with blood		
Group A/pernicious anemia	No	Yes
Associated with *H. pylori*	Yes	Yes

Complications of Gastric Surgery

Early complications	Late complications
Hemorrhage	Recurrent ulcer
Stomal obstruction	Fistula
Leaking	Stump carcinoma syndrome
Gastrojejunal blow out (4th day)	Small stomach syndrome
Abdominal distention due to paralytic ileus	Nutritional deficiency
Peritonitis	Gastrojejunal intussusception
Postoperative pancreatitis	Gastrojejunocolic fistula
	Gall stones
	Early and late dumping
	Malignant change
	Postvagotomy diarrhea

OBSTRUCTIVE JAUNDICE

History

1. Duration of jaundice
2. *Progressive*: Malignancy, primary biliary cirrhosis (PBC), primary sclerosing cholangitis (PSC)
3. *Intermittent*: Periampullary (Associated with melena), ascariasis, CBD stone
4. Continuous
5. Clay colored stools
6. Itching
7. Loss of weight and appetite.

Past Illness

1. Similar illness in the past
2. Any signs/symptoms of liver failure
3. Previous history of biliary tract surgery
4. Drug history (ATT, OCP, anabolic steroids)
5. Silvery stool—periampullary CA.

Personal History

Alcoholism.

Family History

Hemolytic jaundice runs in family (sickle cell anemia) storage disease, gallstone disease, biliary stricture.

Treatment History

Previous abdominal surgery
Blood transfusion—HBsAg.

General Examination

1. Jaundice
2. Excoriation
3. Shininess of nail
4. Pallor
5. Migratory thrombophlebitis
6. Virchow's node
7. Pedal edema
8. Bradycardia
9. Features of liver failure.

ABDOMINAL EXAMINATION

Inspection

1. Abdominal distension
2. Skin over abdomen for scratch mark
3. Umbilicus shape
4. Pulsation and peristalsis
5. Dilated veins—caput medusae.

Palpation

1. Local rise of temperature and tenderness
2. Guarding and rigidity
3. Palpable GB
4. Any mass or organomegaly
5. Free fluid.

Percussion

Shifting dullness, fluid thrill, Puddle's sign.

Auscultation

Bowel sounds.

System Examination

Thyroid and Breast Examination

Examination of Lymph Nodes

Left supraclavicular lymph node (LSCL) enlargement—Troisier's sign.

Investigations

1. Blood, TC, DC, Hb
2. Bilirubin—conjugated increased in obstructive jaundice
3. HbsAg—in case of jaundice
4. Liver function test—serum alkaline phosphatase
5. Serum amylase—elevated in pancreatitis (within 12 hours)
6. Coagulation profile—prothrombin time
7. Urine—urobilinogen
8. USG abdomen—dilatation of CBD in obstructive jaundice, stones, HSM
9. X-ray abdomen—Visualize gallstones
10. Barium meal follow through
    a. Gas under diaphragm
    b. To rule out pancreatitis
11. Aspiration of peritoneal fluid

12. Endoscopic retrograde cholangiopancreatography (ERCP), magnetic resonance cholangiopancreatography (MRCP), CT or MRI
13. Laparoscopy.

Treatment

Conservative Management

1. IV fluid—dextrose
2. Mannitol to prevent hepatorenal syndrome
3. Parenteral antibiotics
4. Avoid hepatotoxic drugs
5. Ryle's tube aspiration if GI bleed
6. Diuretics
7. Vitamin K 1 amp at least for 3 days—100 mg I/m/IV
8. Oral neomycin/metronidazole to sterilize the GIT
9. Adequate calories
10. Give drug which increase the GI motility.

Common Causes of Obstructive Jaundice

1. Gallstones
2. CA gallbladder
3. Hydatid cyst
4. LNs in porta hepatis
5. Stricture of biliary tree
6. Worms—ascariasis, liver fluke
7. CA head of pancreas, periampullary CA
8. Cholangiocarcinoma.

Gallstones

1. Cholesterol stones
   a. Solitary
   b. Cholesterol only
   c. Stones are soft
2. Pigment stones
   a. Multiple
   b. Calcium bilirubinate
   c. Hard and coral like, small
3. Mixed stones
   a. Multiple
   b. Major component—cholesterol bilirubinate, $CaPO_4$, $CaCO_3$, Ca palmitate and protein
   c. Soft and faceted.

Investigations for Gallstones

1. USG is the first investigation
2. MRCP is the best noninvasive investigation
3. ERCP is the gold standard for diagnosing common bile duct (CBD) stones.

Classification of Choledochal Cyst

Type 1: Characterized by fusiform dilatation of the bile duct and is the most common type.
Type 2: Appears as a diverticulum protruding from the wall of the CBD.
Type 3: Dilatation of the biliary tract within the duodenum; also known as choledochocele.
Type 4a: Multiple dilatation of extrahepatic and intrahepatic bile ducts.
Type 4b: Multiple dilatation involving only the extrahepatic bile ducts.
Type 5: Multiple dilatation of the intrahepatic bile ducts; also known as Caroli's disease.

Risk Factors of Cholangiocarcinoma

1. Primary sclerosing cholangitis
2. Choledochal cyst
3. Ulcerative colitis
4. Clonorchis sinensis infection
5. Chronic typhoid carriers.

Important Triads

1. *Saints triad*: Gallstone; diverticulosis of colon; hiatus hernia
2. *Charcot's triad*: Jaundice; pain and fever
3. *Virchow's triad*: Changes in blood flow; changes in vessel wall; hypercoagulability

4. *Hutchinson's triad*: Hutchinson's teeth (notched upper incisors); interstitial keratitis; nerve deafness
5. *Alport's syndrome*: Progressive renal failure; sensory neural deafness; ocular anomalies
6. *Kwashiorkor*: Edema; growth retardation; mental changes (apathy, listlessness, lethargy)
7. *Behcet's syndrome*: Recurrent oral ulcers, genital ulcers, iridocyclitis (+ skin lesions make a tetrad)
8. *Whipple's triad*: Symptoms of hypoglycemia; serum glucose > 45 mg/dL; relief with ingestion of glucose
9. *Hypernephroma*: Hematuria; pain and renal mass
10. *Trotter's triad*: Conductive deafness; immobility of homolateral soft palate; trigeminal neuralgia
11. *Gradenigo's triad*: 6th nerve palsy; deep seated retro-orbital pain; persistent ear discharge
12. *Hemobilia*: Biliary colic; obstructive jaundice; melena or occult blood in stool.

Ranson's Prognostic Signs of Acute Pancreatitis

At admission	During the initial 48 hours
Age > 55 years	Hematocrit > 10 points
WBC > 16,000/mm^3	Blood urea nitrogen elevation > 5 mg/dL
Blood glucose > 200 mg/dL	Serum calcium < 8 mg/dL
Serum LDH > 350 IU/L	Arterial PCO_2 < 60 mm Hg
Serum AST > 250 IU/dL	Base deficit > 4 mEq/L
	Estimated fluid sequestration > 6L

Criteria for Gallstone Pancreatitis

At admission	During the initial 48 hours
Age > 70 years	Hematocrit fall > 10 points
WBC > 18,000/mm^3	Blood urea nitrogen (BUN) elevation > 2 mg/dL
Blood glucose > 220 mg/ dL	Serum calcium < 8 mg/dL
Serum LDH > 400 IU/L	Base deficit > 5 mEq/L
Serum AST > 250 U/dL	Estimated fluid sequestration > 4L

Complications of Gallstones

1. In the gallbladder
   a. Silent stones
   b. Acute and chronic cholecystitis
   c. Empyema
   d. Gangrene
   e. Perforation
   f. Mucocele
   g. Carcinoma.
2. In the bile duct
   a. Cholangitis
   b. Obstructive jaundice
   c. Acute pancreatitis
3. In the intestine
   Acute intestinal obstruction.

Indication for Common Bile Duct Exploration

1. History of Charcot's triad—pain, intermittent jaundice, fever
2. USG proven stones in CBD
3. Dilated CBD (>1 cm)
4. OTC stone filling defect
5. Palpable stone in CBD.

Indications for Cholecystectomy

1. Cholelithiasis
2. Diverticulitis of GBs
3. Cholesterosis
4. Cholecystitis
5. Chronic typhoid carriers
6. Porcelain GB
7. Empyema of GB
8. Mucocele
9. As a part of Whipple surgery
10. CA of GB.

Complications of Cholecystectomy

1. Postcholecystectomy syndrome
2. Hemorrhages from hepatic artery
3. Waltman Walter syndrome
4. Stricture of CBD
5. Injury to liver.

Preoperative Preparations of Cholecystectomy

1. Consent
2. Anesthetic check up
3. CVS respiratory, LFT
4. Coagulation profile
5. Drugs—broad spectrum antibiotics, subcutaneous heparin.

Indications for Choledochotomy

Absolute indications (high suspicion of CBD calculi)
1. Palpable CBD stones
2. Jaundice with cholangitis
3. Demonstration of stones by intraoperative cholangiography
4. Dilatation of CBD > 12 mm.

Relative indications (low suspicion of CBD calculi)
1. Jaundice without cholangitis
2. History of pancreatitis
3. Dilated CBD
4. When on aspiration bile is white
5. A dilated cystic duct.

Postoperative Care

1. Removal of T tube after 10 days
2. After testing for patency of T tube by injecting radiopaque dye (tube cholangiogram)
3. White bile—due to obstruction of large duct this is mainly mucous coming along with bile.

Causes of Gallstones

1. Metabolic
   a. Drugs—OCP
   b. Obesity
   c. Increased bile salt—ileal disease
   d. Cholestyramine therapy
   e. Increase in age.
2. Infection
   H. pylori infection.
3. Bile stasis
   a. Estrogen therapy
   b. Long-term parenteral therapy.
4. Hemolysis
   a. Hereditary spherocytosis
   b. Sickle cell anemia
   c. Thalassemia
   d. Malaria.

ABDOMINAL LUMP

Right Hypochondrium

1. Liver
   a. Congenital Riedel's lobe
   b. Amoebic hepatitis and abscess
   c. Suppurative pyelophlebitis
   d. Suppurative cholangitis
   e. Gumma of liver
   f. Hydatid cyst
   g. Carcinoma of the liver
   h. Melanotic carcinoma of liver
   i. Cirrhosis of liver.
2. Gallbladder
   a. Mucocele
   b. Empyema
   c. CA of head of pancreas
   d. CA of common bile duct
   e. CA of gallbladder.
3. Subphrenic space
   Subphrenic abscess

4. Pylorus of stomach and duodenum
   a. CA
   b. Subacute perforation of peptic ulcer.
5. Hepatic flexure of colon
   a. Intussusception
   b. Hypertrophic tuberculosis
   c. Carcinoma of part of colon.
6. Parietal swelling
   a. Swelling of skin and subcutaneous
   b. Parietal abscess.

Epigastrium

1. Parietal swelling
2. Intra-abdominal swelling
   a. Liver and subphrenic abscess
   b. Subacute perforation of peptic ulcer
   c. Transverse colon—Intussusception
   d. Hyperplastic TB
   e. Omentum
   f. Abdominal aorta
   g. Retroperitoneal sarcoma and teratoma
   h. Congenital pyloric stenosis
   i. Carcinoma stomach
   j. Diverticulitis
   k. Neoplasms
   l. Pancreas
   m. Lymph nodes.

Left Hypochondrium

1. Parietal swelling
2. Intra-abdominal swelling
   a. Spleen
      i. Hemolytic anemia (hereditary spherocytosis, acquired hemolytic anemia)
      ii. Idiopathic thrombocytopenic purpura
      iii. Porphyria
      iv. Egyptian splenomegaly
      v. Felty's syndrome
      vi. Leukemia
      vii. Tumors and cysts
   b. Stomach
   c. Left lobe of liver
   d. Splenic flexure of colon
   e. Tail of pancreas
   f. Left subphrenic space
   g. Left kidney
   h. Left suprarenal gland.

Lumbar Region

1. Parietal swelling
   a. Lumbar abscess
   b. Lumbar hernia.
2. Intra-abdominal swelling
   a. Ascending or descending colon
   b. Right or left kidney.

Umbilical Region

1. Parietal swelling
   a. Umbilicus
      i. Congenital polyp or adenoma
      ii. Umbilical hernia
      iii. Postoperative or incisional hernia

b. Rectus sheath
    i. Hematoma
    ii. Desmoid tumor
    iii. Abscess
2. Intra-abdominal swelling
    a. Small intestine and mesentery—matted coils of intestine with tuberculous mesenteric lymphadenitis
    b. Tumors of small intestine
    c. Cysts of the mesentery
    d. Retroperitoneal connective tissue—retroperitoneal cyst, lymphoma and sarcoma.

Right Iliac Region

1. Parietal swelling
2. Intra-abdominal swelling—appendicular lump
3. Ileocecal region
    a. Hyperplastic ileocecal tuberculosis
    b. Crohn's disease or regional ileitis
    c. Actinomycosis
    d. Amoebic typhlitis
    e. CA of cecum
    f. Impaction of round worms
4. Other swellings
    a. Lymph nodes
    b. Retroperitoneal sarcoma
    c. Kidney—undescended or dropped
    d. Retained or undescended testis
    e. Urinary bladder—retention of urine, huge diverticulum of bladder
    f. Tubo-ovarian mass, pyosalpinx, cyst and abscess of the broad ligament fibroid, ovarian cyst
    g. Iliac artery aneurysm
    h. Iliac abscess and iliopsoas cold abscess
    i. Gallbladder—hydrops
    j. Pelvic abscess.

Hypogastrium

1. **Parietal swelling**—urachal cyst
2. Intra-abdominal swelling
    a. Urinary bladder—retention of urine
    b. Tubo-ovarian mass
    c. Ovarian tumor and cyst
    d. Pelvic abscess
    e. Uterus—pregnancy and fibroid
    f. Ruptured tubal gestation
    g. Broad ligament cyst
    h. Pelvic bones.

Left Iliac Region

1. *Parietal swelling*: Cold abscess
2. *Intra-abdominal swelling*: Diverticulitis and CA.

Types of Colectomy

Right Hemicolectomy

1. Terminal ileum
2. Ascending colon
3. Proximal 1/3rd of transverse colon (Ileocolic, right colic, right and left branch of middle colic).

Extended Right Hemicolectomy

1. Terminal ileum
2. Ascending colon
3. Proximal 2/3rd of transverse colon (Ileocolic, right colic, right and left branch of middle colic).

Left Hemicolectomy

1. Distal 1/3rd of transverse colon
2. Splenic flexure
3. Descending colon
4. Sigmoid colon (Inferior mesenteric artery).

Most Common Sites

1. *Crohn's disease*: Terminal ileum
2. *Amoebic colitis*: Sigmoid colon
3. *Typhoid ulcer*: Terminal ileum
4. *Tuberculous ulcer*: Terminal ileum
5. *Ulcerative colitis*: Rectum
6. *Volvulus*: Sigmoid colon
7. *Polyps in Peutz-Jeghers syndrome*: Jejunum
8. *Peptic ulcer*: 1st part of duodenum
9. *Gastric ulcer*: Lesser curvature
10. *Hirschsprung's disease*: Rectum
11. *Bleeding in angiodysplasia*: Right colon
12. *Colon carcinoma*: Rectosigmoid.

Hepatocellular Carcinoma

1. Hepatocellular carcinoma (HCC) is more common in males (about 4 times)
2. 60 to 90% arise in cirrhotic liver
3. Cirrhosis with the maximum risk of developing HCC—postnecrotic cirrhosis
4. Cirrhosis with the lowest risk for HCC — alcoholic cirrhosis
5. Hepatocellular carcinoma is the most common primary malignancy of the liver
6. Most common hepatic neoplasms are metastasis
7. Most common benign neoplasm of liver—hemangiomas
8. Most common primary hepatic malignancy in children—hepatoblastoma.

Treatment Options for Hepatocellular Carcinoma

1. Surgical
   a. Resection
   b. Orthotopic liver transplant.
2. Ablative
   a. Percutaneous ethanol injection
   b. Percutaneous acetic acid injection
   c. Thermal ablation (cryotherapy, radiofrequency ablation, microwave).
3. Transarterial
   a. Embolization
   b. Chemoembolization
   c. Radiotherapy.
4. Combination transarterial/ablative
5. External beam radiation
6. Systemic
   a. Chemotherapy
   b. Hormonal therapy
   c. Immunotherapy.

Congenital Anomalies of Vitellointestinal Duct

1. Umbilical fecal fistula—due to persistence of entire vitellointestinal duct
2. Umbilical sinus—when the duct is obliterated at the intestinal end but communicates with the umbilicus at the distal end
3. Meckel's diverticulum—when the duct is obliterated at the umbilicus but persists at its intestinal end
4. Umbilical cyst or vitelline cyst—when both ends are occluded but the tract in between persists
5. Fibrous band—the entire tract may be obliterated, but a fibrous band may persist between the ileum and the umbilicus.

Causes of Retroperitoneal Fibrosis

Benign

1. Idiopathic (Ormond's disease)
2. Chronic inflammation
3. Extravasation of urine
4. Retroperitoneal irritation by leakage of blood or intestinal content
5. Aortic aneurysm
6. Trauma
7. Drugs—chemotherapeutic agents, methysergide, beta adrenoreceptor antagonists.

Malignant

1. Lymphoma
2. Carcinoid tumors
3. Secondary deposits (especially from carcinoma of stomach, colon, breast and prostate).

Stomas

1. May be colostomy or ileostomy
2. May be temporary or permanent
3. Temporary or defunctioning stomas are usually fashioned as loop stomas
4. An ileostomy is spouted and colostomy is flush
5. Ileostomy effluent is usually liquid whereas colostomy effluent is usually solid
6. Ileostomy patients are more likely to develop fluid and electrolyte problems
7. An ileostomy is usually sited in the right iliac fossa
8. A temporary colostomy may be transverse and be sited in the right upper quadrant
9. End colostomy is usually sited in the left iliac fossa
10. All patients should be counseled by a stoma care nurse before operation
11. Complications include skin irritation, prolapsed, retraction, necrosis, stenosis, parastomal hernia and bleeding.

Indications for Enteral Feeding

1. Protein energy malnutrition with inadequate oral intake
2. Dysphagia, except for fluids
3. Major trauma (including surgery) when return to required dietary intake is prolonged
4. Inflammatory bowel disease
5. Distal, low output(< 200 mL) enterocutaneous fistulas
6. To enhance adaptation after massive enterectomy.

Contraindications for Enteral Feeding

1. Small bowel obstruction or ileus
2. Severe diarrhea
3. Proximal small intestinal fistulas
4. Severe pancreatitis.

Complications of Enteral Feeding

Related to Feeding Tube

1. Malposition
2. Dislodgement/migration
3. Aspiration
4. Peritonitis
5. Fistula formation
6. Intestinal obstruction
7. Tube fracture/blockade.

Related to Feeding Regime

1. Feed intolerance (diarrhea, vomiting)
2. Hyperglycemia
3. Enteric infection.

Indications for Parenteral Nutrition

1. Proximal intestinal fistula
2. Inflammatory bowel disease (especially in the preoperative period)
3. Massive intestinal resection (particularly if < 100 cm of small bowel remains)
4. Ileus
5. Severe pancreatitis.

Complications of Parenteral Nutrition

Related to the Feeding Catheter

1. Arterial, pneumothorax, venous, thoracic duct, stellate ganglion, brachial plexus, cardiac perforation
2. Air embolus
3. Catheter related infection
4. Infective endocarditis
5. Central venous/cardiac thrombosis
6. Thrombotic catheter occlusion
7. Catheter migration or embolus.

Related to the Feeding Regime

1. Hyperglycemia
2. Hypoglycemia
3. Hypertriglyceridemia
4. Hyperchloremic acidosis
5. Electrolyte abnormalities
6. Trace element and vitamin deficiency states.

Acute Abdomen

Investigation of Acute Abdomen

Imaging tests	Indications/signs
Chest radiography (erect)	Gas under diaphragm
Anterior radiograph (supine)	Dilated bowel or gas pattern; gas inside or outside bowel; ?obstruction, closed loop or bowel wall edema
Intravenous urography (IVU)	Renal colic, ?ureteric obstruction by stone
Ultrasound	Ascites; cholecystitis/biliary colic; abscess; ?obstruction–dilated fluid filled bowel
Focused high resolution ultrasound	Diverticulitis; appendicitis; bowel wall thickening/abscess
CT scan	Severe pancreatitis; diverticulitis; abscess; small bowel obstruction; bowel infarction
Focused CT scan	Appendicitis; ureteric colic

PERIPHERAL VASCULAR DISEASE AND GANGRENE

History

Age and Sex

1. Old age—atherosclerosis
2. 20–40 years male—TAO
3. Young women—Raynaud's disease
4. Middle age—diabetic arteriopathy.

Clinical Features

1. Duration
2. Onset-bilateral or unilateral
3. Claudication
4. Claudication distance
5. Pain
6. Effect of heat and cold
7. History of fracture of bones, vascular heart disease, diabetes, impotence **(Leriche syndrome)**.

Past History

1. TB, vasculitis and ulceration
2. Bronchial asthma → steroid therapy → immunosuppression → **ulcer**
3. Diabetes mellitus → **diabetic ulcer**
4. Hypertension → atherosclerosis → **Martorell's ulcer**.

Personal History

Smoking.

General Examination

PICCLE

Vitals
Pulse-irregularly irregular—embolism.

Local Examination

Inspection

1. Appearance of limb—pale or cyanosed
2. Wasting
3. Conditions of nail—brittle, broken or lost
4. Skin—color, loss of hair.

Buerger's Postural Test

Vascular angle between 30° and 90°—**positive** (ischemia)
(no pallor or guttering of veins at 90°)—vascular angle > 90°—**Negative** (Normal)
Vascular angle < 30° (severe ischemia).

Capillary Filling Time

1. Normal—remains pink during elevated position
2. Ischemic leg—first pallor when elevated and gradually become pink in horizontal position
3. Severe ischemia—20–30 sec to become pink in horizontal position.

Venous Refilling

1. Normal limb—gradual collapse or guttering of veins above 90°, refilling of veins within 5 sec
2. Ischemic limb—collapse below 10°.

Examination of Gangrene

1. Extent
2. Color
3. Type (dry or wet)
4. Line of demarcation
5. Limb above gangrenous area.

Palpation

1. Local rise of temp and tenderness
2. Capillary filling
3. Venous refilling
4. Crossed leg test **(Fuchsig's test)**
5. Gangrenous area—type, crepitus, limb above gangrenous area.

Palpation of Blood Vessels

Neurogenic Examination

Sensation of gangrenous area.

Examination of Lymph Nodes

Auscultation

Continuous machinery murmur—AV fistula.

Provisional Diagnosis

Peripheral arterial occlusive disease probably due to atherosclerosis, origin—below the level of knee with healing nonspecific ulcer of right foot.

Investigations

1. Blood routine (routine examination)
2. Urine routine (routine examination)
3. FBS, PPBS
4. Serum cholesterol, lipoproteins, triglycerides
5. Arteriography, ECG, X-ray chest
6. USG, Doppler—determination of blood velocity.

Plethysmography

1. Measures blood flow
2. Good noninvasive technique.

Oscillometry

Detect arterial pulsations at different levels of limb.

Signs of Ischemia

1. Thinning of skin
2. Diminished growth of hair
3. Shininess and brittle nail.

ABPI—ankle brachial pressure index
>1: Normal *<0.9*: Obstruction *<0.3*: Imminent necrosis.

Brown's Vasomotor Index

= (Rise of skin temp – rise of mouth temp)/Rise of mouth temp
Operation is only advised when index is > 3.5.

Signs of Gangrene

1. Loss of temperature
2. Loss of color
3. Loss of pulsation
4. Loss of function
5. Loss of sensation.

Classification

Grade	Boyd	Fontaine
I	Walk-pain-continue to walk without pain	No pain
II	Pain during walking continue to walk with pain	Intermittent claudication
III	Pain during walk takes rest	Rest pain
IV	Pain at rest due to ischemia of nerves	Gangrene

Dry gangrene	Wet
Slow onset	Sudden onset
Progress slow	Rapid progress
Edema absent	Edema present
Mummification present	Absent
Line of demarcation—well	Not well
Arterial occlusion only	Both arterial and venous occlusion
Not infected	Usually infected
Example: Atherosclerosis	Example: 1. Embolism, 2. DM, 3. Buerger's disease, 4. Raynaud's disease.

Other Test in Peripheral Vascular Disease

1. **Allen's test**—to know the patency of radial and ulnar arteries
2. **Branham's sign/Nicoladoni's sign**
   a. AV fistula, aneurysm
   b. Apply pressure proximal to fistula
      i. Reduction in size of swelling
      ii. Disappearance of bruit
      iii. Falling pulse rate
      iv. Pulse pressure returns normal
3. **Cold and warm water test**
   Raynaud's disease
   Cold water—white hand
   Warm water—blue due to cyanotic congestion.
4. **Elevated arms test**
   Seen in thoracic outlet syndrome
   Normal—no difficulty
   Abnormal—numbness in fingers, pain in shoulders.
5. **Adson's test**
   +ve in cervical rib
   Scalenus anticus syndrome.

Causes of Gangrene

1. Secondary to arterial obstruction from disease
   a. Thrombosis of atherosclerotic artery
   b. Embolus from the heart in arterial fibrillation or coronary thrombosis

   c. Arteritis with neuropathy in diabetes
   d. Buerger's disease
   e. Arterial shut down Raynaud's disease
   f. Arterial injections, e.g. thiopentone toxic drugs.
2. Infective
   a. Abscess
   b. Gangrene
   c. Gangrene of scrotum.
3. Traumatic
   a. Direct injury (knife, bullet)
   b. Crushing injury
   c. Physical
   d. Heat, irradiation, electrical.
4. Venous
   Varicose vein.

Relationship of Clinical Findings to Site of the Disease

1. Aortoiliac obstruction—claudication in both buttocks, thighs and calves. Femoral and distal pulses absent in both limbs. Bruit over aortoiliac region. Impotence common.
2. Iliac obstruction—unilateral claudication in thigh and calf and sometimes buttock. Bruit over iliac region. Unilateral absence of femoral and distal pulses.
3. Femoropopliteal obstruction—unilateral claudication in calf. Femoral pulse palpable with absent unilateral distal pulses.
4. Distal obstruction—femoral and popliteal pulses palpable.
5. Ankle pulses absent—claudication in calf and foot.

Treatment of Gangrene

1. **General**
   a. Correct congestive cardiac failure (CCF)
   b. Anemia to improve oxygenation
   c. Nutritious diet
   d. Diabetic control
   e. Nonaddictive analgesics.
2. **Local**
   a. Keep limbs absolutely dry
   b. Limb must not be heated
   c. Protection of pressure areas
   d. Minor surgical toilet—lifting of crust, removal of hard devitalized skin
   e. Antibiotics.
3. **Drugs**
   a. Vasodilators (not so useful in atherosclerotic disease)
   b. Nicotinic acid used in thromboangiitis obliterans (TAO)
   c. Other drugs—pentoxifylline-rheological agent 400 mg TID
   d. Aspirin—150 mg/day
   e. Cilostazol—50–100 mg.

Treatment of Peripheral Vascular Disease

1. **Conservative**
   a. Explanation and advise—within 6 months improvement occurs due to development of collaterals
   b. Lifestyle modifications—stop smoking, regular exercise, diet
   c. Care of feet
   d. Heel raise—to improve claudication distance
   e. Head end elevation—Buerger's position.
2. **Medical**
   a. Control of diabetes and hypertension
   b. Drugs
   c. Analgesics.

3. **Surgical**

Direct	Indirect
Stenting (short segment)	Sympathectomy—lumbar
Grafting (long segment)	Or chemical
Transluminal angioplasty	Omentopexy
Thrombolysis	Ilizarov

SALIVARY GLAND

Parotid Gland

History

1. Components of swelling
2. Onset
3. Exact site
4. Duration
5. Growth
   a. Sudden increase in size of both parotid gland with considerable pain the case probably acute **parotitis**
   b. Generalized enlargement of all major salivary glands including lacrimal glands—**Mikulicz's syndrome** and if it is associated with dry eyes and generalized arthritis—**Sjögren's syndrome**
   c. Slow growing tumor—**pleomorphic adenoma**
   d. Rapid painful growth malignant transformation of adenoma
   e. Slow growing painless tumor in the lower part of parotid gland at the lower border of mandible—**adenolymphoma**
6. Complaints of pain
   a. Excruciating pain slight swelling and redness—parotid abscess
   b. Colicky pain during meals—obstruction of parotid gland
7. Complaints of watery discharge
   a. Sinus discharge from glands or its duct—parotid fistula.

Inspection and Palpation

1. Swelling
2. Site of parotid gland—below, behind, and slightly in front of the lobule of ear
3. Swelling obliterates the angle below the lobule of ear
4. Fixity of swelling—asking the patient to clinch his teeth mobility of the swelling is tested over contracted muscle
5. Deep lobe of parotid gland—bimanual examination with one finger of one hand inside his mouth just in front of tonsil and behind the 3rd molar tooth and one finger of the other hand externally behind the ramus of mandible is necessary for palpation of the deep lobe.
6. Skin over the parotid gland—parotid abscess—skin brawny, edematous which pits on pressure; fluctuation is a very late feature of parotid abscess; skin is warm and extremely tender
7. Duct—parotid (Stensen's duct) runs superficial to masseter muscle opens on the buccal surface of cheek opposite the crown of the upper second molar tooth.
8. Suppurative parotitis—gentle pressure over the gland will cause purulent saliva to course out of the orifice of the duct
9. Malignant growth—if blood comes out
10. Fistula.

Examination of Facial Nerve

Facial nerve involved in malignant growth.

Examination of the Lymph Nodes

Preauricular, parotid and submandibular group involved.

Movements of the Jaw

Malignant growth restricts the movement.

Classification of Salivary Gland Tumors

Type	Subgroup	Common example
Adenoma	Pleomorphic or monomorphic	Pleomorphic adenoma, Warthin's tumor
Carcinoma	**Low grade** acinic cell Ca	Adenoid cystic carcinoma
Carcinoma	**High grade** adenocarcinoma	Squamous cell carcinoma
Nonepithelial tumors		Hemangioma, lymphangioma
Lymphomas	Primary and secondary	Non-Hodgkin's lymphoma
Secondary tumors	Local, distant	Tumors of head and neck, skin and bronchus
Unclassified tumors		
Tumor like lesion	Solid lesion	Adenomatoid hyperplasia, benign **Lymphoepithelial lesion**
Tumor like lesion	Cystic lesions	Salivary gland cysts

Ducts of Salivary Glands

1. *Parotid gland*: Stensen's duct (opens at the upper 2nd molar tooth)
2. *Submandibular gland*: Wharton's duct (opens into the papilla just lateral to the frenulum)
3. *Sublingual gland*: Ducts of Rivinus.

Pleomorphic Adenoma (Mixed Tumor)

1. Most common
2. Called mixed—cartilage besides epithelial cells.
3. Epithelial and myoepithelial components in varied pattern—in abundant matrix of mucoid, myxoid or chondroid supporting tissue.
4. Presented as lobulated and painless swelling over parotid region neither adherent to skin nor to masseter muscle.
5. Firm but variable in consistency
6. Facial nerve remains free
7. Small pseudopods may protrude and left behind after enucleation so recurrence occurs in 5–50% of cases.

Malignant transformation suggested by:
1. Becomes painful
2. Starts growing rapidly
3. Feels stony hard
4. Gets fixed to the masseter and mandible deeply or to the skin superficially.

Involve facial nerve—an important feature
1. The cervical LN are enlarged
2. Movement of jaw may be restricted.

Papillary Cystadenoma Lymphomatosum (Warthin's Tumor)

1. Fife to fifteen percent of males above 40 years
2. Always occur in lower portion of parotid overlying the angle of mandible
3. Slow growing swelling over the angle of jaw
4. Consistency soft often fluctuate but not translucent
5. Regional LNS are not enlarged
6. Encapsulated and no malignant transformation.

Carcinoma of Parotid Gland (Adenocarcinoma, Epidermoid, Undifferentiated Carcinoma)

1. > 50 years of age
2. Males and females equally affected
3. Rapidly enlarging swelling in parotid region
4. Painful later, pain radiate to ear
5. On examination skin infiltration, skin becomes tethered and irregular surface, indistinct margin
6. Consistency firm to hard
7. Facial paralysis due to infiltration
8. LN enlarged and hard.

Superficial Parotidectomy

1. Lazy S incision
2. Back of parotid gland identified to expose the facial nerve
3. Sternomastoid retracted and greater auricular nerve divided
4. Second avascular plane opened in front of tragus
5. Facial nerve identified and dissected along its length
6. Facial branches dissected out starting with upper division freeing superior lobe
7. Cut facial nerve branches can be repaired immediately with a cable graft harvested from great auricular nerve.

Complications of Parotid Gland Surgery

1. Hematoma formation
2. Infection
3. Temporary facial nerve weakness
4. Transection of facial nerve and permanent facial nerve weakness
5. Sialocele
6. Facial numbness
7. Permanent numbness of the ear lobe associated with great auricular nerve transection
8. Permanent facial weakness after radical parotidectomy (Frey's syndrome).

Submandibular Salivary Gland

History

Swelling in the submandibular region with colicky pain—stone in submandibular duct and the swelling is tense and painful.

Local Examination

Inspection

Patient asked to suck a little lime or lime juice—swelling appears
Inspection of submandibular duct (Orifices are situated on either side of the frenulum linguae)
1. Orifice inflamed or swollen—stone in duct
2. Extrudation of pus on slight pressure—salivary gland inflammation.

Palpation

1. Submandibular gland palpated bimanually
2. Presence of calculi is also appreciated by this examination
3. This examination also differentiates an enlarged salivary gland from enlarged salivary lymph nodes
4. Swelling of the lymph node may be primary or secondary
5. For secondary involvement look inside the mouth.

Investigation

X-ray: Stone in the salivary gland or duct stones radiopaque.

Sialography

1. It is the contrast X-ray examination of the salivary ducts and glands
2. Also known as pyelography
3. Indications—salivary duct stones and strictures; chronic sialadenitis; tumors of salivary glands
4. Contraindications—contrast allergy; acute sialadenitis.

Treatment—Excision

Important anatomical relations of the submandibular glands

1. Lingual nerve
2. Hypoglossal nerve
3. Anterior facial vein
4. Facial artery
5. Marginal mandibular branch of facial nerve.

Developmental Disorders

1. Duct atresia
2. Ectopic/aberrant salivary gland tissue—**Stafne bone cyst**
3. Invagination into the bone on the lingual aspect of the mandible by ectopic lobe of the juxtaposed submandibular gland.

Inflammatory Disorders of Salivary Gland

1. Acute submandibular sialadenitis—viral, e.g. mumps; bacterial secondary to obstruction
2. Chronic submandibular sialadenitis—obstruction or trauma.

Complications for Salivary Gland Excision

1. Hematoma
2. Wound infection
3. Marginal mandibular nerve injury
4. Lingual nerve injury
5. Hypoglossal nerve injury
6. Transection of nerve to mylohyoid muscle producing submental skin anesthesia.

Calculi Common in Submandibular Gland than Parotid Gland

1. Higher mucin content
2. High Ca and PO_4 content
3. Nondependent drainage of secretions
4. Long and tortuous course of submandibular duct.

Indication for Submandibular Gland Excision

1. Sialadenitis
2. Stones proximal to the lingual nerve
3. Salivary tumors.

Sublingual Gland

Common Disorders of Sublingual Glands

Cysts (Ranula)

1. Ranula—mucous extravasation cyst arising from sublingual gland. It produce a characteristic translucent swelling that takes on the appearance of a frog's belly (ranula)
2. Resolve spontaneously
3. Require normal surgical intervention
4. Excision of the cyst and affected sublingual gland
5. Incision drainage result in recurrence
6. Plunging ranula (retention cyst)
7. Present with dumbbell shaped swelling
8. Soft fluctuant and painless in the submandibular or submeatal region of the neck.

Rx: Excision via cervical approach removing cyst and submandibular glands.

Minor Salivary Gland

Common Disorders of Minor Salivary Gland

Cyst

1. An extravasation cyst is one of the most common salivary gland disorder
2. Trauma to the overlying mucosa
3. Painless swelling and translucent

Rx: Surgical excision including overlying mucosa and the affected gland.

Tumors

1. Ninety percent malignant
2. Common site—upper lip, palate, retromolar region.

VARICOSE VEIN

What is Varicose Vein?

Dilated tortuous superficial elongated veins of lower limb due to valvular or vessel wall deformity resulting in retrograde backflow.

History

Age: Middle age group

Sex: 10:1—Female: Male

Occupation: Prolonged standing.

Clinical Features

1. Dilated veins over lower limb
2. Dull aching pain—towards the end of the day
3. Associated symptoms—itching, hyperpigmentation, ulceration
4. History of fever, trauma, bleeding
5. History of constipation, mass abdomen, micturition problems.

Past History

History of surgery, orthopedic procedure, breathlessness, immobilization, chest pain, DM, TB, HTN.

Personal History

Smoking.

Obstetric History

Multiparity: Proximal obstruction of vein, OCP (alter viscosity of blood).

Family History

Collagen vascular disease (Prune Belly syndrome).

General Examination

PICCLE.

Vitals

Local Examination

Inspection

1. *Long saphenous vein*: Dilated veins seen on the medial aspect of lower limb starting from in front of medial malleolus to medial side of knee and along medial side of thigh upwards to saphenous opening.
2. *Short saphenous vein*: Dilated veins seen on the lateral aspect of lower limb starting from behind lateral malleolus upwards in the posterior aspect of the leg and ends in popliteal fossa
3. *Skin of limbs*: Color, hyperpigmentation, scar, brittleness of nail, stretched and shiny—due to DVT, ulceration and hair loss
4. Impulse on coughing at saphenofemoral opening—*Morrissey's test.*

Palpation

Temperature and tenderness.
Edema and skin thickening.
Trendelenburg test 1: Positive saphenofemoral incompetence.
Trendelenburg test 2: Positive perforator incompetence.
Tourniquet test (remove from below): Positive in all perforator sites.

1. Just over saphenofemoral junction
2. Just below middle of thigh
3. Upper part of leg
4. Palm breadth above ankle joint

Modified Perthe's (tourniquet at saphenofemoral junction and ask to walk for 5 min → pain → DVT): Negative.
Schwartz's test (tap at a prominent part of the veins, feel impulse at SFJ): Positive.
Morrissey's test (elevate the limb to 30°, feel the impulse on cough at SFJ): Positive.
Fegan's test (feel the vein after emptying → depressions): Positive arterial pulses—all pulses are present.

Percussion

Schwartz's test.

Auscultation

No hum or bruit—AV fistula.

Examination of Regional Lymph Nodes

No lymph node enlargement.
Other limb normal.

Examination of Abdomen

No local rise of temperature, no tenderness, soft, no mass, lymph nodes, fluid thrill or shifting dullness.

Provisional Diagnosis

Primary/secondary varicose vein left/right leg involving long/short saphenous system with saphenofemoral/perforator incompetence with features of complications and with evidence of deep vein thrombosis.

Investigations

1. Blood and urine routine
2. ECG specific
3. *Doppler study*: Venous system
4. Duplex US imaging B mode
5. Chest X-ray
6. USG abdomen
7. Photoplethysmography
8. Venogram.

Treatment

1. Conservative management
2. Injection sclerotherapy
3. Surgery.

Conservative Management

1. Elevation of leg and rest
2. Elastic crepe bandage.

Indications
Pregnancy, pelvic tumor, positive perthe's test, AV fistula.

Injection Sclerotherapy

Indications: Below knee varicosity, recurrence after surgery.
Sclerosant: Ethanolamine oleate 5%, sodium tetradecyl sulfate, hypertonic saline, polidocanol, phenol (5%) in almond oil or peanut oil, tetracycline.
MOA: Aseptic thrombosis and fibrosis.

Surgeries

1. Trendelenburg's operation
2. Stripping
3. Subfascial ligation of Cocket and Dodd
4. SEPS—subcutaneous endoscopic perforator surgery
5. Hook phlebectomy—multiple perforators
6. New—Laser coagulation.

Anatomy

Tributaries of Great Saphenous Vein

Sole
1. Medial marginal vein (below knee)
2. Anterior vein of leg
3. Posterior arch vein.

Thigh
1. Accessory saphenous vein
2. Anterior cutaneous vein of thigh.

Just before piercing cribriform fascia
1. Superficial epigastric
2. Superficial external pudendal
3. Superficial circumflex iliac.

Just before termination
Deep external pudendal.

Perforators

1. *Dodd*: Mid thigh perforator
2. *Boyd*: Gastrocnemius perforator
3. *Cocket*: Lower leg perforator
4. *May or Kuster*: Ankle perforators.

Causes of Varicose Veins

1. Primary
2. Secondary
   a. Pregnancy
   b. Pelvic tumor
   c. Ascites
   d. DVT
   e. AV fistula.

Latest Classification of Varicose Veins

Clinical-Etiology-Anatomy-Pathophysiology (CEAP) Classification

Clinical Presentation

1. *Grade 0*: No varicosity
2. *Grade 1*: Subcutaneous flares, thread veins, reticular veins
3. *Grade 2*: Varicose veins
4. *Grade 3*: With edema
5. *Grade 4*: With pigmentation
6. *Grade 5*: Healed ulceration
7. *Grade 6*: Active ulceration.

Etiology

1. Congenital
2. Primary
3. Secondary.

Anatomical

1. Superficial
2. Deep
3. Perforators.

Pathology

1. Reflux
2. Obstructive
3. Combined.

Complications

1. Hemorrhage
2. Calcification of veins
3. Equine deformity
4. Eczema
5. Marjolin's ulcer
6. Phlebitis
7. Periostitis
8. Hyperpigmentation
9. Lipodermatosclerosis
10. Venous ulcer.

Mechanism of Venous Ulceration

1. Fibrin cuff hypothesis
2. White cell trapping hypothesis.

Treatment of Varicose Ulcer

Bisgard's regime

1. Elevation
2. Elastic crepe bandage
3. Active exercises
4. Heel down first—gait
5. Trendelenburg operation after ulcer heals
6. If secondary infection—antibiotics.

MALIGNANT MELANOMA

1. Malignant tumor arising from melanoblasts
2. Etiopathogenesis—UV rays
3. Age and sex—common in females
4. Genetic factors—familial dysplastic nevus syndrome
5. Trauma
6. Pre-existing mole
7. Immunosuppression—renal transplantation, leukemia
8. Most malignant type of melanoma—nodular type
9. Least malignant type of melanoma—lentigo maligna
10. Most common site of melanoma in males—trunk and back
11. Most common site of melanoma in females—lower extremity (knee to ankle)
12. Most common site of lentigo maligna melanoma—face, neck
13. MC site of acral lentiginous melanoma—palms, soles, subungual region.

Pathological Grading of Malignant Melanoma

I. **Clark's level of invasion** (Used only in T1 tumors)
   Level 1: Tumor confined to basement membrane
   Level 2: Tumor extending to papillary dermis
   Level 3: Tumor reaches the interface between papillary dermis and reticular dermis
   Level 4: Tumor reaches the reticular dermis
   Level 5: Tumor invades subcutaneous fat.

II. **Breslow's thickness**
   Stage 1: Thickness less than 0.75 mm (epidermis)
   Stage 2: 0.76 to 1.49 mm (papillary dermis)
   Stage 3: 1.50 to 3.99 mm (papillary dermis)
   Stage 4: > 4 mm.

Clinical Features

1. Change in pre-existing mole
2. Nonhealing ulcer
3. Satellite nodule.

Differential Diagnosis

1. Pigmented basal cell CA
2. Histiocytoma
3. Nevus
4. Kaposi's sarcoma
5. Cavernous hemangioma.

Investigations

1. **Specific**
   a. Excision biopsy
   b. FNAC—from the nodes can be taken.

2. **Nonspecific**
   a. X-ray chest—cannon ball appearance
   b. USG abdomen—secondaries in liver
   c. X-ray of bone—osteolytic lesion.

Treatment

1. Wide excision with excision biopsy—1 cm healthy margin (lesion 2–4 cm)
2. Clarke's level 3 lesion—wider excision—2 cm of healthy margin
3. Subungual malignant melanoma—amputation of digit
4. Malignant melanoma of choroids—enucleation of eyes
5. Amputation
6. Palliative—radiotherapy.

Advanced Malignant Melanoma—Rx

1. Radiotherapy
2. Systemic chemotherapy—cisplatin, vinblastine, bleomycin
3. Immunotherapy—alpha interferon, interleukin 2, monoclonal antibodies
4. Surgery or CO_2 laser excision
5. Hormone therapy
6. Isolated limb perfusion with melphalan
7. Prognosis—poor.

SIGNS in a mole when it becomes malignant.

Major sign: Change in size, shape, color

Minor sign: Inflammation, crusting or bleeding, sensory change, diameter > 5 mm.

Types of Melanoma (NASAL)

1. **N**odular—worst prognosis
2. **A**cral lentiginous—palms and soles
3. **S**uperficial spreading—most common
4. **A**melanotic (desmoplastic)
5. **L**entigo maligna melanoma (Hutchison's melanotic freckle)—elderly.

When to Suspect Melanoma

1. **A**symmetry
2. **B**order irregularity
3. **C**olor variation
4. **D**iameter more than 6 mm
5. **E**levation.

Breslow's Staging

1a: Thickness < 0.75 mm
1b: Thickness between 0.76 and 1.49 mm
2a: Thickness between 1.50 and 3.99 mm
2b: Thickness > 4 mm
3a: Any of the above + node < 3 cm
3b: Any of the above + node > 3 cm/3 or more nodes
4: Any of the above + any node + mL distant metastasis.

Spread

1. Local—continuity, contiguity
2. Lymphatic
3. Blood spread.

Management of Lymph Nodes

1. Lower limb—ilioinguinal block dissection
2. Sentinel lymph node mapping with isosulfan blue.

CARCINOMA OF TONGUE

Precancerous Condition

1. Chronic superficial glossitis
2. Smoking pipes and cigars
3. Syphilis
4. Sessile papilloma
5. Plummer-Vinson syndrome.

Clinical Types

1. Fungating or warty type
2. Fissure or cracked type
3. Frozen type
4. Ulcerating or excavating type
5. Nodular type.

Clinical Features

1. Fungating growth or ulcer
2. Ankyloglossia—cannot protrude tongue
3. Growth in posterior third of tongue—alteration of voice and dysphagia
4. Profuse salivation
5. Dysphagia and fetor.

Diagnosed by

1. Palpation
2. Laryngoscopy.

Spread

1. Locally
2. Lymphatic spread
3. Blood spread.

Causes of Death

1. Inhalation bronchopneumonia due to aspiration
2. Cancerous cachexia and starvation
3. Hemorrhage from primary growth
4. Asphyxia.

Treatment

1. Wide excision
2. Partial glossectomy
3. Hemiglossectomy
4. Total glossectomy
5. Commando's operation.

CARCINOMA PENIS

Premalignant Lesions

1. Genital warts—**Buschke-Lowenstein tumor**
2. Erythroplasia of Queyrat or Paget's disease of penis
3. Leukoplakia
4. Bowen's disease
5. Chronic balanoposthitis.

Etiology

1. Phimosis
2. Carcinoma is common in population who do not practice circumcision due to smegma.

Clinical Features

1. Nonhealing ulcer
2. Foul smelling discharge—blood stained
3. Hematuria
4. Recent phimosis.

Spread	Investigations
Direct spread	Wedge biopsy
Lymphatic spread	FNAC of lymph nodes
Sentinel lymph node biopsy	

Treatment According to Stage

Stage 1: Growth confined to prepuce—Circumcision
Growth involving glans—Partial amputation with 2 cm margin
Stage 2: Tumor involving penile shaft—(1) Partial amputation, (2) Total penectomy with perineal urethrostomy
Stage 3: Mobile regional nodal metastasis with stage1/2—(1) Sentinel lymph node biopsy, (2) Ilioinguinal block dissection
Stage 4: Tumor beyond penile shaft, fixed regional lymph nodes or distant metastasis—Radiotherapy [external (4000-6000 rads) and interstitial (radium wires/tantalum wires)] + chemotherapy (cisplatin, MTX, bleomycin).

Radiotherapy

Indications

1. Young patients who want sexual life
2. Fixed/ulcerated inguinal metastasis
3. Patient refuses surgery.

Complication: Radionecrosis of penis.

FOURNIER'S GANGRENE

1. Idiopathic gangrene of scrotal skin
2. Uncommon vascular disaster of infective origin
3. Sudden appearance of scrotal swelling
4. Onset of gangrene leading to exposure of scrotal contents
5. Testis not involved due to thick *tunica albuginea*
6. 50% cases idiopathic.

Etiology

1. Trauma
2. Infection
3. Instrumentation.

Organism

1. Hemolytic streptococci
2. *E. coli*
3. *Staphylococcus*
4. *Clostridium welchii.*

Treatment

1. Ampicillin/gentamicin/cephalosporins
2. Wide excision of necrotic scrotal skin followed by skin grafting.

SWELLINGS OF NECK

Anatomically

1. Lateral swelling
   a. Submandibular triangle
      i. Lymph node enlargement (LNE)
      ii. Enlarged submandibular salivary glands
      iii. Submandibular sialadenitis
      iv. Deep or plunging ranula
      v. Extension of growth from jaw
   b. Carotid triangle
      i. Aneurysm of carotid artery
      ii. Carotid body tumor
      iii. Branchial cyst
      iv. Bronchogenic carcinoma
      v. Thyroid swelling deep to sternocleidomastoid
      vi. Sternomastoid tumor may develop in newborn
   c. Posterior triangle
      i. Enlarged supraclavicular LN
      ii. Cystic hygroma
      iii. Pharyngeal pouch
      iv. Subclavian aneurysm
      v. Aberrant thyroid
      vi. Cervical rib
      vii. Lipoma (Dercum's disease)
2. *Midline swellings (From above downwards)*:
   a. Ludwig's angina
   b. Enlarged submental LN
   c. Sublingual dermoid
   d. Lipoma in submental region
   e. Thyroglossal cyst
   f. Subthyoid bursitis
   g. Goiter of the thyroid isthumus and pyramidal lobe
   h. Enlarged LN and lipoma in the substernal space of Berns
   i. Retrosternal goiter
   j. Thymic swelling.

Clinically

1. Acute swellings
   a. Cellulitis
   b. Boils
   c. Carbuncle
   d. Ludwig's angina
   e. Acute lymphadenitis.
2. Chronic swelling
   a. Cystic—branchial cyst
   b. Thyroglossal cyst
   c. Dermoid cyst
   d. Cystic hygroma
   e. Sebaceous cyst
   f. Cystic adenoma of thyroid gland
   g. Cold abscess.

3. Solid swellings
   a. Swelling arising from thyroid
   b. Bronchogenic CA
   c. Sternomastoid tumor.
4. Pulsatile swelling
   a. Aneurysm of carotid or subclavian artery
   b. Carotid body tumor
   c. LN swelling lying in close proximity to carotid artery to elicit transmitted pulsations
   d. Few primary toxic goiter
   e. Meningocele.

Discussion

Branchial Cyst

1. Probably develops from vertical remnants of second branchial cleft
2. Lined by squamous epithelium
3. Contains thick turbid fluid with cholesterol crystals
4. Usually present in the upper neck in early or middle adulthood
5. Found at the junction of upper third and middle third of sternomastoid muscle anteriorly
6. Fluctuant and transilluminant and soft
7. If infection occurs erythematous and tender and difficult to differentiate from tubercular abscess
8. Diagnosed by USG and FNAC
9. Treatment—complete excision.
   a. Fluctuation positive
   b. Transillumination negative
   c. Reducibility negative
   d. Compressibility negative.

Differential Diagnosis (DDs)

1. Submandibular gland swellings
2. Plunging ranula
3. Cystic hygroma
4. Cervical LN enlargement
5. Carotid body tumor.

Branchial Fistula

1. May be unilateral or bilateral
2. Represent persistent second branchial cleft
3. External orifice—lower third of neck anterior border of sternocleidomastoid (SCM)
4. Internal orifice—anterior aspect of the posterior faucial pillar behind tonsil tract is lined with ciliated columnar epithelium. It passes through the bifurcation of the common carotid artery.
5. There may be small amount of recurrent mucous or mucopurulent discharge onto the neck
6. **Treatment**—stepladder pattern dissection with multiple incision along the course of the tract.

Cystic Hygroma

Features

1. Soft, cystic
2. Fluctuation positive
3. Impulse on cough present
4. Partially compressible
5. Brilliantly transilluminant
6. Usually present in the neonate or early infancy may present at birth (may be so large to obstruct the labor)
7. Occurs due to sequestration of portion of jugular lymph sac
8. Lying soft and partially compressible. Multiloculated swelling hence partially compressible.
9. Increase in size when child coughs or cries

10. Filled with clear lymph and lined by a single layer of epithelium with a mosaic appearance
11. *Treatment*:
    a. Excision early stage
    b. Sclerotherapy.

Common Sites

1. Posterior triangle—most common
2. Cheek
3. Axilla
4. Groin
5. Mediastinum.

ULCER

History

1. Duration
2. History of trauma, fever, pain, discharge
3. History of swelling preceded by ulcer
4. History of syphilis, leishmaniasis.

General Examination

PICCLE and vitals.

Local Examination

Inspection

1. Site, size, shape, number
2. Edge
    a. Undermined (TB)
    b. Punched out (syphilitic)
    c. Rolled out (squamous cell CA) (rodent ulcer)
    d. Sloping (healing and venous)
    e. Raised and pearly white beaded
3. Floor
    a. Slough
    b. Discharge
    c. Granulation tissue
4. Surrounding area
5. Whole limb.

Palpation

1. Local rise of temperature and tenderness
2. Site, size, shape, number
3. Edge, margin
4. Base—on which ulcer rests
5. Depth
6. Bleed—on tough
7. Relations with deeper structure
8. Surrounding skin.

Examination of Regional Lymph Nodes

Examination of Vascular Insufficiency

Examination of Peripheral Nerve

Investigations

1. Blood and urine (routine examination)
2. *Urine*: Sugar, ketone bodies
3. FBS, PPBS
4. Pus culture and sensitivity (C and S)
5. X-ray chest to rule out TB
6. FNAC for lymph nodes

7. *Wedge biopsy*: Marjolins, malignant ulcer
8. Lipid profile
9. Blood urea, serum creatinine—RFT
10. X-ray of affected limb
11. ECG and Doppler.

Phases of Ulcer

1. Stage of extension
   a. Slough
   b. Induration
2. Stage of transition
   a. Red granulation tissue
   b. Less induration
3. Stage of repair
   a. Granulation tissue
   b. Fibrous tissue.

Ulcer: Painless and Painful

Painless	Painful
Trophic painless	Arterial painful
Syphilitic	Tropical
Epithelioma	Meleney's
Marjolins	Martorell
Chronic venous ulcer	Inflammatory

Classification of Ulcers

1. Clinical
   a. Spreading
   b. Healing
   c. Callous/chronic ulcer (> 6 weeks).
2. Pathologically
   a. Nonspecific
      i. *Traumatic*: Mechanical (dental ulcer)
         - Physical (X-ray, electrical burns)
         - Chemical (caustics)
      ii. *Arterial*: Atherosclerosis
         - Buerger's disease
         - Raynaud's syndrome
      iii. Venous—varicose ulcer
      iv. Neurogenic—bedsore
          Perforating ulcer
      v. *Associated with malnutrition*: Trophic ulcer
      vi. *Associated with diseases*: Gout, DM, anemia
   b. *Specific*: TB, syphilis, leprosy, actinomycosis
   c. *Malignant*: Epithelial, basal cell, malignant melanoma.

Factors Affecting Healing of Ulcer

Systemic	Local
1. DM a. Immunosuppression b. Neuropathy c. Microangiopathy	1. Infection
2. TB	2. Foreign body
3. Jaundice	3. Sequestrum

Contd...

Contd...

4. Uremia	4. Lack of rest
5. Arterial insuffiency a. TAO b. Senile c. Atherosclerosis	5. Involvement of bone, muscle, nerve, joint
6. Venous ulcer	6. Too frequent dressings
7. Malignancy	
8. AIDS	

Diagnosis

Nonhealing/healing ulcer of **site** (foot) with **risk factors** (diabetes, hypertension, atherosclerosis) with healthy/nonhealthy **granulation tissue** with or without features of **malignancy.**

Discussion

Grading of diabetic foot ulcer and treatment

Grade	Features	Treatment
0	No skin lesion—foot at risk (flat foot, hallux valgus, liable to injury)	Care of foot, shoes, keep foot dry, avoid injuries
1	Superficial ulcerations (full thickness of skin)	Local dressing and antibiotics
2	Deep ulcerations (up to tendon, bone, muscle)	Drainage and let out pus
3	Definitive involvement of bone or joint cavity (osteitis, osteomyelitis)	Liberal wound debridement
4	Portion of foot gangrenous—fore foot gangrenous (local gangrene)	Partial amputation
5	Whole foot gangrene	Major amputation

Granulation tissue

Healthy	Nonhealthy
Pinpoint	Flabby
Painless	Painful
Pink	Pale
Bleed on pressure	Exuberant

Ulcer causing organisms

1. Staphylococci
2. Streptococci
3. *E. coli*
4. *Proteus*
5. *Pseudomonas.*

Principles of Ulcer Management

1. Determine the etiology
2. Accurate assessment of ulcer
3. Identify and correct comorbid factors
4. Treat underlying causes
5. Adequate drainage and desloughing
6. Avoid adherent dressings.

Basic Requirements of the Ideal Ulcer Dressings

1. Maintain high humidity between wound and dressing
2. Absorbent, removes excess exudate
3. Nonadherent, allowing easy removal without trauma at dressing change
4. Safe and acceptable to patient (nonallergic)
5. Permit gaseous exchange but impermeable to microorganisms
6. Cost effective.

General Treatment

1. Control of diabetes
   a. *Plain insulin*: Short acting initially and then shift to long acting
   b. Change to oral hypoglycemic agents (after wound healing)
2. *Control of infection*: Broad spectrum antibiotics (change antibiotics according to C and S)
3. *Local treatment of diabetic foot*:
   a. Podiatry—Foot care
   b. H_2O_2 or eusol or iodine solution initially then betadine solution
   c. Metronidazole ointment
   d. Cellulose containing **Salutyl** ointment
   e. Packing
   f. Daily dressing of ulcer
   g. Large ulcer—skin grafting from same leg—split skin graft.

Types of Procedures

1. *Debridement*: Spreading ulcer with slough
2. *Skin grafting*: Healing ulcer
3. *Incision (I) and drainage (D)*: Abscess
4. *Disarticulate toe*: Gangrene toe
5. *Excision of metatarsal bone*: Involvement of metatarsals
6. *Forefoot amputation*: Gangrene confined to toe
7. *Multiple fasciotomy*: Spreading cellulitis
8. *Amputation below knee and above knee*: Spreading cellulitis with gangrene.

Skin Grafts

Skin grafts	Components	Donor site	Use
Partial thickness **(Thiersch Graft)**	Epidermis + available thickness of dermis	Thigh	Large area of skin defects and burns
Full thickness **(Wolfe graft)**	Epidermis + all of dermis	Postauricular, supraclavicular and groin	Repair of defect in face
Composite graft	Skin + fat + cartilage	Pinna of ear, skin and cartilage	Nasal defect, amputated finger tip pulp in children

Examples of Wounds and Reconstruction

Wounds	Reconstruction
Congenital:	
Cleft lip	Local flaps
Syndactyly	Local flaps with or without skin flaps
Hypospadias	Local flaps with or without skin flaps
Giant nevus	Tissue expansion + local flaps
Developmental:	
Breast asymmetry	Tissue expansion
Bell's palsy	Free tissue transfer
Infection: Fournier's gangrene	Skin graft
Trauma:	
Burns	Skin graft
Scar revision	Tissue expansion + flaps
Nasal loss	Local or distant flaps
Open tibial fracture	Fasciocutaneous flap, muscle flap, free flap
Hand or digit amputation	Microvascular reimplantation
Pressure sores	Local flaps, vacuum assisted closure (VAC) therapy

Contd...

Contd...

Neoplasia: Skin cancer Oral cancer Breast cancer	 Local skin flap Free tissue transfer Free or distant (pedicled) flaps tissue transfer

Split Skin Graft versus Full Thickness Graft

Split skin graft	Full thickness graft
Donor site factors	
Large area available	Smaller area
Donor site heal spontaneously	Donor site must be closed
Donor site reusable	Donor site scars
Recipient factors	
Poor color match	Good color match
Easily abraded	Abrasion resistant
Inferior cosmetic result	Good cosmetic result
More reliable take	Less reliable take
Shiny texture, inelastic	Normal texture, elastic

Definitions of Infected States

1. SSSI (superficial surgical site infection)—is an infected wound
2. SIRS (systemic inflammatory response syndrome)—is the body systemic response to an infected wound
3. MODS (multiple organ dysfunction syndrome)—is the effect that the infection has on the whole body
4. MSOF (multiple system organ failure)—is the end stage of uncontrolled MODS.

Classification of Surgical Wounds

Clean Wound (Class 1)

Include those in which no infection is present; only skin microflora potentially contaminate the wound. No hollow viscous is entered. No inflammation. For example, Hernia repair, breast biopsy.

Clean/Contaminated Wounds (Class 2)

Include those in which a hollow viscous such as the respiratory, alimentary or genitourinary tracts with indigenous bacterial flora is opened, but under controlled circumstances without significant spillage of contents. No inflammation. For example, Cholecystectomy, elective GI surgery.

Contaminated Wounds (Class 3)

Include open accidental wounds encountered early after injury, those with extensive introduction of bacteria into a normally sterile area of the body due to major breaks in sterile technique (e.g. Open cardiac massage); uncontrolled spillage of viscous contents such as from intestine. Inflammation is present. For example, Penetrating abdominal trauma, large tissue injury, enterotomy during bowel obstruction.

Dirty (Class 4)

Include traumatic wounds in which a significant delay in treatment has occurred and in which necrotic tissue is present. Includes wounds in which pus is present. Includes those wounds created to access a perforated viscous accompanied by a high degree of contamination. Severe inflammation is seen. For example, Perforated diverticulitis, necrotizing soft tissue infection.

Use of Antibiotics as Prophylaxis of Surgical Site Infection's

1. *Class 1*: Controversial, most surgeons do not give
2. *Class 1d*: Prophylactic antibiotics given
3. *Class 2*: Prophylactic antibiotics given
4. *Class 3 and 4*: Prophylactic as well as therapeutic.

Suggested Prophylactic Regimens for Operations at Risk

Type of surgery	Organisms encountered	Prophylactic regimen suggested
Vascular	*Staphylococcus epidermidis* *Staphylococcus aureus* Aerobic gram negative bacilli	3 doses of flucloxacillin with or without gentamicin, vancomycin or rifampicin
Orthopedic	*Staphylococcus aureus/epidermidis*	1 to 3 doses of a wide spectrum cephalosporin or gentamicin beads
Esophagogastric	Enterobacteriaceae Enterococci (Including anaerobic/ viridans streptococci)	1 to 3 doses of a 2nd generation cephalosporin and metronidazole in severe contamination
Biliary	Enterobacteriaceae (*E. coli*) Enterococci (*Streptococcus faecalis*)	1 dose of 2nd generation cephalosporin
Small bowel	Enterobacteriaceae Anaerobes (mainly bacteroides)	1 to 3 doses of 2nd generation with or without metronidazole
Appendix/colorectal	Enterobacteriaceae Anaerobes (mainly bacteroides)	3 doses of a 2nd generation cephalosporin with metronidazole

VARICOCELE

Definition

1. Veins of pampiniform becomes dilated and tortuous
2. Common side—left side.

Causes (Why Left Side is Common than Right Side)

1. Left testicular vein drains into left renal vein—high venous pressure
2. Total length of testicular vein more on left side (left vein drains at a higher level)
3. Left testicular vein arches over left renal vein
4. Loaded sigmoid colon press upon testicular vein
5. Left renal vein is nut cracked between abdominal aorta and superior mesenteric artery
6. Left suprarenal vein drains into left renal vein—due to adrenalin.

Note: Varicocele may be secondary to renal cell carcinoma blocking the renal vein by venous permeation. Always palpate the abdomen and renal angle for any mass in case of varicocele.

Presenting Complaint

1. Aching or dragging pain after prolonged standing
2. Swelling which appears on standing and disappears on lying down with scrotum elevated.

Signs

1. Impulse on coughing is more like a thrill
2. Veins felt like **"bag of worms"**
3. After occluding superficial inguinal ring and asked to stand veins form below
4. Blow test is positive.

Grading of Varicocele

1. *Grade 1*: On Valsalva
2. *Grade 2*: On palpation
3. *Grade 3*: On inspection.

Surgery Indications

1. Painful
2. Infertility
3. Large swelling
4. Medically unfit for job.

Treatment

1. Conservative
   Scrotal support and reassurance
2. Surgical
   a. Classical varicocele operation
   b. Laparoscopic
   c. Scrotal approach
   d. Palomo's approach.

HERNIA

History

1. *Age*: Young individuals: Indirect inguinal hernia (IIH)
   Old age: Direct inguinal hernia (DIH)
2. *Occupation*: Strenuous work, smoking.

Complaints

1. *Pain*: Dragging and aching type of pain worse as day passes.
2. Lump
   a. Swelling in the groin
   b. How did it start?
   c. Where did it first appear?
   d. What was the size and extent when it was first seen?
   e. Does it disappear automatically on lying down?
3. Systemic symptoms—colicky abdominal pain, vomiting, abdominal distention, constipation.
4. Other symptoms—persistent coughing of chronic bronchitis, frequency of micturition, urgency—benign hypertrophy of prostate (BHP).

Past History

1. Appendicectomy
2. Similar illness.

Family History

Collagen vascular disease, Prune Belly syndrome.

General Examination

PICCLE and Vitals

Local Examination

Inspection

1. Swelling (always examine in standing position)
   a. Size
   b. Shape-indirect inguinal hernia—pyriform or ovoid
   c. Position—medial part of inguinal region
   d. Extent—from inner part of inguinal ligament down to scrotum
2. Visible pulsations or peristalsis present or not
3. Expansile impulse on coughing.

Palpation

1. Local rise of temperature or tenderness
2. Size and shape
3. Position and extent
4. To get above the swelling.
5. Consistency
   a. *Doughy and granular*: **Omentum**
   b. *Elastic*: **Intestine**
6. Relation of swelling to testis and spermatic cord
7. Impulse on coughing—absent in strangulated and incarcerated hernia
8. **Ziemann's technique**—if impulse felt on.
   a. Index finger over deep inguinal ring 1/2 inch above the mid-inguinal point (midpoint between anterosuperior iliac spine and pubic symphysis)—indirect inguinal hernia **(IIH)**
   b. Middle finger over superficial inguinal religion—direct inguinal hernia **(DIH)**
   c. Ring finger over saphenous opening 4 cm below and lateral to pubic tubercle—**femoral hernia**
9. Reducibility
10. Invagination test
    Little finger or index finger
    a. Directed backwards/upwards— Direct hernia (DH)
    b. Backwards outwards/oblique and laterally— Indirect hernia (IH)
11. Ring occlusion test
    Thumb on deep inguinal ring
    a. Direct hernia (DH)—bulge medial to occlusing finger (+ve)
    b. Indirect hernia (IH)—not find access (-ve).

Percussion

1. Resonant contains intestine—enterocele
2. Dull contain omentum or extraperitoneal fatty tissue.

Auscultation

Peristaltic sound—enterocele.

Examination of Testis, Epididymis and Spermatic Cord

Examination of Regional Lymph Nodes

Examine the Tone of Abdominal Muscles

Malgaigne's bulgings—abdominal muscles weak.

Examination of Abdomen

Examination of Respiratory System

Cardiovascular System

CNS

Diagnosis

1. Side
2. Complete/incomplete
3. Type—IIH, DIH, femoral hernia (FH)
4. Complications (with or without).

Gormall's Test

In case of child with small inguinal hernia, the child is held from back by both hands of the clinician on the abdomen. The abdomen is pressed and child is lifted up making the hernia apparent.

Named Hernias

1. *Richter's hernia*: A portion of circumference of bowel strangulated
2. *Littre's hernia*: Meckel's diverticulum
3. *Maydl's hernia*: (Hernia-en-W)-retrograde strangulation—2 loops of bowel remain inside
4. *Amyand's hernia*: Appendix
5. *Pantaloon hernia*: Direct and indirect hernia combined
6. *Beclard's hernia*: Femoral hernia through the opening of the saphenous vein.

Investigations

1. To assess the general condition
2. Complete blood picture; urine routine examination; chest X-ray (CXR); ECG; pulmonary function test; USG abdomen; sigmoidoscopy
3. Specific—herniography—inject radiopaque dye and take X-ray.

Complications of Hernia

1. Irreducible
2. Obstruction
3. Strangulation
4. Inflammation
5. Incarceration.

Treatment

1. *Herniotomy*:
   Excision of the sac alone.
   Done in infants, young adults with good posterior wall; congenital hernia.
2. *Herniorrhapy*: Herniotomy with reinforcement of posterior wall
   a. **Bassini's** repair
   b. **Shouldice** repair
   c. Upper and lower flaps of transversalis fascia (double breasting)
   d. Conjoint tendon—inguinal ligament
   e. Upper flap of external oblique aponeurosis—inguinal ligament
3. *Hernioplasty*:
   a. **Lichtenstein** repair (Tension free)
   b. Prolene darning
4. *Other surgeries*:
   a. **Kuntz** operation
   b. **Andrew's** operation
   c. **McVay's** operation
   d. **Nyhus** repair.

Short Surgical Procedures

1. *TAPP*: Transabdominal preperitoneal repair
2. *LEP*: Laparoscopic extraperitoneal repair
3. *IPOM*: Intraperitoneal only mesh repair
4. *PEER*: Percutaneous endoscopic external ring repair.

Complications of Surgery

1. Hemorrhage
2. Recurrence
3. Injury to testicular nerve, pampiniform plexus
4. Injury to femoral vessels, bladder
5. Injury to cord structures
6. Injury to ilioinguinal nerve
7. Rejection of mesh and mesh migration
8. Scar formation
9. Desmoid formation
10. Neuroma formation
11. Neuralgia
12. Osteitis pubis.

Gilbert and Rutkow Classification

1. Normal deep ring} Ih
2. Deep ring < 2 finger width} Ih
3. Deep finger > 2 finger width} Ih
4. Herniation through Hesselbach triangle} Dh
5. Herniation through punctum in Hesselbach triangle} Dh
6. Combined hernia/pantaloon hernia
7. Femoral hernia.

Types of IIH

1. ***Bubonocele***—confined to inguinal canal
2. **Funicular**—upper part of testis
3. **Complete/vaginal/scrotal**—up to bottom of testis.

Mechanisms Preventing Hernia in Inguinal Region

1. Obliquity of the inguinal canal
2. Shutter mechanism of arched fibers of inferior oblique (IO) and transversus abdominis (TA)
3. Sphincteric action of TA and IO at deep inguinal ring
4. Ball valve action of cremasteric muscle
5. Fibers of IO entering to deep inguinal ring
6. Conjoint tendon in front of Hesselbalch's triangle.

Contents of Inguinal Canal

1. Spermatic cord
2. Ilioinguinal nerve
3. Genital branch of genitofemoral nerve
4. Round ligament in females
5. Vestigial remnant of processes vaginalis.

Contents of Spermatic Cord

1. Vas deferens
2. Testicular nerve
3. Artery to vas
4. Cremasteric artery
5. Pampiniform plexus of veins
6. Lymphatics
7. Sympathetic nervous system
8. Genital branch of genitofemoral nerve
9. Processus vaginalis.

Layers of Hernial Sac (DIH)

1. Skin—Two layers of superficial fascia
2. External oblique aponeurosis—Conjoint tendon
3. Fascia transversalis—Peritoneum.

Layers of Hernial Sac (IIH)

1. Skin—Two layers of superficial fascia (fatty and membranous)
2. External spermatic fascia—continuation of external oblique aponeurosis
3. Cremasteric muscle and fascia—continuation of internal oblique
4. Internal spermatic fascia—derived from fascia transversalis
5. Extraperitoneal fat—peritoneum.

Nyhus Classification

1. Indirect hernia + normal deep ring
2. Indirect + wide deep ring
3. Posterior wall defect
   a. Direct
   b. Indirect
   c. Femoral.
4. Recurrent
   a. Direct
   b. Indirect
   c. Femoral
   d. Combined.

HYDROCELE

Classification

1. Congenital
   a. Patent processus vaginalis
   b. Present since birth
   c. Disappears on lying down
   d. Direct communication between tunica vaginalis (TV) sac and peritoneal cavity
   e. Associated with TB peritonitis.
2. Acquired
   a. Primary
      i. Idiopathic
      ii. Enormous swelling of scrotum
      iii. Fluid surrounds the testis and makes it impalpable
   b. Secondary
      i. Acute epididymo-orchitis, syphilis, malignancy
      ii. Lymphatic obstruction, postherniorrhaphy, trauma.

Etiology

1. Defective absorption by tunica vaginalis
2. Excessive production of fluid
3. Interference with drainage by the lymphatic vessels.

Other Types of Hydrocele

1. Infantile hydrocele : Tunica and processus vaginalis are distended up to the deep inguinal ring
   No communication with peritoneal cavity
2. Funicular hydrocele : Funicular process is closed just above the tunica vaginalis
3. Hydrocele of canal of nuck : In females at the site of round ligament
4. Hydrocele of hernial sac : Neck of hernial sac closed by adhesions/plugged with omentum
5. Encysted hydrocele of cord : Cystic swelling in the inguinal or inguinoscrotal region
   Fluctuation test, translucency test positive
   No impulse on coughing
   Testis felt separately
   Traction test present.

Differential Diagnosis

1. Hematocele
2. Pyocele
3. Epididymal cyst
4. Testicular tumor
5. Spermatocele
6. Chylocele
7. Filariasis.

Local Examination

1. Can get above the swelling
2. Fluctuation test positive
3. Transillumination test positive
4. Dull on percussion
5. Reducibility negative for vaginal hydrocele
6. Testis not palpable in primary hydrocele.

Investigations

1. Blood and urine (routine examination)
2. Doppler to rule out varicocele
3. Aspiration—diagnostic
4. Scrotal USG
5. Sperm count before surgery.

Treatment

1. *Lord's plication of TV sac*: Small sac with thin wall
2. *Jaboulay's eversion procedure*: Moderate sac
3. *Subtotal excision*: Large sac with thin wall
4. *Aspiration*: Elderly and those unfit for surgery.

Complications of Hydrocele

1. Rupture
2. Hernia of hydrocele sac
3. Hematocele
4. Calcification of sac wall
5. Infection
6. Atrophy of testis.

Surgery

OSCE

Spotters

1. Incisional hernia—Rx
2. Two characteristic features of colon
3. Common cause of intestinal obstruction
4. Differentiating features between small intestine and large intestine
5. Why radiotherapy after surgery in CA breast.

Drugs

1. Adrenaline, atropine—dose, uses, complications and lifesaving indication
2. Metronidazole.

Instruments

1. Ryle's tube—metabolic abnormalities in gastric outlet obstruction (GOO)
2. T tube indication and T tube cholangiogram
3. Stapler device—uses
4. Lung holding forceps
5. Nasogastric tube
6. Needle holder—uses
7. Foley's catheter—2 uses
8. FNAC needle—use; FNAC stain
9. Suture materials.
10. Sinus forceps (Hilton's method) I and D.

Absorbable suture materials

1. Plain and chromic catgut—derived from submucosa of jejunum of sheep
2. Chromic catgut is catgut with chromic salt
   Absorption time Plain catgut—7 days
   Chromic catgut—21 days
3. Vicryl-polyglactic acid—absorbs within 90 days
4. Dexon-polyglycolic acid—like vicryl
5. Maxon-polyglyconate—monofilament
6. PDS—Poly Dioxanone suture—monofilament
7. Monocryl-polyglecaprone—monofilament.

Nonabsorbable suture materials

1. Silk
2. Polypropylene—prolene
3. Polyethylene—ethylene
4. Nylon
5. Steel.

Specimens

1. Partial gastrectomy specimen—indications
2. Commando's operation
3. Colon—indications of colectomy
4. Gastrectomy
5. Seminoma testis
6. Radical gastrectomy specimen—indications
7. Small intestinal polyp
8. Sigmoid volvulus—predisposing factors
9. Cholangiogram—surgery, findings and condition
10. Orchidectomy specimen—tuberculous orchitis
11. Cholecystectomy specimen—types of gall stones, opaque stones
12. Mesenteric cyst—types; what is pseudomesenteric cyst
13. Hemimandibulectomy specimen—indication, types of CA in alveolar region, anatomical parts of mandible.

X-rays

1. X-ray intestinal obstruction—2 findings
2. Free gas under diaphragm—conditions
3. Submandibular sialography
4. J stent in abdominal X-ray
5. T tube cholangiography
6. Double J stent
7. Intussusception—types
8. Small intestinal obstruction
9. ERCP showing stone and dilated biliary tree
10. Sigmoid volvulus—X-ray findings, Rx, sigmoidopexy
11. X-ray intestinal obstruction with perforation—read the X-ray; identify the loop involved
12. Barium meal follow-through intestinal obstruction distal to jejunum
13. Barium swallow
14. Barium enema.

SURGICAL PROCEDURES

Thyroidectomy

Surgical removal of the thyroid gland. Based on the amount of thyroid tissue removed there are different types of thyroidectomies:

1. *Isthmusectomy* = removal of isthmus
2. *Lobectomy* = removal of a single (right/left) lobe

3. *Hemithyroidectomy* = isthmus + one lobe
4. *Subtotal thyroidectomy* = removal of thyroid gland leaving behind some amount of thyroid tissue (8 g in nontoxic and 4 g in toxic goiters)
5. *Total thyroidectomy* = entire thyroid gland removed
6. *Near total thyroidectomy* = attempted total with preservation of the parathyroid gland and its blood supply and recurrent laryngeal nerve (RLN), leaves a small amount of thyroid gland.

Position (P)

Supine with pillow under the shoulder to extend the neck. Head end with 15° elevation to prevent venous engorgement in the head and neck area.

Anesthesia (A)

1. General anesthesia
2. Can be done under local anesthesia

Incision (I)

Kocher collar incision—transverse incision 2 finger breadth above the suprasternal notch from the anterior border of one SCM muscle to the other.

Procedure

1. The transverse incision cuts through the **skin, subcutaneous tissue** and **platysma:** The two flaps are raised, the superior one up to the thyroid cartilage and the lower one up to the suprasternal notch. Hold the flaps with Jolle's self-retaining retractor.
2. Vertical incision on the **investing layer of deep fascia**.
3. Pull aside the strap muscles.
4. Vertical incision on the **pretracheal fascia.**
5. Look for and ligate and cut the **middle thyroid vein**. Being a short one it bleeds when the thyroid is pulled.
6. Deliver the thyroid. If any difficulty in delivering the thyroid, cut the strap muscles transversely.
7. Ligate and cut the **superior thyroid pedicle (artery and vein)**, close to the gland, as the external laryngeal nerve is away near the gland.
8. Ligate and cut the **inferior thyroid pedicle (vein only)**, as away as possible from the gland, as the RLN is near the pedicle when it approaches the gland.
9. Remove the required amount of gland after placing appropriate clamps (2 nos.) and cut between them and suture the gland with chromic catgut.
10. Close all layers.
11. Place **suction drainage** before closing and bring it out through a separate stab incision. Remove drain when the secretions stop (usually 48 hours). Oral feeds can be started the next day.

Postoperative

Sedation, IV glucose/saline.

Complications

1. Hematoma (management—open the suture and let out the blood immediately or endotracheal intubation and take to theater)
2. Respiratory distress
3. Infection
4. Hypothyroidism
5. Wound complication—keloid, hypertrophic scar
6. RLN injury (and external laryngeal nerve)
7. Thyroid storm
8. Hypoparathyroidism
9. Stitch granuloma.

Tracheostomy

It is a surgical procedure in which a small opening is made on the anterior wall of the trachea and is converted into a stoma on the skin surface.

Indications

1. *Acute upper airway obstruction*: Trauma, acute infections, neoplasms, congenital abnormalities, laryngeal edema, laryngeal nerve palsies and foreign bodies.
2. *Potential upper airway obstruction*: Major surgeries of oral cavity, pharynx, larynx and neck.
3. *Protecting the lower airway*: To prevent aspiration of saliva as in unconscious patient, respiratory muscle paralysis, etc.
4. Artificial respiration (long-term).

Types

1. Emergency
2. Elective
3. Permanent.

P : Supine with a pillow under the shoulders to extend the neck—the trachea is thereby brought forward.
A : LA/GA
I : Vertical incision from cricoid cartilage to the suprasternal notch, preferred in emergencies or transverse incision 2 finger breadth above the suprasternal notch, preferred in elective procedure—leaves a cosmetically better scar.

Procedure

1. After incision tissues cut in midline.
2. Strap muscles pulled aside or cut.
3. Thyroid isthmus pulled aside or cut.
4. A few drops of 4% lignocaine injected into trachea to suppress cough when the trachea is incised.
5. Fix the trachea and open it with a vertical incision in the region of the 2nd and 3rd or 3rd and 4th rings. Do not cut the 1st ring as this will cause perichondritis of cricoid and resultant stenosis.
6. Introduce the tracheal dilator and widen the opening. Convert the vertical opening into a circular one.
7. Introduce a tracheostomy tube of an appropriate size. When in position the tubes should be retained by double tapes passed around the patient's neck with a reef knot on either side or stitch the flanges of the tube directly to the underlying neck skin.

Postoperative

1. Suction—efficient, sterile-as often as required.
2. Humidification + oxygen
3. Warm well ventilated room
4. Take care of the tube and patient—put plastic tube until day 10 (postoperative—when tract is well formed, change to metal tube—else cough in early stages will push it out)
5. Physiotherapy.

Complications

Early	Intermediate	Late
Bleeding	Tracheitis	Large vessel erosive hemorrhage
Apnea	Tracheobronchitis	Tracheal laryngeal stenosis
Pneumothorax	Tracheal crusting	Tracheoesophageal fistula
Injury RLN	2° bleeding	Decannulation problems
Injury esophagus	Tube block/displacement	Wound complications
Blood aspiration	Wound infection	Aspiration of cannula fragments

Advantages

1. Reduces anatomical dead space.
2. Reduces the work of breathing.
3. Increases alveolar ventilation
4. Patient can talk and eat with tube in place (unlike endotracheal tube).

Disadvantages

1. Loss of air conditioning done in the upper respiratory tract (URT).
2. Desiccation of the tracheal epithelium, loss of ciliated cells and metaplasia.
3. Mucus dries up and blocks the tube.

Circumcision

Indications

1. Religious
2. Phimosis and paraphimosis
3. Carcinoma penis stage I
4. Balanitis
5. Unable to retract prepuce for sexual intercourse
6. Splitting of an abnormally tight frenulum.

P : Supine
A : LA/SA/GA—LA is preferred, xylocaine 1 or 2% without adrenaline to the root of penis.

Procedure

1. With 2 hemostats the prepuce is held at 3 o'clock and 9 o'clock positions and pulled forwards.
2. A longitudinal incision is made at the 12 o'clock position at the distal end on the prepuce up to the corona
3. At the corona the incision is extended to either side parallel to the coronal sulcus
4. The skin and subcutaneous tissues are removed
5. Bleeding from the frenular artery is possible and therefore should be ligated with a 'figure of 8' ligature
6. The skin is then sutured to the mucous membrane.

Complications

1. Bleeding
2. Infection
3. Injury to urethra and stricture.

Postoperative

Avoid erection as it causes increased vascularity and hemorrhage. For this give tranquillizers.

Hydrocele

Abnormal collection of serous fluid in some part of processus vaginalis usually tunica.
Indication: Discomfort to the patient by a large hydrocele.
P : Supine
A : SA/LA/GA—Preferred is LA—take 10 cc of 1% lignocaine, add 10 cc water to make it 0.5% dose. Dose = 7 mL/kg. 2 to 3 cc is infiltrated direct into the center of cord by holding the root of cord in between (b/w) thumb and index finger and injected perpendicularly. Any pain during traction of cord is prevented by this. 4 to 5 cc is injected along the line of incision. (Basically lignocaine into the cord and the line of incision).

Vertical Incision (Some Prefer Horizontal)

Procedure

1. *Lords plication*: Done when the sac is small and thin walled.
   Incision: Deliver the hydrocele—remove the fluid—put a few placating (6 nos.) sutures using catgut, so that the tunica vaginalis is ruffed up (or skirted) and sutured onto itself.
2. *Jaboulay's procedure*: Used for slightly larger hydroceles. Here instead of plicating the tunica vaginalis its everted and sutured onto itself behind the testis.
3. *Excision and eversion*: Done in very large or thick walled hydrocoeles. Here the fluid is removed and then a part of the sac is removed. The free end of the remaining tunica is sutured to prevent bleeding.
   After all procedures all layers except skin sutured in one layer with catgut. Skin in another layer with nonabsorbable suture.

Complications

1. Hematoma
2. Torsion of the testis
3. Infection
4. Pyocele
5. Injury to the testis
6. Recurrence.

Hernia

Protrusion of the viscus or part of a viscus through the wall that contains it. Hernia is prevented by:
1. Spincteric action of deep inguinal ring
2. Obliquity of inguinal canal
3. Shutter like action due to the placing of abdominal muscles in different directions.

Indications

1. Emergency—strangulation, obstruction
2. Elective

P : Supine
A : SA/LA/GA
I : Half inch above the inguinal ligament an oblique incision along the medial two-third.

Types of Procedures

1. *Indirect hernias in children*: Reduce contents and herniotomy. No other procedure is needed as the canal will develop normal obliquity as the child grows.
2. *Indirect hernias in adults*: Reduce the contents, twist the sac, place transfixing sutures and cut the excess sac. If the posterior wall is weak, then proceed with hernioplasty or herniorrhaphy.
3. *Direct hernias-herniorrhaphy—Bassini's repair*: Wherein the conjoint tendon is sutured to the inguinal ligament with an absorbable continuous suture.
   Modified Bassini's repair: Use continuous nonabsorbable sutures. The first suture is passed through the periosteum of the pubic tubercle (this is called master or key suture).

Hernioplasty

1. *Darning*: Where a continuous series of figure of 8s are used to strengthen the posterior wall.
2. **Prolene mesh.**

Procedure

1. Skin incision, cutting through the skin, superficial fascia (both the Camper's fatty layer and Scarpa's membranous layer), external oblique aponeurosis which is cut along the line of fibers.
2. Ligate bleeding vessels.
3. Extend the incision in the external oblique aponeurosis, up to and opening the superficial ring.
4. If the sac anterosuperior to the cord it is indirect hernia; direct inguinal hernia lies behind the cord.
5. Using a gauze separate the spermatic cord and the hernial sac.
6. Hold the cord with a cord holding forceps.
7. Isolate the sac up to the deep inguinal ring with slow dissection. You know that you have reached the deep ring when you see the extraperitoneal fat.
8. Feel for the width of the deep ring—is it lax and wide open?
9. The sac is opened in case of indirect hernia and not opened in the direct hernia. Reduce the contents if any and then complete the procedure as mentioned under the heading 'types of procedure'. In direct hernia do a herniorrhaphy or hernioplasty.
10. Close the external oblique aponeurosis with catgut after placing the cord in the inguinal canal. Close the superficial fascia with catgut. Close the skin with nonabsorbable sutures.

Complications

1. Bleeding
2. Infection
3. Injury to the vas deferens
4. Injury to the testicular artery—atrophic testes.
5. Injury to the ilioinguinal nerve—anesthesia over the medial side of the inguinal canal
6. Osteitis pubis

7. Postherniorrhaphy hydrocele—due to lymphatic obstruction
8. Recurrence.

Vasectomy

Permanent sterilization of male by removing a part of both vas deferens.
A = LA.

Procedure

1. Scrotum is cleaned, shaved before the operation
2. Local anesthetic
3. Tiny incision on one side
4. Locate the vas deferens (vas)
5. Vas isolated and drawn out through incision, clamped at 2 sites near each other
6. Segment between the clamps (approximate 5 mm) is removed
7. Ligate the tube—clip/cauterize/suture
8. Repeat on the other side after placing vas back in the scrotum
9. Do not suture the small incision on the scrotum.

Postoperative

1. Warn about the complications numbers 1, 2, 6
2. Advice alternate contraceptives
3. Analgesics and antibiotics
4. No bath for 1 day
5. Scrotal support for 2 weeks
6. No heavy work for 3 weeks
7. Report if bleeding, pain
8. Psychological support—else can cause impotence and other psychosomatic problems.

Complications

1. Takes 12–16 weeks to be effective, i.e. 30–40 ejaculations
2. Needs testing of sperms in semen to assess success.
3. Pain
4. Wound infections
5. Hematoma
6. Spontaneous recanalization, therefore follow-up up to 3 years required.
7. Autoimmune response to sperms, therefore reversal of vasectomy may fail.
8. Sperm granuloma—painful swelling in 10–14 days postoperative. About 1 cm in size. Subsides on its own.

Failure rate of 0.15/100 person years.

No Scalpel Vasectomy

Locate the vas. Hold in place with a clamp. Tiny puncture with a special instrument. Puncture is gently stretched till opening is large enough to deliver the vas. Rest of the procedure as above. No suture.

Recurrence

Caused by:
Preoperative: Chronic cough, constipation.
Operative: Bad surgical technique (tight sutures, using absorbable sutures, wrong type of hernia operation), hematoma and infection, missed pantaloon hernia.
Postoperative: Infection, bleeding, poor general condition, heavy work within 3 months of operation.

Mastectomy

Surgical removal of the breast.

Types of Mastectomy

1. *Lumpectomy*: Removal of the lump with 1 cm margin
2. *Quadrantectomy*: Removal of the mass with 3 cm margin
3. *Radical mastectomy*: Breast + pectoralis major + pectoralis minor + LN up to level 3
4. *Extended radical mastectomy*: Radical mastectomy + en bloc removal of internal mammary LN
5. *Super radical mastectomy*: Radical mastectomy + remove of mediastinal LN
6. *Modified radical mastectomy*: Similar to radical but the structures preserved are:
   a. Pectoralis major (this is always preserved in modified radical)
   b. Pectoralis minor (based on what is done to this muscle, there are different types of modified radical—given below)
   c. Cephalic vein and axillary vein
   d. Long thoracic nerve
   e. Thoracodorsal nerve
   f. Medial and lateral pectoral nerves
   g. Subscapular nerve
7. *Patey*: P minor is removed to facilitate the removal of level 1, 2, 3 LN in axilla
8. *Scanlon*: P minor is divided but not removed to facilitate the removal of level 1, 2, 3 LN in axilla
9. *Auchincloss*: P minor is neither removed nor divided—only retracted—level 3 LN cannot be removed (basically, this is what we call SM+AD).

Simple mastectomy: Only the breast is removed. Axillary sampling may be included in it.
Total mastectomy: Same as simple mastectomy.
Toilet mastectomy: When the tumor presents as a fungating mass the entire breast with the overlying skin is removed. The defect created may be later closed by placing a skin graft. It is usually a palliative procedure.

Indications

CA breast—stage 1, stage 2 and stage 3 (following—neoadjuvant chemotherapy)
P : Supine with arm abducted.
A : GA
I : Elliptical incision, directed transversely or obliquely, enclosing the nipple and areola.

Procedure (Modified Radical)

1. Make incision
2. Use electrocautery for forming the upper and lower flaps
3. Start dissection of breast medially. Elevate the breast sharply off the pectoralis fascia. Ligate bleeding vessels
4. As we move laterally, we encounter the clavipectoral fascia. Cut it and enter the axilla
5. Remove the enlarged LN, or those nodes stained by the sentinel node technique
6. Cut and ligate the tributaries of the axillary vein from the breast
7. Place a rubber drain
8. Close the subcutaneous tissue and skin.

Complications

1. Bleeding
2. Infection
3. Flap necrosis
4. Edema of arm
5. Lymphangiosarcoma (Stewart-Treves syndrome).

Parotidectomy

1. Superficial parotidectomy : Superficial lobe, which lies above the fasciovenous plane of Patey is removed facial nerve preserved
2. Conservative total parotidectomy : Both lobes removed. Facial nerve preserved

3. Radical parotidectomy : Both lobes + facial nerve + LN
4. Enucleation : Resection of the tumor alone.

Preoperative

1. Informed consent
2. Nerve stimulation test and functioning of the facial nerve is confirmed
3. Nondepolarizing muscle relaxants to be used during surgery—only then the intraoperative stimulation of the facial nerve can be done to test and see if its intact
4. Hypotensive anesthesia to be used during the surgery—these glands are very vascular

A : GA/LA
P : Supine with head turned to one side
I : S-shaped incision. Starting in front of the ear lobes which is curved below the ear lobe up to the mastoid and then directed down towards the neck.

Procedure (Superficial Parotidectomy)

1. Infiltrate the incision line with lignocaine and adrenaline
2. Make the incision and raise flaps along the preparotid fascia
3. Blood—free plane anterior to the external auditory meatus (EAM) is opened and proceed in an inferior direction
4. Identify the facial nerve trunk and trace all the branches
5. With gentle traction and further dissection towards the periphery, mobilize the gland and resect the superior lobe
6. As we dissect and approach the ends of the facial nerve branches, we come across the Stensen's duct, which is ligated and cut
7. Vacuum drain is placed
8. Wound closed in layers.

Complications

1. Infections
2. Bleeding
3. Facial nerve injury
4. Greater auricular nerve injury—ear lobe anesthesia
5. Salivary fistula
6. Frey's syndrome.

Complete removal of the parotid gland will reveal the parotid bed

1. *Vein*: Internal jugular vein
2. *Arteries*: Internal and external carotid arteries
3. *Muscles*: Styloglossus, stylopharyngeus and stylohyoid all along with the attached styloid process
4. *Nerves*: Cranial nerves IX, X, XI, XII.

Deep Fascia of Neck

Investing layer

Horizontal: Posterior attachment starts with the ligamentum nuchae and C7 spine, passes anteriorly, dividing to enclose the trapezius and the SCM and meets similar fascia of the opposite side in the midline.

Vertical: Superior attachments starts from the occipital protuberance and superior nuchal line of occipital bone, mastoid part of temporal bone and cartilaginous part and lower border of zygomatic arch. Proceeds downwards, divides to enclose the parotid gland and then attaches to the lower border of mandible, proceeds further enclosing the submandibular gland and terminates by attaching to the spine and acromion of scapula, upper border of clavicle and suprasternal notch.

Pretracheal Fascia

Horizontal: Arises from beneath the SCM, forms the anterior wall of the carotid sheath, splits to enclose the thyroid gland and meets similar fascia of the opposite side in the midline. Ligament of Berry is derived from the fascia (this ligament extends from the medial surface of the lobes of the thyroid to the cricoid cartilage).

Vertical: Attached to hyoid bone in the midline and oblique line of the thyroid cartilage, encloses the thyroid gland and enters thorax and joins the apex of the pericardium.

Prevertebral Fascia

Horizontal: Arising from beneath the SCM, forms posterior wall of the carotid sheath, covers the cervical vertebra and muscles and meets the similar fascia of opposite side in the midline.

Vertical: Base of the skull above to the anterior longitudinal ligament of the upper 3 thoracic vertebra.

Instruments

1. *Artery forceps (Hemostat)*—also called Spenser Wells artery forceps. It has a rachet and 2 blades with uniform serrations used to control bleeding, not only from arteries but from veins and capillaries.
2. *Mosquito forceps*—smaller version of artery forceps used in repair of harelip, cleft palate or other plastic surgery operations.
3. *Allis tissue holding forceps*—used to hold tough structures like fascia, aponeurosis, etc. Used to hold the duodenum for duodenal closure during gastrectomy but with caution as it causes trauma.
4. *Sinus forceps*—artery like forceps with no ratchet in Hilton's method of drainage of abscess, once the incision is made the forceps is thrust into cavity and by opening the blades the loculi are broken.
5. *Babcock's forceps*—it does not have any teeth and has a ratchet and triangular expansion with fenestrations at the operating end used to hold intestines during anastomosis and resection.
6. *Dissecting scissors*—also called Mayo's scissors or tissue scissors. Does not have ratchet and operating end is sharp used to dissect tissue planes during operations and to cut and divide important structures.
7. *Dissecting forceps*—it is a toothed forceps used to pick individual layers such as serosa, seromuscular layers and mucosa during anastomosis.
8. *Needle holder*—used to hold the curved needles which are used to suture the parts.
9. *Deavor's liver retractor*—used to retract liver during vagotomy, cholecystectomy or gastrectomy also to retract the kidney upwards during lumbar sympathectomy.
10. *Humby's knife (skin grafting knife)*—used to take skin graft.
11. *Proctoscope*—used to visualize the rectum and anal canal. In painful conditions like fissure in ano proctoscopy is contraindicated used to diagnose hemorrhoids, Ca rectum or rectal ulcers. Hemorrhoids can be injected and pelvic abscess can be drained into the rectum with the help of a proctoscope.
12. *Right angled forceps (Lahey's forceps)*—useful in ligating the major vascular pedicles, i.e. (superior thyroid pedicle in thyroidectomy, cystic artery in cholecystectomy, lumbar veins in lumbar sympathectomy).
13. *Tracheal dilator*—its peculiarity is that when the handle is opened, the operating end is closed and when the handle is closed the operating end is open used in postoperative period when the tube has to be changed due to blockage.
14. *Metal tracheostomy tube*—two tubes—inner long and outer short tube; has no cuff. Used as permanent tracheostomy tubes.
15. *Cuffed tracheostomy tube*—made of polyvinyl chloride cuff prevents leakage of air and prevents acid aspiration syndrome (Mendelson's syndrome).
16. *Foley's self retaining urinary catheter*—latex with silicon coating. There is a bulb and before inflating make sure that the catheter is in the urinary bladder and not in urethra. Used to drain peritoneal fluid as in biliary peritonitis. Inflated bulb compresses the prostatic bed and controls the bleeding after prostatectomy.
17. *Ryle's tube (nasogastric tube)*—there is a lead shot at the end of the tube its position is confirmed by pushing 5–10 mL of air and auscultating in the epigastrium or by aspirating the gastric juice. Life saving use is in acute gastric dilatation, used to aspirate in intestinal obstruction or pyloric stenosis, used in the diagnosis of gastrointestinal hemorrhage, used to feed coma or tetanus patients.
18. *Kehr's T tube*—in cholecystectomy whenever the bile tube is incised, it is sutured after inserting the T tube, presence of T tube may prevent peritonitis due to biliary leakage in cases of residual stones blocking the lower end of CBD. T tube cholangiography done after 7–10 days and T tube is removed after the following criteria are fulfilled:
    a. The dye flows freely into the duodenum
    b. No filling defects in CBD
    c. After clamping the tube for 24 hours there is no abdominal pain or fever
    d. Patient passing normal colored stools.

TRIADS

1. *Beck's triad*—in cardiac tamponade—muffled heart sounds, distended neck veins, hypotension
2. *Borchardt's triad*—in gastric volvulus—acute epigastric pain, violent vomiting, inability to pass Ryle's tube
3. *Charcot's triad*—in ascending cholangitis—intermittent fever, pain, jaundice
4. *Cushing's triad*—in raised intracranial pressure—increased BP, bradycardia, decreased respiratory rate
5. *Triad of congenital diaphragmatic hernia*—respiratory distress, apparent, dextrocardia, scaphoid abdomen
6. *Dieulafoy's triad*—in appendicitis—hypersensitiveness of skin, reflex muscular contraction, McBurney's tenderness
7. *Galezia triad*—Dupuytren's contracture, retroperitoneal fibrosis, Peyronie's disease of penis
8. *Mackler's triad*—in Boerhaave's syndrome—vomiting, chest pain, subcutaneous emphysema
9. *Murphy's triad*—in acute appendicitis—RIF pain, vomiting, rise in temperature
10. *Triad of portal hypertension*—Splenomegaly, esophageal varices, ascites
11. *Pancoast's triad*—in pancoast tumor—excruciating pain in the arm, Horner's syndrome, erosion of ribs
12. *Saint's triad*—diverticulosis of colon, gallstones, hiatus hernia
13. *Triad of renal cell carcinoma*—anemia, hematuria, mass in loin
14. *Tillaux's triad*—in mesenteric cyst—soft fluctuant swelling in umbilical region, freely mobile in direction perpendicular to mesentery, zone of resonance all around
15. *Virchow's triad*—decreased blood flow, change in vessel wall, increased blood coagulability.

Signs in Surgery

1. *Ballances' sign*—in splenic injury dullness on the left side will no shift
2. *Berry's sign*—absence of carotid artery pulsation in thyroid malignancy
3. *Blumberg sign*—rebound tenderness in peritonitis due to inflamed organ behind it
4. *Boston's sign(Von Graefe's sign)*—lid lag in thyrotoxicosis
5. *Branham sign*—elicited in A-V fistula
6. *Chvostek's sign*—tapping over facial nerve in front of ear lobe causes muscular twitching on that side
7. *Cobra head sign (Adder head appearance)*—radiological sign in ureterocele
8. *Cullen's sign*—discoloration of the umbilicus and surrounding skin in hemoperitoneum
9. *Crow foot sign (Mercedes-Benz sign/Seagull's sign)*—radiological sign in cholelithiasis
10. *Courvoisier's law*—in a patient with obstructive jaundice, if gallbladder is palpable it is not due to gallstones
11. *Cowen's sign*—in response to light on one eye there is jerky constriction of contralateral pupil in Grave's disease
12. *Claw's sign*—radiological (barium) diagnostic of intussusception
13. *Dalrymple's sign*—retraction of upper eyelid and palpebral opening is so wide to see upper sclera in Grave's ophthalmopathy
14. *Double bubble sign*—radiological sign in duodenal obstruction
15. *Enroth's sign*—fullness of eyelids in Grave's orbitopathy
16. *Flare's sign*—precursor of varicose ulcer is a splay of fine venules courses from the medial malleolus and spreads out to be lost beneath the thick skin of heel.
17. *Grey Turner's sign*—skin discoloration in the left flank in acute hemorrhagic pancreatitis
18. *Hamilton Bailey's sign*—a sausage shaped mass with concavity towards the umbilicus which is felt to harden as a wave of peristalsis commences and seen in intussusception
19. Harvey's sign
20. Hamman's sign
21. Joffroy's sign
22. Kocher's sign
23. Kanavel's sign
24. Kehr's sign
25. McBurney's sign
26. Murphy's sign
27. Möbius sign
28. Omega sign
29. Pemberton's sign
30. Pointing sign
31. Rat tail sign
32. Rovsing's sign
33. Setting sun sign
34. Stellwag's sign
35. Trail's sign
36. Tinel's sign
37. Tanyol's sign
38. Troisier's sign
39. Trousseau sign
40. von Graefe's sign
41. Vermooten's sign
42. Wimberger's sign.

3 CHAPTER Orthopedics

STAGES AND PHASES OF FRACTURE HEALING

Stages of Fracture Healing (Frost, 1989)

1. Stage of hematoma
2. Stage of granulation tissue
3. Stage of callus
4. Stage of remodeling (formerly called consolidation)
5. Stage of modeling (formerly called remodeling).

Phases of Fracture Healing

1. *Reactive phase*
   a. Fracture and inflammatory phase
   b. Granulation tissue formation
2. *Reparative phase*
   a. Callus formation
   b. Lamellar bone deposition
3. *Remodeling phase*: Remodeling to original bone contour.

Complications of Fracture

1. Hypovolemic shock
2. Fat embolism syndrome
3. Infection—osteomyelitis
4. Delayed and nonunion
5. Shortening
6. Stiffness of joints
7. Myositis ossificans
8. Injury to major blood vessels, muscles, tendons and joints
9. Adult respiratory distress syndrome
10. Crush syndrome
11. Compartment syndrome
12. Malunion
13. Avascular necrosis
14. Sudeck's dystrophy.

Common Nerves Injured in Fractures

Injury	Nerve
Shoulder dislocation	Axillary
Supracondylar fracture of humerus	Radial or median
Monteggia fracture dislocation	Posterior interosseous
Knee dislocation	Peroneal
Humeral shaft fracture	Radial
Elbow medial condyle	Ulnar
Hip dislocation	Sciatic

Bone Remodeling is Affected by

1. *Mechanical factors (Wolff's law)*: Removal of external stresses lead to bone loss and vice versa.
2. *Piezoelectric changes*: Compression side is electronegative stimulating osteoblast and tension side is electropositive stimulating osteoclast.
3. *Hueter-Volkmann law of epiphyseal pressures*: Increase in pressure across the epiphysis will decrease the growth and decrease in pressure across epiphysis will increase the growth.

Compartment Syndrome

Common in the deep flexion compartment of forearm—common muscles involved are flexor digitorum profundus (FDP) and flexor digitorum longus (FDL). Muscle is the most susceptible tissue to rise in intracompartmental pressure where as nerves can withstand ischemia longer.

Causes

1. Ischemia due to injury to main vessel.
2. Edema inside osteofascial space producing increased space inside the compartment.

Indications for Fasciotomy

1. When intracompartmental pressure > 30 mm Hg.
2. IC pressure >20 mm Hg when patient is unconscious or > 8 hours after injury.

Eaton test: Stretching of fingers by extension produce increasing pain.
Chronic (c/c) compartment syndrome: Anterior compartment of legs in athletes.
Volkman's ischemic contracture: Complications of untreated compartment syndrome.

Nonunion

The process of fracture healing comes to a stand before its completion (not before six months).

Etiology

1. Soft tissue interposition between fragments
2. Segmental fractures with impaired blood supply to middle fragment
3. Comminuted fracture
4. Open fracture
5. Infected fractures
6. Pathological fractures
7. Inadequate immobilization
8. Insecure fixation and premature weightbearing.

Classification

1. Hypervascular nonunion
   a. Elephant foot type
   b. Horse hoof type
   c. Oligotrophic type.
2. Avascular nonunion
   a. Comminuted
   b. Gap atrophic
   c. Torsion wedge.

Radiological Features

1. Fracture line is visible
2. No bridging callus
3. Fracture ends are rounded, smooth and sclerotic
4. Medullary cavity may be obliterated.

Clinical Features

1. Abnormal movement
2. Tenderness at fracture site
3. Increasing deformity.

Treatment

1. Bone grafting with or without internal fixation
2. Excision of fragments without loss of function
3. Ilizarov's external fixation method.

Malunion

The fracture has anatomically malunited with angulation, rotation, or over riding of the fragments.

Etiology

1. Improper treatment
2. Unchecked muscle pull
3. Excessive communication.

Features

1. Deformity
2. Shortening of limb
3. Limitation of movements.

Treatment

1. Osteoclasis (refracturing the bone)
2. Corrective osteotomy
3. Redoing fracture surgically (internal fixation with suitable implants)
4. Excision of protruding bone.

Bone Grafting

It is the procedure of transplanting bone from a donor area to a recipient area.

Indications

1. In the treatment of nonunion of fractures
2. Arthrodesis of joints—to achieve fusion between joint surfaces
3. For filling cavities in bone.

Types

1. Autograft—the same person
2. Allograft—a different person
3. Xenograft—a different species.

Ilizarov's Technique—Uses

1. Nonunion
2. Deformity correction
3. Arthrodesis
4. Limb lengthening
5. Osteomyelitis
6. Nonhealing ulcers, e.g. thromboangiitis obliterans (TAO).

Order of Reimplantation (BEFAN-YS)

1. Bone
2. Extensor tendon
3. Flexor tendon
4. Arteries
5. Nerves
6. Vein
7. Skin.

Shoulder Dislocation

Anterior Dislocation

1. *Most common*: Anterior
2. *Types*: Subcoracoid, subglenoid, subclavicular, intrathoracic
3. *Causes*: Shallowness of the glenoid socket, extraordinary range of movement, ligamentous laxity or glenoid dysplasia, vulnerability during stressful activities

4. *Clinical tests*: Hamilton ruler test, Callaway test, Dugas test, Bryant's test (anterior axillary fold at a lower level)
5. *Methods of reduction*: Hippocrates, Stimsons, Kocher's.

Posterior Dislocation

1. *Causes*: Electric shock, convulsions
2. *Types*: Subacromial, subglenoid, subspinous
3. Adduction internal rotation deformity, medial rotated head looks like an electric bulb in X-ray.

Recurrent Dislocation

1. Capsular pouch
2. *Bankart's lesion*: Avulsion of anterior rim of glenoid with labrum
3. *Hill-Sachs lesion*: Indentation fracture over the posterolateral aspect of the humeral head—anteroposterior (AP) in internal rotation
4. *Dead arm syndrome*: Patient will be reluctant to use abduction + ER position for fear of dislocation.

Treatment

1. Bankart's repair
2. Putti-Platt—subcapsularis advancement and capsular coverage
3. Bristo—coracoid transfer to anterior glenoid.

Inferior Dislocation — Luxatio Erecta

Hyperabduction force with humerus as lever and acromion as fulcrum, humeral head is lifted into subglenoid position. There will be severe soft tissue injury and neurovascular damage. It is rare.

Supracondylar Fracture of Humerus

1. Most common fracture in children around the elbow
2. Types—Extension type 95%; Flexion type
3. Three bony point relation is maintained
4. Gartland classification—type 1 undisplaced, type 2 displaced—posterior cortex intact, type 3 displaced—no contact
5. Causes—bony architecture is weak in this area, bone is remodeling, less cylindrical, metaphysic is just distal to 2 fossae-coronoid and radial and cortex is thin
6. Treatment—undisplaced-immobilize in plaster of Paris (POP); displaced- closed manual reduction (CMR) + Dunlop traction, CMR + percutaneous pinning, ORIF with K wire.

Salter Harris Epiphyseal Injuries

1. Type 1 Salter Harris epiphyseal injury the fracture is through the physeal plate and causes a gap in the epiphyseal plate
2. Type 2 is a triangular fragment of metaphyseal bone seen called Thurston-Holland sign commonly seen in distal radius fracture
3. Type 3 and 4 epiphyseal injury causes joint incongruity
4. Type 3 is through physis and epiphysis
5. Type 4 is metaphysis, physis and epiphysis classically in the lateral condyle fracture of humerus
6. Type 5 injury plate is crushed and the reserve zone is damaged and so growth disturbance
7. Rang in 1996 added type 6 injury of perichondrial ring which carries significant risk of growth disturbance.

Monteggia Fracture

1. Fracture upper-third of the ulna with dislocation of the radial head
2. Treacherous lesion—dislocation often missed
3. Anterior dislocation of radial head is the most common
4. Posterior interosseous nerve palsy
5. Needs surgery
6. In children ulna may look normal.

Colles' Fracture

Transverse fracture at cortical calcaneus junction of the distal end of radius. It may be associated with following injuries:

1. Fracture of styloid process of ulna
2. Rupture of ulnar collateral ligament
3. Rupture of triangular cartilage of ulna
4. Radio-ulnar subluxation.

Clinical Features

1. Pain, swelling and irregularity near the wrist
2. Dinner fork deformity of wrist and hand
3. Limitation of palmar flexion.

X-ray Shows

1. Dorsal displacement and tilt
2. Lateral displacement and tilt
3. Impaction.

Treatment

Closed manipulative reduction under anesthesia and immobilized by below elbow plaster slab with forearm pronated, wrist in slight palmar flexion and ulnar deviation.

Complications

1. Malunion
2. Stiffness of fingers and wrist
3. Sudeck's atrophy.

Galeazzi's Fracture (Fracture Dislocation)

1. Fracture of lower-third of radius with dislocation or subluxation of distal radioulnar joint
2. Radius fracture angulated medially and anteriorly
3. Dorsal dislocation of ulna
4. Confirmed by X-ray
5. *Treatment*: Closed manipulative reduction under anesthesia and plaster, with forearm in supination
6. *Complications*: Malunion, deformity and limitation of supination and pronation.

Scaphoid Fracture

1. Most common carpal bone fracture
2. Most common carpal injury to be missed
3. *Location*: Waist—65%, proximal pole—25%, distal 1/3—10%
4. Radiographic evidence of fracture will appear only in 2 weeks unless displaced
5. A bone scan has 98% specificity and 100% sensitivity to diagnose A/C scaphoid fracture
6. Complication—nonunion, avascular necrosis, secondary osteoarthritis of wrist
7. Even though waist fracture are more common, proximal pole fracture results in AVN and nonunion.

Other Upper Limb Fracture

1. *Smith fracture*: Reverse of Colles'; complication—garden spade deformity
2. *Barton's fracture*: Intra-articular fracture of dorsal margin of the distal radius
3. *Chauffeur fracture*: Lorrie or Hutchinson's fracture: intra-articular fracture at the base of the radial styloid
4. *Bennett's fracture*: Fracture at base of the first metacarpal bone with subluxation or dislocation of carpometacarpal joint
5. *Game Keeper's thumb*: Ulnar collateral ligament injury
6. *Mallet finger*: EDC avulsion from base of P3
7. *Rugger Jersey finger*: Avulsion of FDP.

Tenosynovitis

Inflammation of thin synovial lining of tendon sheath.

Types

1. *Irritative synovitis*: Pain and swelling seen in the tendon of hand. Treatment by rest, analgesics, and ultrasonic therapy. Local hydrocortisone infiltration in severe cases.
2. *Infective synovitis*: Infection of synovial lining of tendon by pyogenic (flexor tendon of hand) or tubercular bacteria (sheath of flexor tendons of forearm at the level of wrist)
   Treatment: Analgesics—anti-inflammatory drugs and antibiotics.

Dislocation of Hip

1. *Types*: Posterior (most common)/dashboard injury, anterior, central
2. *Complications*: Sciatic nerve injury—10-20%; vascular injury—superior gluteal artery; fracture shaft of femur; AVN—40%; secondary OA; myositis
3. *Reduction methods*: Stimson's, Allis, Bigelow's and classical Watson-Jones method
4. *Attitudes and deformities*: Posterior dislocation (flexion, adduction, internal rotation); anterior dislocation (flexion, abduction, external rotation).

Fracture Neck of Femur

1. Types—intracapsular fracture and extracapsular fracture
2. Classification—Garden; Boyd; Delbets classification (children)
3. Clinical Features—complete external rotation of lower limb
4. Most common complication of fracture neck of femur (NOF) are nonunion and avascular necrosis (AVN).

Abduction and External Rotation Deformity

1. Synovitis hip
2. Anterior dislocation
3. Chondrolysis.

Adduction and Internal Rotation

1. Tuberculous arthritis
2. Congenital dislocation of hip (CDH)
3. Posterior dislocation
4. Protrusion acetabuli- rheumatoid arthritis (RA).

Adduction and External Rotation

1. Perthe's
2. Slipped capital femoral epiphysis (SCFE)
3. Irregular dislocation—rupture of ileofemoral ligament.

Spinal and Lower Limb Fractures

1. *Jefferson's fracture*: Burst fracture of atlas due to axial loading on the head
2. *Hangman's fracture*: Traumatic spondylolisthesis of C2 vertebrae
3. *Clay Shoveller's fracture*: C7 spinous process fracture
4. *Pott's fracture*: Bimalleolar fracture
5. *Cotton's fracture*: Trimalleolar fracture
6. *Dupuytren's fracture*: Per injury complete diastasis of tibiofibular syndesmosis, medial malleolus fracture, fracture fibula
7. *Maisonneuve fracture*: Per injury with partial diastasis, medial malleolar # or medial ligament injury, proximal fibular fracture
8. *Whiplash injury*: Hyperextension injury
9. *Footballer's ankle*: Torn anterior capsule of ankle joint

10. *Le Fort-Wagstaffe fracture*: Avulsion fracture from anterior cortex of lateral malleolus due to avulsion of anterior tibiofibular ligament
11. *Tillaux fracture*: Avulsion from the anterolateral aspect of lower tibia due to anterior tibiofibular ligament. SH type 3
12. *Triplane fracture*: Due to external rotation violence. Combination of SH 2 and 3 injury of the lower tibia
13. *Lis Franc's fracture*: Tarsometatarsal dislocation with fracture base of 2nd metatarsal
14. *Jones fracture*: Fracture base of 5th metatarsal.

Seddons Classification

1. Neuropraxia
2. Axonotemesis
3. Neurotemesis.

Pelvic Injuries—Tile's Classification

1. *Type a*: Stable
2. *Type b*: Rot
3. *Type c*: Rotationally and vertically unstable.

Sunderland's Classification

1. Conduction in the axon
2. Continuity of axon
3. Endoneurial tube and its contents
4. The funiculus and its contents
5. Entire nerve trunk
6. Sixth grade McKinnon and Dellon in 1988 is neuroma in continuity.

Typical Deformities

Nerve	Deformity
Radial nerve	Wrist drop
Median nerve	Pointing index
Lateral popliteal nerve	Foot drop
Brachial plexus	Policeman tip hand
Ulnar nerve	Claw hand
Median nerve	Ape thumb
Long thoracic nerve	Winging of scapula
Posterior interosseous nerve	Finger drop
Ulnar nerve	Benediction hand

Brachial Plexus Injuries—Classification

1. Open injuries of brachial plexus
2. Closed injuries of brachial plexus—supraclavicular (supraganglionic and infraganglionic); infraclavicular and postanesthetic palsy
3. Radiation injury to brachial plexus
4. Obstetric palsy.

Frozen Shoulder

1. Etiology unknown
2. Sudden onset, sometimes following trauma—very painful
3. Usually in middle aged women
4. Loss of external rotation is diagnostic
5. Passes through painful, stiff then resolving phases
6. Usually recovers spontaneously in 1–3 years
7. Calcific tendonitis is a differential diagnosis.

Tennis Elbow

1. Usually follows a period of overactivity
2. Tenderness is distal and anterior to lateral epicondyle
3. Forced palmar flexion and pronation against resistance reproduces the pain
4. Local injection may help
5. Surgery gives good results in most cases.

Congenital Talipes Equinovarus—CTEV (Clubfoot)

Characterized by foot plantar flexed at ankle, inverted at subtalar joint and adducted at forefoot.

Pathological Anatomy (Medial Talonavicular Dislocation)

1. Medially dislocated navicular bone and rotated in it is longitudinal axis
2. Head of talus looks downwards, laterally and plantar-flexed
3. Contracted spring ligament
4. Inverted calcaneum
5. Soft tissue on posterior aspect of ankle and medial aspect of foot are contracted
6. Capsules of subtaloid, talonavicular, naviculocuneiform joints are contracted.

Clinical Features

1. Equinus deformity at ankle
2. Varus deformity at subtaloid joint
3. Adduction deformity at tarsometatarsal joints
4. Small foot with poorly developed heel
5. Prominent lateral malleolus
6. Wasting of calf.

Treatment

Principle
1. Treatment should begin in the first few weeks of life
2. *Components of deformity corrected in the following sequence*:
   a. Forefoot adduction
   b. Inversion Equinus.
3. Minimum force in correction gives a better functioning foot.

Conservative
1. *In the first three weeks*: Mother is taught to mold the infant foot twice a day
2. *Three weeks to 3 months*: The surgeon manipulates the foot once in two weeks and position maintained by plaster of Paris cast
3. Maintenance of correction
   a. By below knee splints
   b. Special clubfoot boots.

Surgical
1. Soft tissue operations
   a. Posteromedial soft tissue release
   b. Complete subtaloid release.
2. *Bone operations*: Lateral wedge resection and calcaneocuboid fusion.

External fixatives
Ilizarov external fixation or Joshi apparatus.

Congenital Dysplasia of Hip

1. One in 1000 live birth, left hip more commonly involved
2. First born female baby, breech presentation—oligohydramnios
3. Asymmetrical thigh or gluteal fold (u/l); b/l widening of perineum
4. Waddling gait, lordosis, positive telescopy, vascular sign of narath +ve
5. Limited abduction, Galeazzi's sign +ve (Allis)
6. Trendelenburg test +ve, ortolani and Barlow test +ve in neonates
7. *X-ray*: Perkins line, shenton line broken, Hilgenreiner's line and Von Rosen sign +ve
8. *Splints*: Pavlik Harness, Von Rosen splint, Barlow splint, Frejka pillow, Craig and Aberdeen splint, Dennis Brown abduction splint
9. *Causes*: Genetically determined joint laxity, hormonal joint laxity, breech presentation
10. *Pathology*: Femoral head nucleus appear late, acetabulum late and sloping, fibrocartilaginous labrum/limbus folded to cavity, capsule elongated, femoral neck anteverted.

Genu Valgum (Knock Knee)

1. Physiological (3–6 years)
2. Increased intermalleolar distance (8 cm)
3. Increased incidence of dislocation of patella
4. *Bilateral (B/L) causes*: Rickets, tumors, trauma, infections
5. *Unilateral (U/L) cause*: Bone dysplasia-Morquio
6. *Treatment*: Conservative (mermaid splint); Osteotomy (Mc Evans, Physeal stapling).

Genu Varum (Bow Legs)

1. Physiological 0–1.5 years
2. Increased intercondylar distance (6 cm)
3. Seen in achondroplasia, Blount's disease, osteogenesis imperfect.

Perthe's Disease (Coxa Plana, Pseudocoxalgia)

1. Osteochondritis of epiphysis of upper end of femur
2. Commonly in boys in the age group of 5–10 years.

Etiology

Mild trauma, metabolic disturbances or inflammation.

Pathology

Avascular necrosis of head of femur.

Clinical Features

1. Pain in hip radiating to knee
2. Limitation of movements with muscle spasm

Radiological Feature

Collapse and sclerosis of epiphysis of femoral head.

Treatment

1. Prevention of deformity of femoral head and promotion of containment of head inside acetabulum
2. Bed rest with skin traction

3. Walk with a weight relieving caliper
4. Surgical—femoral osteotomy, containment osteotomy.

Complications

1. Incongruity between femoral head and acetabulum
2. Secondary osteoarthrosis of hip joint

   Prognosis is poor when:

   a. Age more than 9 at the time of diagnosis
   b. More than half of epiphysis is avascular
   c. Loss of containment of head inside acetabulum
   d. Seen in girls.

Common Osteochondritis

1. *Perthes' disease*: Femoral head
2. *Panner's disease*: Capitulam
3. *Kienbock's disease*: Lunate bone
4. *Osgood-Schlatter disease*: Tibial tubercle
5. *Sever's disease*: Calcaneal tuberosity
6. *Kohler's disease*: Navicular bone
7. *Freiberg's disease*: Metatarsal head
8. *Scheuermann's disease*: Ring epiphysis of vertebrae
9. *Calve's disease*: Central bony nucleus of vertebral body.

Osteomyelitis

It is the inflammation of bone and bone marrow caused by infective organisms.

Osteomyelitis—Causes

1. Most common cause of bone and joint infection is from hematogenous
2. Most common cause of hematogenous osteomyelitis is *Staphylococcus aureus*
3. Most common organism causing osteomyelitis in children under 3 years is hemophilus
4. Organism causing osteomyelitis in sickle cell anemia is *Salmonella*.

Acute Osteomyelitis

1. Common site—distal end of femur and proximal end of tibia
2. Most common causative organism—*Staphylococcus aureus.*

Clinical Features

Acute pain and swelling at the end of bone.

On examination

1. Diffuse swelling, warmth, and tender over affected area
2. Unable to move the limb—pseudoparalysis
3. A palpable fluctuant abscess may present.

Investigation

1. Increased WBC count with high polymorphs
2. Raised ESR
3. Blood culture
4. X-ray—patchy areas of destruction and slight periosteal reaction at metaphysis.

Differential Diagnosis

1. Acute poliomyelitis
2. Acute septic arthritis
3. Acute rheumatic arthritis.

Treatment

1. Affected part must be rested in a splint
2. Parenteral broad spectrum antibiotics
3. Surgical drainage of abscess under general anesthesia
4. Pus sent for smear, culture and sensitivity to antibiotics
5. Antibiotics treatment for 4–6 weeks
6. Limb immobilized in plaster without weightbearing.

Complications

1. Septicemia
2. Pyemia
3. Acute pyogenic arthritis
4. Growth plate disturbances—shortening, lengthening or deformity of limb
5. Pathological fracture
6. Chronic osteomyelitis.

Chronic Osteomyelitis

Persisting pyogenic infection of bone of more than 6 weeks.

Reasons

1. Delayed and inadequate treatment
2. Type and virulence of organism
3. Reduced host resistance.

Clinical Features

1. Discharge of pus and small sequestra from sinuses
2. Pain, swelling, fever
3. Thickened irregular bone
4. Adjacent joint may be stiff.

Radiological Findings

1. Sclerosis of cortical bone
2. Bone cavity
3. Sequestrum.

General Management

Identify causative organism by culture from swab of the pus and give appropriate antibiotics.

Surgical Management

1. Sequestrectomy—removal of sequestrum
2. Saucerization—drainage by deroofing of cavity
3. Curettage
4. Excision of infected bone
5. Amputation.

The Cierny and Mader Classification of Chronic Osteomyelitis—Treatment Guidelines

1. Stage 1—medullary
   a. Cancellous bone only involved
   b. Remove involved bone
   c. Pack with antibiotic loaded implant
   d. Graft at 6–8 weeks
   e. No stabilization required.
2. Stage 2—superficial
   a. Cortical bone only involved
   b. Excise involved cortex
   c. Provide soft tissue cover
   d. Stabilize if more than one-third of the cortex involved.
3. Stage 3—localized
   a. Cortical and cancellous bone involved
   b. Radical excision
   c. Staged reconstruction using graft
   d. Stabilization often needed.

4. Stage 4—diffuse
   a. Most of bone and soft tissues involved in a segment
   b. Radical excision required, leaves segmental defect
   c. Stabilization with external fixator required.

Complications

1. Pathological fracture
2. Deformity
3. Shortening
4. Lengthening
5. Bone defects
6. Muscle fibrosis—joint stiffness.

TB Spine

1. Sites—paradiscal (most common); central (concertina collapse); anterior (serrated margin); posterior (spinal tumor syndrome)
2. Pathognomic radiological feature is disk narrowing
3. First symptom in tuberculous cord compression is spasticity
4. Most common site in spine is dorsolumbar
5. MC route of infection is hematogenous
6. MC variety is paradiscal
7. MC presenting symptom is back pain.

Bony Ankylosis

1. Pyogenic arthritis
2. Ankylosing spondylitis
3. Late stage of RA
4. TB with secondary infection.

Fibrous Ankylosis

1. TB
2. Rheumatoid arthritis (RA)
3. Osteoarthritis
4. Idiopathic chondrolysis.

Sequestrum

1. Sandy
2. Flaky
3. Feathery
4. Kissing
5. Ring
6. Tubular.

CLASSIFICATION OF TUMORS OF BONE

1. *Bone forming tumors*:
   a. Benign—osteoid osteoma, osteoma, osteoblastoma
   b. Intermediate—aggressive osteoblastoma
   c. Malignant—osteosarcoma
2. *Cartilage forming tumors*:
   a. Benign—osteochondroma, chondroma, chondroblastoma, chondromyxoid fibroma
   b. Malignant—chondrosarcoma
3. *Giant cell tumor*: Osteoclastoma
4. *Marrow tumors*: Malignant—Ewing's sarcoma, plasma cell tumor, multiple myeloma, lymphoma
5. *Vascular tumors*:
   a. Benign—hemangioma, glomangioma
   b. Malignant—angiosarcoma
6. Others
   a. Benign—neurilemmoma, neurofibroma
   b. Malignant—malignant fibrous histiocytoma liposarcoma, adamantinoma, undifferentiated sarcoma.

Age Specific and Site Specific Tumors/Lesions

1. *Epiphysis*: Chondroblastoma, giant cell tumor, degenerative cyst in osteoarthritis (OA)
2. *Metaphysis*: Osteochondroma, enchondroma, osteogenic sarcoma, unicameral bone cyst, aneurysmal bone cyst (ABC)
3. *Diaphysis*: Ewing's sarcoma, adamantinoma, fibrous dysplasia, osteoid osteoma, lymphoma
4. *0–5 years*: Osteomyelitis, metastatic neuroblastoma, leukemia, eosinophilic granuloma
5. *6–20 years*: Unicameral bone cyst (UBC), ABC, Ewing's, osteomyelitis, osteogenic sarcoma, chondroblastoma, chondromyxoid fibroma, fibrous dysplasia and osteoid osteoma
6. *20–40 years*: Giant cell tumor (GCT)
7. *> 40 years*: Metastasis, multiple myeloma, chondrosarcoma.

Osteosarcoma

1. Second most common primary malignant bone tumor
2. Commonly affects metaphysic
3. Five to twenty years boys commonly affected
4. Commonly seen around knee
5. Other sites—proximal femur, proximal humerus
6. *Classification*: Primary osteosarcoma (intramedullary, juxtacortical, parosteal, periosteal); secondary osteosarcoma (postradiation, Paget's, multiple enchondromatosis, multiple osteochondromatosis, irradiation, fibrous dysplasia) and based on histomorphology (osteoblastic, chondroid, fibroblastic, telangiectatic)
7. Most common type is primary medullary
8. Most common presenting feature is pain
9. Most common site of metastasis is lung with cannon ball mets
10. Most common site is distal end of femur—50%, proximal tibia—20%,proximal humerus—10%
11. X-ray-sclerotic and lytic lesions, sunburst appearance, Codman's triangle, expansile lytic lesion—telangiectatic osteosarcoma.

Ewing's Sarcoma

1. Common in late childhood and early adult life
2. Diaphysis and metadiaphysis commonly affected in long bone, scapula and ilium
3. Small round cell neoplasm
4. Differential diagnosis—osteomyelitis, onion peel appearance in X-ray
5. Most common malignant tumor with multicentricity
6. Most common site is femur (22%)
7. Most common presenting symptom is painful hot swelling
8. Most common malignant tumor of flat bones
9. Tumor melts by radiotherapy like snow and chemosensitive
10. Radiotherapy + chemotherapy+ surgery- Marcove-Rosen regime
11. Periosteal response in exuberant and may consist of multiple layers of new bone which gives para-amino salicylic acid positive.

Osteoclastoma (Giant Cell Tumor)

1. Eccentric expansile epiphyseal lytic lesion in skeletally mature patients
2. Egg shell crackling and no periosteal reaction
3. X-ray—soap bubble appearance
4. Differential diagnosis—chondroblastoma
5. Treatment
   a. Curettage alone
   b. Curettage and bone graft or bone cement or cryosurgery

c. Resection and reconstruction with arthrodesis or prosthesis
d. Resection and replacement with allograft or autograft
e. Excision of bone if expendable
f. Therapeutic embolization
g. Radiotherapy if inaccessible areas (spine)
h. Chemotherapy if metastasis
i. Amputation as the last option.

Multiple Myeloma

1. Multiple punched out lytic lesions
2. Bone marrow examination > 30% plasma cells
3. X-ray—punched out lytic lesion with generalized osteoporosis
4. Bone scan gives cold spot in myeloma lesions
5. Anemia, raised ESR, albumin/globulin (A/G) reversal, serum Ca^{2+} elevated with normal SAP, BJP in urine
6. Serum and urine electrophoresis shows M band
7. Bone pain is the most common symptom
8. Bone lesions are lytic in nature and rarely associated with osteoblastic new bone formation
9. Extramedullary plasmacytomas are found in submucous lymphoid tissue of nasopharynx and PNS
10. Treatment of plasmacytomas is radiation therapy
11. Lytic beveled lesions are seen in skull X-rays.

Spotters

1. Cubitus varus deformity
2. Supracondylar malunion (gun stoke deformity)
3. Nonunion—3 conditions causing nonunion of humerus
4. Genu valgum
5. CTEV-management (3 procedures), define resistant, neglected CTEV
6. C/C osteomyelitis
7. Anterior dislocation of shoulder
8. Discoid meniscus, cyst of lateral meniscus.

X-rays

1. X-ray pelvis—dislocation of pubic bone—important complications
2. X-ray upper limb—subperiosteal bone formation differential diagnosis (D/D)
3. Intertrochanteric fracture management
4. Supracondylar fracture management
5. Fracture neck of femur—types of fracture, blood supply, causes of nonunion, attachment of capsule
6. Spiral fracture shaft of femur—immediate complications
7. Fracture greater trochanter
8. Colles' fracture
9. Brodies abscess (radiolucent area in distal end of radius)
10. Shenton's line
11. Fracture pelvis complications
12. Tumors—osteosarcoma; osteoclastoma; Ewing's sarcoma.

Usual Tests Asked

1. *Adson's test*: For thoracic outlet syndrome
2. *Ape thumb*: For median nerve injury

3. *Barlow's test, Ortolani's test and Galeazzi's sign*: Congenital dislocation of hip
4. *Bryant's test*: Anterior dislocation of shoulder
5. *Chvostek's sign*: Tetany
6. *Claw hand and froment sign*: Ulnar nerve injury
7. *Cozen's test*: Tennis elbow
8. *Drawer test*: Anterior for anterior cruciate ligament (ACL) and posterior for posterior cruciate ligament (PCL)
9. *Foot drop*: Common peroneal nerve injury
10. *Gower's sign*: Muscular dystrophy
11. *Kanavel's sign*: Infection in ulnar bursa
12. *Lasegue's test*: Disk prolapse
13. *McMurray's test*: Meniscus injury
14. *O'donoghue triad*: Triad of MCL, ACL and medial meniscus injury
15. *Thomas test*: Hip flexion deformity
16. *Tinel's sign*: Detecting improving nerve injury
17. *Wrist drop*: Radial nerve injury
18. *Runner's knee*: Patellar tendonitis.

Instruments

1. *Periostium elevator (Farabeuf)*: To elevate the periosteum (thick fibrous covering). Periosteum is elevated in all operations as all important structures are outside the periosteum. Periosteum is not lifted in some operations such as excision of osteochondroma.
2. *Bone lever-used*: To lever out a bone from the depth of the wound; to retract the soft tissues.
3. *Bone nibbler-used*: For nibbling the bone. Some common nibblers are straight nibbler (for general use); curved nibbler (for spinal use); double action nibbler (rounger) (straight or curved).
4. *Bone cutter*: Used for cutting of bones into small pieces, e.g. for bone grafts one part of cutting end is spoon shaped and has a long lever arm.
5. *Osteotome*: Cutting a bone which is deep. Both edges are beveled (O)—osteotome. Common osteotomes are McMurray's osteotomy for fracture of neck of femur; corrective osteotomies for deformities such as genu valgum (knock knees); genu varum (bow legs).
6. *Bone chisel*: Like an osteotome only 1 surface is beveled (C)—chisel; used for removing protruding bone or leveling a bone surface, e.g. for leveling callus, removing osteochondroma.
7. *Mallet*: Used for hammering osteotome, chisel, etc.
8. *Bone curette*: Used for curetting a cavity in the bone or for removing fibrous tissue. Curettage is done for benign tumors such as enchondroma, giant cell tumor, infections such as tubercular cavity of the bone, osteomyelitis and also to scoop out the bone graft.
9. *Bone gouge*: Concave bladed chisel. Used for cutting on round bony surfaces or for making a round hole in the bone, e.g. iliac crest.
10. *Bone AWL*: Pointed thin instrument for making a hole in the bone.
11. *Bone holding forceps*: Different types: Lane's forceps—for holding femur, tibia lion toothed forceps; self-retaining -AO type of forceps.
12. *Plate holding forceps*: Hold bone together with plate; two types Arbeitsgemeinschaft für Osteosynthesefragen (AO) self-retaining forceps; Lowman's clamp.
13. *Kirschner's wire (martin)*: Thin straight steel wire of diameter 1-3 mm. Used for temporary reduction of small bones giving traction, e.g. for giving traction through olecranon for fixing fracture in children for Ilizarov's fixation system.
14. *Steinmann pin (No thread in pin)*: Stout straight steel rod of diameter 3-6 mm used for skeletal traction—common sites being upper end of tibia, supracondylar region of femur and calcaneum.
15. *Denham pin (Middle thread in pin)*: Used in osteoporotic bone.
16. *Shantz pin (Endz thread in pin)*: Used for external fixation.
17. *Bohler's stirrup*: Used for holding a Steinmann pin and applying traction.

Types of Buttress Plates

- L Plate—upper end of tibia
- Ellis Plate—lower end of tibia
- Cobra Plate—lower end of femur or tibia.

Types of Screw

- Cortical Screw
- Cancellous Screw
- Partially Threaded Screw/Lag Screw
- Locking Screw.

Types of Prosthesis

- Austin Moore's prosthesis—two holes
- Thompson prosthesis
- Bipolar prosthesis.

NAILS

1. *Kuntscher's nail (Gerhard)*: Clover leaf shaped—used for internal fixation of fracture of femoral shaft, tibia
   Complications of Kuntscher nailing:
   a. Nail getting stuck
   b. Proximal migration of the nail leading to bursitis
   c. Distal migration of the nail leading to stiffness of the knee
   d. Splintering of cortex while hammering the nail
   e. Infection
2. *Smith-Peterson's nail (SP nail)*: Used for internal fixation of fracture of femoral neck
3. *V nail*: Cross-section is V shaped. It has a bend (Herzog bend). Kuntscher's nail can be converted to V nail. Used for internal fixation of fracture of tibial shaft
4. *Radial nail*: It has a notch called talwaker
5. *Ulnar nail*: No notch.

Plates and Screws

1. *Dynamic hip screw*: Used for internal fixation of trochanteric fractures has two components—lag screw and barrel. Lag screw slides freely into the barrel so there is a controlled collapse at the fracture site
2. *Dynamic compression plate*: Thick plate with oval holes which are staggered
3. Semitubular plate—has central holes and they are circular
4. Recon plates—has hexagonal holes and is thin; used for iliac crest and acetabulam
5. *Angled blade plate*: Used in supra- and intercondylar fracture
6. *Buttress plate*: Small thin plate which can be used for fixation of small fracture
7. Cortical screw—more threads, pitch and lead are less
8. *Malleolar screw*: Self-cutting and self-tapping
9. Cancellous screw—less number of threads, pitch and lead are more
10. Austin Moore prosthesis—It has two fenestrations in the middle. Used for replacement of femoral head in case of fracture of the neck of femur in elderly persons. The prosthesis can be used only without cement. Locking screw—thread at head
11. *Thompson's prosthesis*: Without fenestrations. Indicated in old fracture of femoral neck. Used with or without cement.
12. Jess-Joshi's external stabilizing system; Joshi's fixator is a versatile fixator for stabilizing for all types of fracture of the bones of the hand with possibility of adequate soft tissue care. Uses—CTEV and CIADER (communicated intra articular fracture of distal end of radius).

4 CHAPTER Obstetrics

NORMAL PREGNANCY

First Trimester

Symptoms

1. Amenorrhea
2. Morning sickness—starts arounds 4–6 weeks
3. Hyperemesis gravidarum (Severe vomiting, weight loss, dehydration, acidosis and hypokalemia)
4. Frequency of micturition.

Signs

1. Breast : Montgomery follicles appear
2. Vagina : Bluish discoloration **(Chadwick's or Jacquemier's** sign)
   Increased vaginal pulsation (**Osiander's** sign)
3. Uterus : Changes in size shape and position
   Hegar's sign (6th or 8th week to 12th week)
4. Cervix : Softens by 6–8 weeks of pregnancy.

Second Trimester

Symptoms

Quickening—at the end of week 16.

Signs

1. Skin : Linea nigra
   : Linea albicantes (striae gravidarum)
2. Intermittent uterine contractions—Braxton Hicks sign
3. Active fetal movements
4. Fetal heart sounds—heard from 20th week.

Signs in Normal Pregnancy

1. *Placental sign*: Bleeding at the time of next period
2. *Hartman sign*: Implantation bleeding
3. *Jacquemier's sign (Chadwick's sign)*: Blue hue of the vagina
4. *Osiander's sign*: Increased pulsations through lateral fornix
5. *Goodell's sign*: Cervix becomes soft
6. *Piskacek's sign*: One-half more firm than the other half due to implantation laterally

7. *Hegar's sign*: Upper part of the body of the uterus enlarged and lower part empty
8. *Palmer's sign*: Rhythmic uterine contraction during bimanual examination.

Investigations

1. Urine pregnancy test—bioassay
2. Blood and urine routine (R/E)
3. Blood grouping and Rh typing
4. Human immunodeficiency virus (HIV), hepatitis B antigen (HbsAg), Veneral Disease Research Laboratory (VDRL)
5. USG
6. Glucose challenge test (GCT).

Immunization

Tetanus toxoid is safe and mandatory in India. Usually given at booking visit or at 16–24 weeks followed by second dose 1 month later. In women, immunized within two years, single booster dose is enough.

Drugs

Folic acid 5 mg during 1st trimester (ideally should be started preconceptionally).
Iron and calcium started from 13 weeks onwards. This is continued till three months postpartum.

Diet

Extra 300 kcal/day and 60 g protein/day.
Iron rich foods—green leafy vegetables, jaggery.

Warning Signs in Pregnancy

1. Bleeding per vaginum at any time of pregnancy
2. Headache, blurring of vision, epigastric pain and oliguria are signs of impending eclampsia
3. Severe pedal edema, edema of face and hands
4. Decreased/lost fetal movements
5. Abdominal pain
6. UTI/vulvovaginitis
7. Leaking per vaginum.

Antenatal Checkup—Low Risk

1. Every month up to 28 weeks
2. Every two weeks 28–36 weeks
3. Weekly thereafter.

Wight gain average 500 g/week.
If single scan is only being done a targeted second trimester scan is ideal.

Methods of Induction

1. Medical
   a. Oxytocin
   b. Prostaglandin E2 (Dinoprostone)—0.5 mg
   c. Prostaglandin E1 (Misoprostol)—25 microgram
   d. Mifepristone
2. Surgical—ARM (amniotomy using Kocher's forceps), stripping of membranes
3. Mechanical—Foley.

Complications of Induction

1. Hyperstimulation leading to fetal distress and rupture uterus
2. Traumatic postpartum hemorrhage (PPH)
3. Maternal and fetal infection
4. Iatrogenic prematurity
5. Dysfunctional labor and failed induction
6. Increased cesarean section (CS) rates
7. Water intoxication with oxytocin.

LABOR is the process by which the product of conception are expelled by the mother within the last few hours of pregnancy.

Stages of Labor

Onset of labor is defined as the start of painful uterine contractions accompanied by any one of the following:

1. Ruptured membranes
2. Bloody show
3. Complete cervical effacement.

First Stage (Stage of Cervical Dilatation and Effacement)

1. From the onset of true labor pain to complete dilatation of cervix
2. Primigravida—about 12 hours Prolonged labor—>18 hours
3. Multigravida—about 5-6 hours Prolonged labor—>12 hours.

Phenomena

1. Uterine contractions
2. Mucosanguineous discharge (show)
3. Dilatation of cervical canal
4. Fixation of the head at the brim of the pelvis
5. Rupture of membranes.

Second Stage (Stage of Expulsion)

1. Extends from complete dilatation of cervix to the expulsion of the fetus(es)
2. Primigravida—1-2 hours
3. Multigravida—1/2 to 1 hour.

Third Stage (Stage of Placental Delivery)

Extends from complete expulsion of fetus to the complete expulsion of placenta and membranes and firm contraction and retraction of uterus.

1. Average duration—few minutes to 15 minutes
2. *Phenomena*:
   a. Characteristic uterine contractions
   b. Separation of placenta
   c. Expulsion of placenta
   d. Control of hemorrhage
   e. Permanent contraction and retraction of uterus.

Types of Placental Seperation

1. *Central*: Schultz method
2. *Marginal*: Mathew Duncan's method.

Signs of Placental Seperation

1. Uterus becomes firm and globular
2. Increased bleeding per vaginum
3. Uterus rises in the abdomen as the seperated placenta passes down into the lower segment and vagina pushing uterus up-Schroeder's sign
4. Lenghthening of extravulval part of umbilical cord
5. On pushing uterus cephalad cord does not recede—Kustner's sign.

Active Management of Third Stage

1. Administration of uterotonic agents
2. Controlled cord traction for placental delivery includes cord clamping and cutting (Current evidence shows delayed cord clamping and cutting is beneficial to the baby: WHO)
3. Uterine massage after delivery of placenta.

Definitive indications for early cord clamping

1. Rh iso immunization
2. HIV positive mother
3. Birth asphyxia
4. Preterm/Intrauterine growth restriction (IUGR) fetus—due to risk of hypervolemia.

Fourth Stage

The hour immediately following delivery of placenta is critical and termed as fourth stage, BP, pulse monitored, watch for bleeding p/v, perineum and vagina examined for hematoma at episiotomy site.

Abnormalities of Labor

1. *Prolonged latent phase*: Nullipara > 20 hours and multiparas > 14 hours
2. *Protracted active phase*: Nullipara < 1.2 cm/hr and multipara < 1.5 cm/hr
3. *Secondary arrest of dilatation*: Cessation of dilatation for > 2 hours
4. *Prolonged deceleration phase*: Nullipara > 3 hrs and multipara > 1 hour
5. *Failure to descend*: No descent
6. *Protracted descent*: Nullipara < 1 cm/hr and multipara < 2 cm/hr
7. *Arrest of descent*: Cessation of descent for 1 hour or more
8. *Prolonged second stage*: >2 hours in primigravida > 1 hour in multigravida
9. *Precipitate labor*: Nullipara-dilation and descent > 5 cm/hr, multipara-dilation and descent >10 cm/hr.

Causes

1. Inadequate contraction, unfavorable cervix
2. Malposition/CPD/inadequate contraction.

Mechanism of Labor

Defined as positional changes in the presenting part by which the fetus adjusts itself to and passes through the parturient canal.

1. Engagement
2. Descent
3. Flexion
4. Internal rotation
5. Extension and birth of fetal head
6. Restitution
7. External rotation
8. Expulsion.

Engagement is said to occur when greatest transverse diameter of the presenting part has passed the pelvic inlet.

Crowning: Head is said to be crowned when biparietal diameter stretches the vulval outlet and does not recede in between contractions.

Moulding: Shifting or sliding of the fetal skull bones to accomodate maternal pelvis

1. Grade 1/+ : Obliteration of suture line
2. Grade 2/++ : Reducible overlap
3. Grade 3/+++ : Irreducible overlap.

Asynclitism: Sagittal suture is deflected either anteriorly (Nagele's) or posteriorly (Litzmann's).

Differences between caput succedaneum and cephalohematoma

Characteristics	Caput succedaneum	Cephalohematoma
Incidence	Very common	Less common
Location	Subcutaneous plane	Located over parietal bones, between skull and periosteum
Time of presentation	Maximum size and firmness at birth	Increasing size for 12–24 hours and then stable
Clinical time course	Softens progressively from birth and resolves within 2 or 3 days	Takes 3–6 weeks to resolve
Characteristic findings	Diffuse, crosses suture line	Does not cross the suture line, has distinct margins
Association	None	Linear fracture of skull bone in 5–25%; hyperbilirubinemia

Female Pelvis

Types of Caldwell and Moley's classification

Gynecoid	50%	Round
Anthropoid	25%	Anteroposteriorly oval
Android	20%	Triangular
Platypelloid	5%	Transversely oval

True Pelvis

Boundaries

1. Symphysis pubis
2. Pubic tubercle
3. Iliopubic eminence
4. Sacroiliac articulation
5. Pubic crest
6. Pectineal line
7. Iliopectineal line
8. Anterior border of ala of sacrum.

False Pelvis

Boundaries

Posteriorly : Lumbar vertebrae
Laterally : Iliac fossa
Anteriorly : Anterior abdominal wall.

Diameters of Pelvic Inlet

Anteroposterior Diameters

1. *Obstetric conjugate*: 10.5 cm
   a. Shortest distance from pubic symphysis to middle of sacral promontery
   b. Most important diameter
2. *Anatomic conjugate/true conjugate/conjugata vera*: 11 cm
   Middle of sacral promontery to superior surface of pubic symphysis
3. *Diagonal conjugate*: 12.5 cm
   a. Middle of sacral promontery to subpubic angle
   b. Obstetric conjugate = diagonal conjugate—1.5 cm.

Transverse Diameter—13.5 cm

Widest distance between iliopectineal lines.

Oblique Diameter—12.5 cm

1. Distance between sacroiliac joint of one side to opposite iliopectineal eminence
2. Right oblique diameter extends from right sacroiliac joint to left iliopectineal eminence.

Pelvic Joints

1. Symphysis pubis
2. Secondary fibrocartilaginous joint; no capsule and synovial cavity; articular surface covered with hyaline cartilage
3. Sacroiliac articulation
   Synovial joint; capsule and synovial cavity present; articular surface ilium and sacrum and are not alike.

Fetal Skull

Vertex—quadrangular area.

Boundaries

1. *Anteriorly*: Bregma and coronal suture
2. *Behind*: Lambda and lambdoid suture
3. *Laterally*: Line passing through parietal eminences.

Fontanelle

Anterior Fontanelle

Formed by four sutures—diamond shaped.

Boundaries

1. *Anterior*: Frontal suture
2. *Laterally*: Coronal suture
3. *Posterior*: Sagittal suture

Normally become ossified by 18 months > 24 months is abnormal.

Posterior Fontanelle

Formed by 3 suture lines—triangular shaped.

Boundaries

1. *Anterior*: Sagittal suture
2. *Either side*: Lambdoid suture.

Diameters of Skull and Presentations

Engaging Diameters

	Diameter	Presentation	Measurement
1.	Suboccipitobregmatic	Vertex presentation	9.5 cm
2.	Suboccipito frontal	Vertex presentation	10 cm
3.	Occipitofrontal	Vertex presentation	11.5 cm
4.	Mentovertical	Brow presentation	13.5 cm
5.	Submentovertical	Face presentation	11.5 cm
6.	Submentobregmatic	Face presentation	9.5 cm
7.	Bisacromial	Shoulder	12 cm
8.	Bitrochanteric	Breech	10 cm.

Transverse Diameters

1. Biparietal diameter - 9.5 cm
2. Super subparietal - 8.5 cm
3. Bitemporal diameter - 8 cm
4. Bimastoid diameter - 7.5 cm.

Definitions

1. *Fetal lie* is the relation between longitudinal axis of fetal ovoid and the longitudinal axis of uterine ovoid.
2. *Fetal presentation* is that portion of ovoid which is in relation to lower pole of uterus and which is first to engage in the pelvis when the labor starts.
3. *Fetal position* is the relation of an arbitrarily chosen position of the fetal presenting parts to the four quadrants of maternal pelvis.
4. *Induction of labor* is the artificial initiation of uterine contractions prior to their spontaneous onset beyond the period of fetal viability.
5. *ARM/amniotomy*: Rupturing membrane overlying the cervix using a Kocher's forceps.

6. *Chloasma*: Hyperpigmented patch on cheeks and face.
7. *Labor* is the process by which the product of conception are expelled by the mother after attaining viability.
8. *Normal labor*: Process by which the fetus presenting as vertex is expelled by the natural efforts of the mother when pregnancy has reached term with no complications.
9. *Onset of labor* is defined as the start of painful uterine contractions accompanied by any one of the following:
   a. Ruptured membranes b. Bloody show c. Complete cervical effacement.
10. *Preterm labor*: Spontaneous expulsion of the products of conception after viability and before 37 weeks (term).
11. *Mechanism of labor*: Defined as positional changes in the presenting part by which the fetus adjusts itself to and passes through the parturient canal.
12. *First stage of labor*: From the onset of true labor pain to complete dilatation of cervix.
13. *Second stage of labor*: Extends from complete dilatation of cervix to the expulsion of the fetus(es).
14. *Third stage of labor*: Extends from complete expulsion of fetus to the complete expulsion of placenta and membranes and firm contraction and retraction of uterus.
15. *Fourth stage of labor*: The hour immediately following delivery of placenta is critical and termed as fourth stage, BP, pulse monitored, watch for bleeding p/v, perineum and vagina examined for hematoma at episiotomy site.
16. *Engagement* is said to occur when greatest transverse diameter of the presenting part has passed the pelvic inlet.
17. *Crowning*: Head is said to be crowned when biparietal diameter stretches the vulval outlet and does not recede in between contractions.
18. *PROM*: Spontaneous rupture of membranes before onset of labor.
19. *Preterm premature rupture of membrane (PPROM)*: PROM before 37 weeks.
20. *Partogram*: Graphical record of the progress of labor, whereby cervical dilatation and descent of fetal head is plotted against time.
21. *Antepartum hemorrhage*: Bleeding from the genital tract after fetal viability and before delivery.
22. *Placenta previa*: Placenta located partly or completely in the lower uterine segment.
23. *Abruptio placenta*: Hemorrhage occurring in pregnancy due to separation of normally situated placenta.
24. *Vasa previa*: When fetal vessels in the membranes cross the region of internal os and are ahead of presenting part, the condition is called vasa previa.
25. *Abortion*: The World Health Organization defines it as expulsion or extraction of an embryo or fetus before attaining viability or weighing 500 g or less from its mother.
26. *Ectopic pregnancy*: Pregnancy where implantation occurs in a site other than the uterine cavity.
27. *IUGR*: Fetuses those have failed to attain their own genetic growth potential.
28. *Polyhydramnios*: An excess of amniotic fluid more than 2000 mL/AFI > 25 cm/SDP > 8 cm.
29. *Oligohydramnios*: Amniotic fluid is reduced to AFI < 5 cm/SDP < 2 cm.
30. *GDM*: Carbohydrate intolerance of variable severity with onset/first recognition during present pregnancy.
31. *PIH*: Hypertension arising for the first time after 20 weeks of gestation in the absence of proteinuria.
32. *Pre-eclampsia*: Pregnancy induced hypertension (PIH) in association with significant proteinuria.
33. *Eclampsia*: Seizures that cannot be attributed to any other cause in a patient with pre-eclampsia.
34. *Significant proteinuria*: In pregnancy 300 mg in 24 hours.
35. *Anemia in pregnancy*: Hb below 11g/dL (WHO). Practically in India < 10 g/dL.
36. *Contracted pelvis*: Is one in which any of the essential diameters are so reduced, as to affect the normal mechanism of labor.
37. *Episiotomy*: Surgical incision made over the perineum and vulva during delivery to increase the space available at the perineum and to prevent perineal tears.
38. *Cesarean section*: Delivery of viable fetus through an incision made in abdomen and intact uterus.

MALPRESENTATIONS

Symptoms

1. History of antepartum hemorrhage in present pregnancy
2. History suggestive of hydramnios
3. History suggestive of a pelvic lump like leiomyoma or ovarian tumor in the past.

Obstetric History

1. Any malpresentations in past (due to persistant etiological factor like contracted pelvis, pelvic mass, congenital malformations of uterus)
2. Previous vaginal deliveries—trial of labor, difficult forceps delivery, fetal malformations like neural tube defects (recurs).

Examination (General and Systemic Examination)

1. *Height*: Short stature is suggestive of pelvic contraction
2. *Pallor*: During surgical management.

Abdominal examination

1. Uterine size—in weeks of gestation
2. Fundal height in cm from top of pubic symphysis
3. Abdominal girth at the level of umbilicus
4. Liqour.

Palpation

To determine the number of fetuses, lie, presentation, position, attitude and position of anterior shoulder.

Diagnostic Palpatory Findings in Various Malpresentations

1. **Breech presentation**
   a. Single fetus in a longitudinal lie
   b. Fetal head palpable in fundal area
   c. *Frank breech*: Head in midline and nonballotable
   d. *Complete breech*: Head is on one side of midline and ballotable, pelvic grip reveals fetal breech
   e. Lateral grips—back on one side and fetal limbs on other side
   f. Position of anterior shoulder and fetal heart sounds is higher than or at the level of umbilicus
   g. Transverse lie or oblique lie-single fetus; fundal and pelvic grips are empty
   h. Fetal head palpable in one of the iliac fossa or hypochondria
   i. Fetal back felt along the ant wall of uterus or post or not felt at all
   j. Fundal height is usually less than expected
   k. Position of anterior shoulder and fetal heart sounds are variable.
2. **Face presentation**
   a. Single fetus in longitudinal lie and cephalic presentation
   b. Fetal back—only lower portion is felt (attitude is extended)
   c. Sinciput lies at lower level than the occiput
   d. FHS—heard better on the opposite side to the back of fetus.
3. **Brow presentation**
   a. Same as that of face presentation except degree of extension is incomplete, sinciput at a higher level than in face presentation
   b. Localization of placenta—fetus usually faces the placenta
   c. Fetal parts are not felt well if the placenta is low lying and anterior
   d. Placental soufflé may be heard
   e. Gross fetal malformation
   f. Abnormality of uterine contour.

Pelvic Examination

Confirm the presentation, assess the pelvic size and presence of pelvic tumors.

Investigations

1. Blood R/E and urine R/E
2. Ultrasound scan—congenital malformations of the fetus; position of placenta; uterine abnormalities; amount of liquor amnii; pelvic masses; fetal maturity.
3. X-ray pelvimetry.

Breech

Longitudinal lie where presenting part is podalic pole and denominator is sacrum.

Types

Complete/flexed breech: Universal flexion at thighs and knees.

Incomplete Breech

1. *Extended/frank breech*: Flexion at thighs and extension at knees. Presenting part—buttock
2. *Knee presentation*: Extension at thighs and flexion at knees. Presenting part—knees
3. *Footling presentation*: Extension at thighs and knees; presenting part—foot
4. *Complicated breech*: Breech with any maternal/fetal complication
5. *Uncomplicated breech*: Breech without any maternal/fetal complication.

Breech Incidence

Decreases as gestational age increases:

1. 20% at 28th week
2. 5% at 34th week
3. 3% at term.

Frequency of Different Types of Breech Presentation

1. Frank breech - 64%
2. Single footling - 14%
3. Complete breech - 12%
4. Double footling - 10%.

Causes

Maternal

1. Multiparity
2. Uterine obliquity
3. Placenta praevia
4. Uterine fibroids in lower segment
5. Bicornuate/septate uterus.

Fetal

1. Prematurity—the most common cause
2. Multiple pregnancy
3. Hydrocephalus
4. Polyhydramnios
5. Oligohydramnios
6. Extended legs.

Conduct of Breech Delivery

Criteria for Vaginal Delivery

1. Weight of baby between 2-3 kg
2. No FPD—fetopelvic disproportion
3. Adequate pelvis. Good uterine contraction
4. Good obstetric history (no PIH, Rh-ve mother)
5. If fetus is dead.

Methods of Vaginal Delivery

1. Spontaneous breech delivery
2. Assisted breech delivery
3. Breech extraction.

Management

Mechanism of breech delivery

Engaging diameter—bitrochanteric—10 cm

1. Descent
2. Internal rotation
3. Lateral flexion
4. Delivery-restitution
5. Delivery of shoulders
6. Delivery of head.

Indications for elective CS in breech:

1. Complicated breech
2. Fetal weight < 2500 or > 3500 g
3. Severe IUGR
4. Preterm breech
5. Footling/knee presentation
6. Hyperextended fetal head
7. Previa or abruption placenta
8. Abnormal clinical pelvimetry
9. Suspected fetal jeopardy
10. Oligohydramnios.

External Cephalic Version

Done at 36 weeks.

Presentation other than cephalic is converted by external manipulation into cephalic presentation.

Assisted Breech Delivery

Delivery of breech

1. Breech climbing perineum
2. Liberal episiotomy
3. Baby's back should be always anterior
4. Hold baby by femoropelvic grip
5. Wrap baby in a warm towel to avoid premature breathing efforts by tactile stimulation.

Delivery of Shoulder

Lovset's maneuver:

1. Inferior angle of scapula seen
2. Trunk rotated 180 degree with downward traction
3. Posterior shoulder comes anteriorly and emerges under pubic arch
4. Trunk is rotated in reverse direction 180 degree and anterior shoulder delivered.

Delivery of after Coming Head

1. *Burns Marshall maneuver*: Steady traction on feet and baby swung in an arc towards mother's abdomen
2. *Kristeller maneuver*: Simultaneous suprapubic pressure in Burns Marshall
3. *Mauriceau-Smellie-Veit maneuver*: Fetal body rest on left palm and forearm; index and middle fingers of same hand applied over malar bones to flex head and two fingers of right hand hooked over fetal neck. Downward traction is applied
4. *Piper's forceps*: Best method for delivery of after coming head.

Breech Extraction

1. Cervix fully dilated and fetal distress present
2. Entire fetus delivered vaginally under general anesthesia.

Complications of Breech Delivery

1. PROM and prematurity
2. Cord prolapse and cord compression
3. Congenital anomalies
4. Prolonged delivery and delay in after coming head

5. Intracranial hemorrhage
6. Fracture/dislocation of cervical vertebra
7. Cervical/brachial plexus injury
8. Sternomastoid hematoma
9. Fracture femur/clavicle/humerus.

GESTATIONAL DIABETES MELLITUS

1. Pregnancy is a diabetogenic state
2. Insulin production increases due to beta cell hypertrophy and hyperplasia in normal pregnancy
3. Insulin sensitivity is normal in early pregnancy but as pregnancy advances due to increased production of human placental lactogen, estrogen, progesterone and cortisol increased insulin resistance occurs at peripheral and hepatic level
4. Increased destruction of insulin by kidneys and placenta (insulinase) may play a role
5. Pregnancy is characterized by fasting hypoglycemia and postprandial hyperglycemia
6. In fasting state, there is hypoglycemia and increased breakdown of triglycerides to fatty acid and ketone body
7. This pregnancy induced switch in fuels from glucose to lipids is called accelerated starvation
8. Renal tubular threshold for glucose falls and glycosuria is not diagnostic of impaired glucose tolerance (IGT) in pregnancy.

Types of Diabetes in Pregnancy

1. Pregestational diabetes
2. Gestational diabetes—90%.

Effects of Pregnancy on Overt Diabetes

1. Increased insulin requirement from three months till term and marked fall in puerperium
2. Diabetes becomes difficult to control, wide fluctuations in glucose levels
3. Progression of diabetic retinopathy
4. Worsening of nephropathy.

Indicators of High-Risk Gestational Diabetes

1. History of still birth
2. History of neonatal death
3. History of fetal macrosomia
4. Concomitant obesity or hypertension
5. Development of polyhydramnios pre-eclampsia or fetal macrosomia.
6. Inadequate metabolic control with diet alone.

Risk Factors for Gestational Diabetes Mellitus

1. Previous baby > 4 kg
2. Elderly primi > 35 years
3. Past history of gestational diabetes mellitus (GDM)
4. History of stillbirth or neonatal death
5. Glycosuria
6. Family history of diabetes
7. History of excessive weight gain.

In high-risk patients screening is done at:

1. First antenatal visit
2. 24–28 weeks
3. 32–34 weeks.

Screening

Universal screening with 50 g GCT.

Glucose Challenge Test

Procedure—50 mg oral glucose given irrespective of the last meal and blood sugar estimated after 1 hour if > 140 mg% do GTT. In Indian contest, it will be better to take 130 mg% as cut off value as the incidence of GDM is more in India.

Diagnosis

Glucose Tolerance Test

Procedure—unrestricted diet for past 3 days and fasting overnight. Early morning fasting blood glucose sample collected

1. 100 mg glucose dissolved in water given
2. Blood with urine sample are collected after 1, 2 and 3 hours
3. GDM is diagnosed of any two values abnormal
4. One value abnormal IGT.

GTT (NDDG, Carpenter and Coustan) all values in mg/dL

Time	Carpenter and Coustan	NDDG (plasma)	IMCH, Calicut
Fasting	95	105	90
1 hour	180	190	165
2 hours	155	165	145
3 hours	140	145	125

Case Taking

1. **History of present illness**
   Symptoms: Cause of weight gain, recurrent UTIs
2. **Obstetric history**
   a. Previous history of large baby > 4 kg
   b. Unexplained perinatal death
   c. History of congenital anomalies, abortion
   d. History of diabetes in past pregnancy
3. *Past history*: History of diabetic complications
4. *Family history*: History of diabetes in family
5. *General examination*: Serial weight recording
6. *Vitals*: Blood pressure due to PIH incidence
7. **Abdominal examination**
   a. *Inspection*—abdomen distended
   b. *Palpation*—fundal height more than expected
   c. Umbilical girth more than 100 cm—hydramnios.

Investigations

1. Biweekly blood glucose
2. Serum HbA_{1C} (glycosylated Hb)
3. Glycosylated fructosamine
4. Weight recording
5. Optic fundus examination—to rule out diabetic retinopathy
6. BP recording
7. Renal function test, liver function test
   a. Anomaly scan and fetal echocardiography
   b. Polyhydramnios, macrosomia, IUGR
   c. BPP and fetal weight estimation.
8. *USG*: Early pregnancy for accurate dating.

MANAGEMENT OF GESTATIONAL DIABETES MELLITUS

Medical Management

1. Tight glycemic control
2. Preconception period—advice about timing and control over diabetes

3. Antenatal management—ANC once in 2 weeks up to 28 weeks and weekly after 28 weeks
4. Diet prescription—30 kcal/kg/day divided into 3 meals + 3 snacks. Rich in fiber and low fat
5. Insulin indicated if diet control fails. A mixture of rapid and intermediate acting insulin like mixtard can be given twice daily. Two-third of dose in morning and one-third at night 30 min before meals and no oral hypoglycemic which can cross placenta and cause fetal hypoglycemia. Insulin does not cross placenta
6. Biweekly blood glucose estimation
7. Upperlimb exercises and walking.

Obstetric Management

Antepartum

1. DFMC 32 weeks onwards
2. Antepartum fetal surveillance—NST weekly from 32 weeks and twice weekly after 36 weeks
3. USG
4. Corticosteroids for lung maturity are not contraindicated.

Intrapartum

1. Admit at 37 weeks
2. Never allow to go beyond term
3. Morning dose of insulin skipped in case of induction, elective CS or as soon as spontaneous labor starts
4. Frequent blood sugar monitoring
5. If insulin is needed regular insulin in ringer lactate is given as infusion
6. Wait for spontaneous delivery and terminate at 40 weeks if not on insulin and no complications
7. Termination at 38 weeks if on insulin and no complications
8. If complicated—induction or LSCS-assess the lung maturity before LSCS by L:S ratio
9. Prophylactic antibiotics—must
10. Control ketosis and manage complications.

Postpartum

WHO GTT with 75 g glucose 6 weeks postpartum.

Values

	Normal	IGT	Diabetes
Fasting	<110	110–125	>125
2 hours	<140	140–199	>199

Management of Overt Diabetes

Prepregnancy Care

1. Prepregnancy counseling
2. $HbA_{1C} < 8$
3. Reduce weight in obese
4. Switch to insulin if on oral hypoglycemic
5. Self-administration of insulin (subcutaneous injection)
6. Symptoms of hypoglycemia informed.

Medical

1. Diet as in gestational diabetes mellitus
2. Mixture of intermediate acting and short acting (NPH: Regular insulin = 2:1) is unlikely to be sufficient—3 premeal injections of rapid acting and one intermediate acting insulin at bedtime.

Obstetric

1. *Antepartum fetal surveillance*:
   a. DFMC 28 weeks onwards
   b. NST 32 weeks onwards twice weekly
   c. BPP twice weekly 36 weeks onwards.

2. Admit at 37 weeks
3. Termination at 38 weeks if no complications.

Postpartum Management

1. Adjust the dose of insulin as insulin requirement falls
2. Breastfeeding and antibiotics for control of infection.

LSCS in diabetes

1. Macrosomia
2. Antepartum fetal distress
3. Bad obstetric history (BOH)
4. Complicated GDM
5. Intrapartum fetal distress.

Contraception

1. *Uncomplicated cases*
   a. Combined pills less preferable over progesterone pills
   b. After 2 children postpartum sterilization (PPS) is done
2. *Complicated cases*: Avoid pregnancy by barrier method.

Complications

Maternal

Antepartum

1. Pre-eclampsia
2. Polyhydramnios—due to fetal hyperglycemia and fetal polyuria
3. Preterm delivery
4. Infections, UTI, vulvovaginal candidiasis
5. Ketoacidosis.

Intrapartum

1. Increased incidence of CS
2. Prolonged labor due to big baby
3. PPH atonic due to over distention, traumatic due to big baby, operative interference
4. Genital tract trauma—due to macrosomia
5. Shoulder dystocia.

Risk Factors Associated with Shoulder Dystocia (DOPE)

1. **D** is for diabetes
2. **O** is for obesity
3. **P** is for post-term (also for prior large baby)
4. **E** is for excessive weight gain during pregnancy.

Postpartum

1. Puerperal sepsis
2. Failing lactation
3. Increased maternal morbidity.

Fetal and Neonatal Complications

1. Due to fetal hyperinsulinemia and explained by Pedersen hypothesis
2. Maternal hyperglycemia leads to fetal hyperglycemia which stimulates fetal pancreas to produce more insulin.

Fetal

1. Abortions
2. *Unexplained intrauterine death (IUD)—caused by*:
   a. Pre-eclampsia and diabetic vasculopathy—placental insufficiency
   b. Macrosomia—increased demand

   c. Ketoacidosis—hypovolemia and hypotension
   d. Chronic hypoxia - hyperglycemia mediated chronic aberrations in oxygen transport
      - Increased glycosylated Hb can lead to microangiopathy and hypoxia
      - Insulinemia increases fetal metabolic rate and oxygen requirement
      - Hyperglycemia causing villous edema osmotically.
3. *Congenital malformations*:
   a. Cardiac defect—the most common transposition of great arteries (TGA) and ventricular septal defect (VSD)
   b. Neural tube defects (NTD)—anencephaly, spina bifida
   c. Caudal regression syndrome/sacral agenensis—specific to diabetes
4. Prematurity
5. Macrosomia.

Neonatal

1. Respiratory distress syndrome (RDS)—Lung maturity ↓ hyperinsulinemia -phospholipids ↓ surfactants ↓ respiratory distress syndrome
2. Hypoglycemia and hypocalcemia
3. Polycythemia and hyperbilirubinemia
4. Hyperviscosity syndrome
5. Hypertrophic cardiomyopathy
6. Birth trauma—Erb's and Klumpke's paralysis, fracture clavicle and humerus
7. Hypothermia—large surface area and lose heat rapidly.

Congenital Fetal Anomalies

Caudal regression syndrome:
1. Neural tube defects
2. Sacral agenesis
3. Cardiac anomalies
4. Renal anomalies
5. Anorectal malformations
6. Lower limb hypoplasia.

White's classification of DM complicating pregnancy

Class	Onset	FBS	PPBS	Therapy
A1	Gestational	<105 mg/dL	<120 mg/dL	Diet
A2	Gestational	>105 mg/dL	>120 mg/dL	Insulin

Class	Age of onset	Duration	Vascular disease	Therapy
B	>20 years	<10 years	None	Insulin
C	10–19 years	10–19 years	None	Insulin
D	<10 years	>20 years	Benign nephropathy	Insulin
F	Any	Any	Nephropathy	Insulin
R	Any	Any	Proliferative retinopathy	Insulin
H	Any	Any	Heart	Insulin
T	Any	Any	Prior renal transplantation	Insulin

Glycated Hemoglobin

1. Glycated hemoglobin provides an accurate and objective measure of glycemic control over a period of weeks to months. In diabetes, the slow nonenzymatic covalent attachment of glucose to hemoglobin (glycation) increases the amount in the HbA1 (HbA_{1C}) fraction relative to nonglycated adult hemoglobin (HbA0).

2. HbA_{1C} concentration reflects the integrated blood glucose control over the lifespan of the erythrocyte (120 days), half of the erythrocytes are replaced in 60 days and HbA_{1C} is weighted by changes in glycemic control occurring in the month before measurement (representing 50% of the HbA_{1C} concentration). As HbA_{1C} is affected more by recent than by earlier events, a large shift in blood glucose control is rapidly accompanied by a change in HbA_{1C}, detectable within 2–3 weeks.
3. HbA_{1C} also provides an index of risk for developing diabetic complications.
4. Glycated serum proteins (fructosamine) can be measured and, because of their shorter half-life, give an indication of glycemic control over the preceding 2 weeks.

HbA_{1C}

1. Normal - 5%
2. Controlled DM - 6–7%
3. Uncontrolled DM - 7%.

HYPERTENSIVE DISORDERS OF PREGNANCY

Presenting Complaints

History of visual disturbances, headache, auditory disturbances, epigastric pain (suggestive of severe PIH or impending eclampsia), lower limb edema.

History

1. No history symptom of heart disease, liver disease, deep vein thrombosis, renal disease, chronic hypertension
2. History of PIH in mother of patient, excessive enlargement of uterus, PIH in past pregnancies
3. History symptom of diabetes mellitus
4. History of diminished fetal movements in past pregnancy.

General Examination

1. Severity of edema—facial puffiness/vulval edema
2. Pallor and icterus
3. Systolic and diastolic blood pressure is measured and mean pressure calculated
4. **Mean arterial pressure** : (Systolic + 2 × diastolic pressure)/3
   Diastolic pressure + 1/3 pulse pressure
5. *Excessive weight gain*: Serial weight recording
6. *Obstetric examination*: Number of fetus or IUGR.

Investigations

Hematological Tests

1. Hemoglobin—hemoconcentration
2. Peripheral smear (PS)—hemolysis
3. Lactate dehydrogenase (LDH)—increased
4. Platelet count—thrombocytopenia.

Liver Function Test

1. Bilirubin—increased
2. SGOT/SGPT—elevated
3. Prolonged clotting time, APTT and prothrombin time.

Renal Function Test

1. Urine—albuminuria, glycosuria, evidence of chronic renal disease; 24 hour urine protein
2. Serum uric acid—increased—due to renal tubular dysfunction
3. Serum creatinine and urea-elevated.

Fundoscopy

1. Arteriolar spasm and vascular damage—reversible after delivery
2. Retinal edema⟶Cotton wool exudates⟶Retinal hemorrhages⟶Retinal detachment.

Assess fetal well-being, fetal growth retardation.

Case Discussion

Classification of Hypertensive Disorders of Pregnancy

1. *Gestational hypertension/pregnancy induced hypertension*: Hypertension arising after 20 weeks of gestation in the absence of proteinuria. Blood pressure returns to normal 12 weeks postpartum.
2. *Pre-eclampsia*: PIH with significant proteinuria
3. *Eclampsia*: Convulsive disorder of pregnancy. Seizures that cannot be attributed to any other cause in a patient with pre-eclampsia.
4. *Chronic hypertension*: Hypertension before pregnancy, hypertension detected before 20 weeks of pregnancy (except in gestational trophoblastic disease) and detected after 20 weeks of gestation but persisting 12 weeks postpartum are considered.
5. *Chronic hypertension with superimposed pre-eclampsia*: New onset proteinuria in chronic hypertensive pregnancy.

Mild Pre-eclampsia

Proteinuric PIH with diastolic pressure below 110 mm Hg.

Criteria of Severe Pre-eclampsia

1. Blood pressure > 160/110 mm Hg
2. Proteinuria > 5 g/day
3. Uric acid > 8 mg%
4. Oliguria < 400 mL/day
5. Thrombocytopenia < 100000/mm^3
6. Edema
7. IUGR
8. Head ache/visual disturbance/epigastric pain
9. Increased liver enzymes
10. Increased serum creatinine
11. Pulmonary edema.

Impending/imminent eclampsia

1. Head ache/flashing lights
2. Nausea/vomiting
3. Epigastric/right upper quadrant pain
4. Brisk deep tendon reflexes and ankle clonus.

Predictors of Pre-eclampsia

1. *Mean arterial pressure*: 90 mm Hg or more
2. *Gant's roll over test*: Predict pregnancy induced hypertension. The woman is turned from left lateral to supine position. If there is an increase in the diastolic BP of 20 mm or more, the test is considered positive
3. *Uterine artery Doppler*: Persistence of diastolic notch at 20–22 weeks. Best predictive test.

Alarming Symptoms of Pre-eclampsia

1. Headache
2. Disturbed sleep
3. Diminished urinary output
4. Epigastric pain
5. Blurring or dimness of vision.

Management

Mild Pre-eclampsia

Antihypertensives

1. Alpha methyl dopa	1–2 g/day	3–4 divided doses	Drug of choice
2. Nifedipine	20–40 mg/day	2–4 divided doses	calcium channel blocker (CCB)
3. Hydralazine	50–300 mg/day	2–3 divided doses	Vasodilation

4. Labetalol	200–400 mg/day	2 divided doses	Alpha and beta blockade
5. Atenolol	50–200 mg/day	1–2 divided doses	Beta blocker.

ACE inhibitors are contraindicated.

Maternal monitoring

Rest in left lateral position and avoid added salt.

Daily monitoring

1. Daily BP chart
2. Daily urine albumin
3. Weight chart, input/output chart.

Twice weekly monitoring

1. RFT
2. LFT
3. Uric Acid
4. Platelet count
5. Bleeding time (BT), clotting time (CT) and coagulation profile.

Fetal monitoring

1. Daily fetal movement count (DFMC)
2. Ultrasound to assess fetal wellbeing and IUGR
3. BPP/Modified BPP (Biophysical profile)
4. Doppler velocimetry in IUGR.

Obstetric management

1. Delivery is the only definitive treatment
2. Induced at 38 weeks
3. Antenatal corticosteroids (betamethasone) if preterm
4. Avoid prophylactic ergometrine—cause sudden rise in BP.

Severe Pre-eclampsia

1. Before 24 weeks	Termination
2. After 34 weeks	Termination
3. Between 24–34 weeks	Expectant management.

Expectant management

1. Antihypertensives
2. Monitoring
3. Antenatal steroids.

Indications for termination

1. Impending signs of eclampsia/eclampsia
2. Uncontrolled hypertension
3. Abnormal renal/liver function tests/coagulopathy
4. Hemolysis elevated liver enzymes low platelet count (HELLP) syndrome
5. Abruption
6. Fetal distress
7. Severe IUGR
8. Grade 3 and 4 retinal changes.

Intrapartum

1. Medical
2. BP control
3. Anticonvulsants
4. Fluid management
5. Corticosteroids—for HELLP/preterm.

Obstetric management

1. Avoid prolonged labor
2. Continuous cardiotocogram (CTG) monitoring
3. CS—if associated obstetric indications, failed induction, fetal distress, severe IUGR.

Postpartum management

1. Methergine/ergometrine contraindicated
2. Use oxytocin/PGF2 Alpha
3. Avoid aggressive fluids—Monitor central venous pressure (CVP)
4. $MgSO_4$ continued for another 24 hours
5. Continue antihypertensives and taper doses—nifedipine/atenolol.

Eclampsia

General

1. Left lateral position in a cot with railings
2. Asess airway and clear airways with suction
3. Oxygen
4. Intravenous (IV) line
5. Pulse oxymetry and monitoring oxygen saturation
6. Catheterize bladder and strict I/O chart.

Medical Management

1. Pritchard's regime
2. $MgSO_4$ is the drug of choice
3. Loading $MgSO_4$ 4 g IV over 2–3 minutes; 4 g IM on each buttock
4. Maintainence 4 g IM 4th hourly alternatingly on each buttock.

Prophylactic Anticonvulsant Therapy

1. $MgSO_4$ loading 8 g (4 g, IM on each buttock)
2. Maintainence 4 g 4th hourly alternatingly on each buttock continue till 24 hours after delivery or till symptoms disappear with BP under control or after last seizure.
3. Monitor
   a. Knee jerk : Should be normally present
   b. Urine output : 100 mL in preceding 4 hours
   c. Respiratory rate : Should be normal.

Status Eclampticus

Thiopentone sodium slow IV under supervision of anesthetist.

Obstetric Management

Immediate termination after controlling seizures.

Blood Levels of $MgSO_4$

1. Therapeutic range — $MgSO_4$ 4–8 mEq/L
2. Absent knee jerk — $MgSO_4$ 10 mEq/L
3. Respiratory arrest — $MgSO_4$ 12 mEq/L

Antidote for Mg toxicity—10 mL 10% calcium gluconate IV.

Complications of Pre-eclampsia

1. Maternal
   a. Eclampsia
   b. Abruptio placenta
   c. Cerebral hemorrhage and cerebrovascular accident
   d. Cortical blindness and visual disturbances
   e. Liver failure
   f. Renal failure
   g. HELLP syndrome
   h. DIC and hemorrhage
   i. Pulmonary edema and adult respiratory distress syndrome (ARDS)
   j. Cyanosis
   k. Sudden postpartum collpase.
2. Fetal
   a. IUGR
   b. IUD
   c. Prematurity
   d. Oligohydramnios
   e. Fetal asphyxia.

Complications of Eclampsia

1. *Due to fits*:
   a. Injuries b. Aspiration c. Asphyxia
2. Acute pulmonary edema
3. Acute left ventricular failure
4. Hypostatic and infective pneumonia
5. Cerebral hemorrhage and hyperpyrexia
6. Renal failure with anuria
7. Ketoacidotic shock and dehydration
8. Sepsis with infection
9. Retinal edema with decreased vision or blindness
10. Hepatic necrosis or psychosis.

HELLP Syndrome

Criteria for diagnosis of HELLP syndrome:
1. Hemolysis
   a. Schistiocytes b. SGOT > 72 IU/L
   c. Bilirubin > 1.5 mg/dL d. LDH > 600 IU/L
   e. Absent plasma haptoglobin
2. Elevated liver enzymes
3. Low platelet count
   Less than 1 lakh.

Management

1. Terminate pregnancy
2. Intravenous dexamethasone 12 mg 2 doses 12th hourly
3. Prophylactic anticonvulsant therapy
4. Emergency BP control
5. Blood and blood products.

Pathological Changes in Pre-eclampsia

Kidney : Glomerular capillary endotheliosis
Liver : Periportal hemorrhagic necrosis
Brain : Cerebral edema, thrombosis, hemorrhage
Heart : Subendothelial hemorrhages
Placenta : Failure of cytotrophoblastic invasion into spiral arterioles.

INTRAUTERINE GROWTH RESTRICTION

Symptoms

Cause of failure of fetus to grow adequately.

History

1. History suggestive of PIH; cyanotic heart disease; anemia; sickle cell hemoglobinopathy; restrictive pulmonary disease, collagen vascular disease.
2. History of chronic renal failure.
3. Chronic hypertension; undernutrition; exposure to heavy irradiation in the present pregnancy; addiction to drugs heroin, heavy smoking or alcoholism, decrease or loss of fetal movements.

Obstetric History

Birthweight of previous babies and evidence of IUGR.

General Examination

1. Presence of hypertension, pallor, edema and evidence of malnutrition
2. Serial weight chart; cardiovascular and respiratory symptoms are examined.

Obstetric Examination

1. Fundal height and abdominal girthless than expected; serial fundal height and serial abdominal girth shows a lag in growth
2. Estimation of volume of liquor amnii (reduced in IUGR)
3. Estimation of fetal weight by Johnson's formula.

Investigations

1. Hemoglobin, blood group; VDRL, HIV HbsAg
2. USG-biometry
   a. Serial record of biparietal diameter, length of femur
   b. Abdominal circumference—most sensitive
   c. *Head circumference*: Abdomen circumference ratio
   d. Estimated fetal weight
   e. Amniotic fluid volume assessment
   f. Congenital malformations of fetus
   g. Recent advances like fetal umbilical blood flow rates
   h. Blood flow in descending thoraxic aorta
   i. Uteroplacental blood flow velocity time waveform.
3. Daily fetal movement count (DFMC)
4. Electronic fetal heart rate monitoring (NST and CST)
5. Maternal biochemical test
   a. FBS and PPBS
   b. Blood urea
   c. Serum creatinine
   d. Serum uric acid and proteins
   e. TORCH titer—early onset IUGR
   f. Antiphospholipid antibody (APLA)
6. Bishop's score for inducibility of labor
7. *Amniotic fluid analysis*: Lecithin (L): Sphingomyelin ratio (S).

Diagnosis

Clinical

Decreased maternal weight gain; fundal height and amniotic fluid volume.

Doppler Ultrasonogram

Middle cerebral artery blood flow decreased in symmetrical IUGR.

Umbilical artery

1. Reduced diastolic flow
2. Absent end diastolic flow
3. Reversal of end diastolic flow.

Management

Antepartum Fetal Surveillance

1. Daily fetal movement count (DFMC)
2. Doppler
3. Amniotic fluid volume
4. Nonstress test
5. Biophysical profile and modified biophysical profile.

Obstetric Management

At 36 weeks

Deliver if having reduced fetal growth, severe oligohydramnios or abnormal doppler.

32–36 weeks

1. Try to postpone delivery until 36 weeks if BPP satisfactory
2. Steroids are given for lung maturity
3. Deliver when NST become abnormal and before reversal of end diastolic flow
4. Absent end diastolic flow and steroids given at 34 weeks can be delivered.

Before 32 weeks

1. *In utero* transfer to institution with good neonatal intensive care unit
2. In all cases with gestation less than 36 weeks antenatal are steroids given.

Definitions

Low birth weight (LBW): Birth weight below 2500 g
Small of gestational age (SGA): Weight below 10th centile for their gestational age
Intrauterine growth restriction (IUGR): Fetuses that have failed to achieve their own genetic growth potential.

Classification

1. Constitutional
2. Growth restriction
   a. Symmetrical (type I)—due to intrinsic cause
   b. Asymmetrical (type II)—brain sparing due to extrinsic cause.

Differences between symmetrical and asymmetrical IUGR

Symmetrical	Asymmetrical
Uniformly small	Head larger than abdomen
Ponderal index normal	Ponderal index low
HC/AC and FL/AC normal	HC/AC and FL/AC high
Etiology—intrinsic to fetus	Extrinsic to fetus—chronic placental insufficiency
Total cell number—less	Total cell number normal
Cell size normal	Cell size small
Poor prognosis	Good prognosis

Etiology of IUGR

Fetal

1. Chromosomal defects
2. Congenital anomalies
3. Toxoplasmosis, others (syphilis, varicella zoster, parvovirus B19), rubella, cytomegalovirus and herpes (TORCH) infections
4. Multifetal gestation.

Placental

1. Chronic abruption
2. Abruptio placenta
3. Hypertensive diseases
4. Heart diseases
5. Placental and cord abnormalities.

Maternal

1. Small mothers (genetic and racial factors)
2. Poor nutrition
3. Anemia
4. Maternal diseases (HTN, CVS, renal failure)
5. Maternal infections (TORCH, UTI)
6. Toxins (alcohol, smoking)
8. Unknown—40% of cases.

Complications

Fetal

1. Stillbirths
2. Fetal distress.

Neonatal

1. Metabolic—hypoglycemia, hypothermia, hypocalcemia, polycythemia.
2. Hypoxic—meconium aspiration syndrome (MAS), hypoxic ischemic encephalopathy (HIE), necrotizing enterocolitis, pulmonary hemorrhage.
3. Congenital malformations, chromosomal abnormalities, congenital TORCH infections.

Late Sequelae

1. Impaired neurodevelopment and cerebral palsy (CP)
2. *Barker hypothesis*: Develop diabetes and hypertension in later life.

MULTIPLE PREGNANCY

Incidence of Multiple Pregnancy

1. Hellin's rule
2. Twins 1 in 80
3. Triplets 1 in 80^2
4. Quadruplets 1 in 80^3.

Varieties

Monozygotic (Identical)	Dizygotic
Single ova + 1 sperm	2 ova + 2 sperms
Same sex twins	Sex may be different
25%	75%
Mono chorionic/Dichorionic	Dichorionic diamniotic
Single placenta	2 separate placenta

Zygosity and Chorionicity

1. Zygosity—type of conception
2. Chorionicity—type of placentation
3. Detected postnatally by examining membranes
4. Detected prenatally by USG
   a. Number of sacs—before 10 weeks 1 sac—monochorionic, 2 sac—dochorionic
   b. Placenta—2 placenta dichorionic (DC)
   c. Sex—discordant sex-dichorionic, concordant sex- not always monochorionic
   d. Intertwin membrane—thicker and more echogenic DC

e. Twin peak sign (lambda sign)—DC (chorionic tissue between layers of intertwin membrane)
f. *T sign-monochorionic (MC) (no chorionic tissue between layers of inter twin membrane)*:

Type	Time of division after fertilization
Dichorionic diamniotic (DCDA)	Within 72 hours
Monochorionic monoamniotic (MCDA)	Between 4 and 8 days
Monochorionic monoamniotic (MCMA)	Between 8 and 13 days
Conjoint twins	After 13 days

Twin Presentations in Frequency

1. Both vertex
2. Vertex + breech
3. Both breech
4. Vertex + shoulder
5. Breech + shoulder
6. Both shoulders.

Symptoms

Complains of excessive distention of abdomen (axial edema, varicose veins, difficulty in breathing) or excessive fetal movements or excessive vomiting.

History

1. History of induction of ovulation with gonadotropic hormones or clomiphene citrate
2. History of multiple pregnancy in family on maternal side
3. History of conception within 1 month of stopping oral contraceptive pills
4. History of anemia
5. History of edema feet and painless bleeding per vaginum
6. History of bleeding per rectum (hemorrhoids)
7. History suggestive of cardiorespiratory embarrassment.

General Examination

Pallor, edema and varicose veins in lower extremities, blood pressure and weight.

System Examination

Obstetric Examination

1. Uterine size
2. Fundal height—more than period of amenorrhea
3. Abdominal girth—greater than expected (>100 cm).

Palpation

1. Identification of 2 fetal heads or 3 fetal poles
2. If only 2 poles are palpable the distance between the 2 poles may be too great to be the length of the fetus
3. Fetal heart sounds are audible at two different sites at two different rates differing from each other by 10 beats/min or more are heard by 2 persons at the same time
4. Malpresentations are more common
5. Leiomyomas and ovarian tumors associated with pregnancy are diagnosed by:
   a. Presence of only 2 fetal poles
   b. Absence of two distinct fetal heart sounds on repeated examinations
   c. Immobility and constancy of large and small masses
   d. History of presence of leiomyoma or ovarian tumor prior to present pregnancy.

Investigations

1. Hemoglobin
2. Blood group
3. VDRL
4. Urine analysis
5. USG—number, lie, presentation, position, attitude of the fetus
   a. Localization of placenta and chorionicity
   b. Evidence of twin to twin transfusion syndrome
   c. Congenital malformations of the fetus
   d. Hydramnios
   e. Cord presentation.

Differential Diagnosis

1. Early diagnosis—history, clinical and ultrasonography
2. Prevent preterm birth
3. Early detection of complications.

Management

Antepartum

1. Diet—Increased calories (singleton requirement+ 300 kCal/day), proteins, vitamins and minerals Fe and folate.
2. Frequent ANC—to detect complications early (2 weeks interval).
3. Bed rest in left lateral position from 22 weeks onwards.
4. Fetal growth assessment—clinical and USG for early detection of discordancy and intervention Ideally every 3–4 weeks.
5. Prevent preterm labor (tocolytics in preterm labor) prophylactic tocolytics not recommended—injection betamethasone 12 mg in 2 times 24 hours apart for preterm cases.
6. Admit as early as possible at least 6 week before EDC.

Intrapartum

Type of twins	Time of termination
DCDA	38 weeks
MCDA	36 weeks
MCMA	Elective CS at 32–34 weeks

Route of delivery decided by assessing fetal presentations.

Indications for Elective CS in Multiple Pregnancy

1. First baby nonvertex
2. Conjoint twins
3. Multiple pregnancy + pre-eclampsia, big baby, cord prolapse, uterine inertia, nondilating cervix for 2nd twin, contracted pelvis, placenta praevia, previous scar on uterus, precious baby
4. Monoamniotic twins
5. Chronic twin to twin transfusion syndrome (TTTS)
6. Higher order pregnancies.

Vaginal Delivery

1. Careful fetal monitoring (FHS and CTG)
2. IV line
3. Blood kept cross matched and available
4. Anesthetist informed
5. Exclude cord prolapse after rupture of membranes.

Management of Labor

Delivery of First Baby

1. Liberal episiotomy even if babies are small
2. Do not give ergometrine after delivery of first twin
3. Baby should be handed over to pediatrician.

Delivery of Second Baby

1. Second twin should be delivered within ½ hour (controversial)
2. Do abdominal and vaginal examination after delivery of first twin to assess lie and presentation of 2nd baby
3. Exclude cord prolapse and monitor FHS.

Longitudinal lie

1. Uterine contractions can be augmented by oxytocin and artificial rupture of membrane (ARM) after fixing presenting part
2. Delivered as vertex or assisted breech delivery
3. Vertex at a higher station—high vacuum (only indication of high vacuum in modern obstetrics)
4. In case of fetal distress/abruption/cord prolapse—deliver by vacuum/forceps or breech extraction.

If transverse—external cephalic version/podalic version + ARM (oxytoxin) once head fixes.

If it fails and membranes intact then under general anesthesia (GA) internal podalic version followed by breech extraction (only indication of internal podalic version in modern obstetrics) and manual removal of placenta.

If membranes not intact or IPV not possible do CS for 2nd baby.

Internal Podalic Version

1. Indication—transverse lie in a case of second of twin
2. Condition to be fulfilled—cervix must be fully dilated; liquor must be adequate; fetus must be like
3. External cephalic version—no anesthesia
4. Internal podalic version—general anesthesia
5. Bipolar version—lesser degree placenta previa.

Complications

Maternal

Antenatal

1. Hyperemesis
2. Abortion
3. Anemia
4. Hydramnios-for 2nd sac
5. Pre-eclampsia
6. APH—placenta previa and abruption of 2nd twin
7. Chest pain and palpitation
8. Pressure symptoms—backache, fatigue, lower limb edema, hemorrhoids, varicosity, constipation.

Intrapartum

1. PROM—due to overstretched lower segment and malpresentations
2. Cord accidents—cord entanglement for MCMA twins, cord prolapse
3. Interlocking of twins
4. Increased incidence of vaginal and abdominal operative procedures—malpresentations
5. Obstructed labor and traumatic delivery.

Postpartum

1. Postpartum hemorrhage
   a. Atony of uterine muscles due to over distention
   b. Large area of placenta taking more time to separate and opens multiple sinuses
   c. Implantation of placenta in lower segment which fails to retract

d. Co-existing anemia and PIH
e. Traumatic component is more
2. Infection and sepsis
3. Subinvolution.

Fetal

1. IUGR
2. IUD—more in MC twins due to congenital malformations, TTTS
3. Fetus papyraceous
4. Increased fetal anomalies
5. Preterm delivery and low birthweight
6. Malpresentations
7. Increased perinatal mortality
8. Discordant growth and twin to twin transfusion syndrome (TTTS), acardiac twin, stuck twin
9. Vanishing twin.

Differential Diagnosis of Overdistended Uterus

Early pregnancy
Vesicular mole
Multiple mole

Other
Multiple pregnancy
Hydramnios
Tumors complicating pregnancy
Mistaken date
Large baby

Medical
Ascites
Hepatosplenomegaly
Intra-abdominal tumors

HEART DISEASE COMPLICATING PREGNANCY

Physiological Cardiovascular Changes in Pregnancy

1. *Blood volume*: Increase by 40%
2. *Pulse rate*: Increase by 10% (15 bpm)
3. *Stroke volume*: Increase by 10%
4. *Cardiac output*: Increase by 40%
5. *Blood pressure*: Diastolic pressure falls due to decrease in peripheral vascular resistance
6. *Heart*: Displaced to left and upwards by gravid uterus, eccentric hypertrophy.

CVS Changes Mimicking Heart Disease

1. Increase in HR and ectopics
2. Collapsing pulse due to wide pulse pressure
3. JVP waves prominent
4. Heart size increases
5. Apex beat displaced upwards and laterally
6. S1 loud, presence of S3
7. ESM
8. Pedal edema
9. ECG—left axis deviation and mild ST changes.

Types of Heart Disease

1. *Rheumatic (most common)*: Mitral stenosis most common
2. *Congenital*: ASD most common

Maximum maternal mortality is seen with Eisenmenger syndrome/primary pulmonary hypertension.

New York Heart Association Functional Classification (NYHA)

Class I – No limitation of physical activity
Class II – Symptoms on ordinary physical activity
Class III – Symptoms on less than ordinary physical activity
Class IV – Symptoms at rest

Contraindications for Pregnancy

1. Eisenmenger's syndrome
2. Primary pulmonary hypertension and pulmonary hypertension of any cause
3. Uncorrected severe coarctation
4. Marfan's with aortic involvement
5. Severe MS with complications.

Offer MTP in 1st trimester for these patients.

Symptoms

Complains of palpitation, breathlessness on exertion, syncope, paroxysmal nocturnal dyspnea (PND), orthopnea, edema feet, cough with expectoration.

History

History of cardiac failure in past pregnancy, corrective cardiac surgery prior to present pregnancy with details of operation, drug therapy in present pregnancy (anticoagulants, antibiotic prophylaxis for rheumatic fever, hematinics), fetal movements normal or decreased

History suggestive of anemia, PIH, infections, thyrotoxicosis, infective endocarditis, tachycardia, atrial fibrillation and rheumatic fever in the present pregnancy or in childhood.

General Examination

General condition, temperature, pulse (rate, rhythm, volume) respiratory rate, BP, jugular venous pressure (JVP), pallor, edema feet, hepatomegaly (CCF), splenomegaly (IE), thyroid enlargement, dental caries.

Cardiovascular System

To assess the degree of cardiac dysfunction and to determine the presence of any complication.

Respiratory System

Basal crepitations and evidence of infection.

Obstetric Examination

Evidence of IUGR.

Investigations

To Assess Cardiac Status

Electrocardiography, echocardiography, chest X-ray (PA view), vector cardiography, phonocardiography, Holter monitor studies.

To Assess Complicating Factors

Hemoglobin (Hb), urine (R/E, culture, colony count, antibiotic sensitivity), serum electrolytes, serum uric acid, blood urea nitrogen, X-ray pelvimetry.

Management

Antepartum Management

1. Classify patient as per NYHA
2. Avoid excessive weight gain and sodium intake
3. Prevent anemia and infection
4. Complete cardiology work up
5. Continue rheumatic fever prophylaxis
6. Use of anticoagulants
7. Ensure infective endocarditis (IE) prophylaxis during any surgical procedures
8. Antenatal visits
   Grade 1: Antenatal checkup in outpatient (OP), once in 2 weeks up to 20 weeks
   Grade 2: Weekly after 20 weeks.
9. Medical termination of pregnancy (MTP) (first trimester) and valvotomy (second trimester) in indicated cases
10. Admission
    Grade 1: Admit at 36 weeks
    Grade 2: Admit at 28 weeks
    Grade 3: Admit at 1st visit, hospitalized throughout pregnancy
    Grade 4: Admit at 1st visit, hospitalized throughout pregnancy.

Intrapartum Management

1. Vaginal delivery preferred unless there are obstetric indications
2. Induction avoided unless absolutely necessary
3. Coarctation of aorta is an indication for CS.

First stage
1. Avoid supine position. Left lateral position better. Propped up semi recumbent position is the best.
2. Analgesia—Epidural with fentanyl preferred which is cardiovascularly stable opioid (avoid in cyanotic HD, severe AS and patients on anticoagulants).
3. Sedation—with injection morphine.
4. Pulse oxymetry and oxygen therapy if required.
5. IV fluids must be restricted. 75 mL/hour. Give oral fluids. Keep patient on the dry side.
6. Pulse, BP, respiration monitoring every 30 min.
7. Infective endocarditis prophylaxis—ampicillin 2 g IV and Gentamycin 1.5 mg/kg 30 minutes before procedure. In penicillin allergic vancomycin and gentamicin.
8. Continuous electrocardiography monitoring in cases of pulmonary HTN.

Second stage
1. Avoid lithotomy or dorsal position. Left lateral position preferred
2. Pulse and respiration every 10 min
3. Pudental block in cases epidural not given
4. Outlet forceps should be used to shorten second stage
5. Injection frusemide 40 mg immediately after delivery of baby.

Third stage
1. Methergine is contraindicated. Sudden shifting of blood from uterus to systemic circulation should be avoided.
2. If PPH occurs oxytocin 20 units as IV drip or prostaglandin F2 alpha IM. Avoid ergometrine having properties of fluid retention.

Postpartum Management

1. Continue antibiotics
2. *Contraception*:
   a. Permanent—vasectomy preferred, minilap tubal ligation (TL), interval lap TL
   b. Temporary—barrier contraceptive method of choice—oral contraceptive pills (OCP), intrauterine contraceptive device (IUCD)
3. Early completion of family
4. Correction of heart lesion before next pregnancy
   a. *Grade 1 and 2*: Safe vaginal delivery at term; low forceps or vacuum if 2nd stage is delayed
   b. *Grade 3*: Safe delivery at term; mitral valvotomy
   c. *Grade 4*: Treat cardiac problem before 12 weeks; MTP in cases with bad prognosis.

Complications

Maternal

1. Cardiac failure
2. Infective endocarditis
3. Pulmonary embolism.

Fetal

1. IUGR-cyanotic heart disease
2. Increased chances of CHD.

Factors Precipitating Cardiac Failure

1. Infections
2. Anemia
3. Hypertension
4. Physical and emotional stress
5. Altered physiology due to pregnancy.

Prognostic Factors

Maternal

1. Age > 35
2. Poor socioeconomic status
3. Atrial fibrillation
4. Mitral stenosis (good)
5. Parity.

Fetal

1. Grade 1 and 2 (not much effect)
2. Grade 3 and 4 (mortality 30%)
3. Grade 3 and 4 prematurity (bad).

Rule of 5 (High-Risk Periods)

1. Five weeks of pregnancy—when hemodynamic changes of pregnancy develops.
2. Five months of pregnancy and 5 weeks before expected date of confinement (EDC)—when hemodynamic changes peak and cardiac demands are maximum.
3. Five hours after onset of labor—cardiac output increases by 10–15% with every uterine contraction during labor.
4. Five days after delivery—decreased peripheral resistance with right to left shunting and pulmonary embolization from silent iliofemoral thrombus.

PREVIOUS CESAREAN SECTION

Obstetric History

1. Any previous normal deliveries and their birthweight
2. Any difficult forceps delivery especially after prolonged trial of labor

3. Details of cesarean section in the past:
   a. Indication
   b. Nature of cesarean section—elective/emergency/after trial of labor, after prolonged labor or failed forceps or vacuum delivery
   c. Nature of uterine incision—upper or lower segment
   d. History of postoperative wound infection.

History

1. History suggestive of genital sepsis after cesarian section which weakens the scar
2. Time since last delivery (uterine scars heal in 6 months during which period pregnancy should not be undertaken)
3. History of blood transfusion after cesarian section or hematinic therapy
4. History of any radiological investigations for assessment of uterine scar integrity
5. History of one or more vaginal deliveries after cesarian section
6. History of present pregnancy—history of excessive uterine enlargement as in case of twins, hydramnios
7. History of pain in the area of uterine scar
8. Bladder symptoms
9. History of adequate hematinic therapy.

General Examination

Height, pallor and spine (spinal abnormality can cause pelvic contraction and nonfeasibility of epidural anesthesia).

Abdominal Examination

1. Nature of abdominal scar—vertical or Pfannenstiel's (suprapubic curvilinear)
2. Distortion, puckering, keloid formation, incisional hernia
3. Malpresentations, multiple pregnancy (repeat CS is indicated if any of the fetus is in malpresentation)
4. Estimated fetal weight, engagement of presenting part
5. Scar tenderness looked for just above and parallel to upper border of pubis.

Vaginal Examination

To assess the bony pelvis by Munro-Kerr method.

Investigations

1. Hemoglobin (anemia)
2. Blood group (Rh incompatibility)
3. USG—fetal maturity by various parameters, placental localization, fetal malformations and malpresentations, assessment of uterine scar
4. X-ray pelvimetry.

Indication of Cesarean Section

Absolute Indications

1. Severe degree CPD/contracted pelvis
2. Placenta previa (type 2 posterior, 3 and 4)
3. Pelvic mass causing obstruction
4. Advanced Ca Cx; vaginal obstruction (atresia, stenosis)
5. Lower limb abnormality of mother
6. Brow presentation
7. Previous 2 CS, previous classical CS
8. Multiple pregnancy—higher order pregnancies, conjoint twins, MCMA twins.

Relative Indications

1. Minor degree CPD
2. Antepartum hemorrhage (APH) (placenta previa, type 1, 2 ant, abruptio placenta)
3. Malpresentations—breech, transverse lie, shoulder
4. Failed induction
5. Fetal distress due to meconium
6. Bad obstetric history
7. Dystocia
8. Previous CS—maternal complications
9. Features of scar dehiscence
10. Hypertension (HTN)—severe pre-eclampsia with unfavourable Cx
11. Eclampsia uncontrolled.

Elective Cesarean Section (CS)—Conditions

1. Previous CS—classical
2. Previous 2 CS
3. Previous CS with twins
4. Previous CS with dysfunctional labor
5. Previous CS with past date
6. Previous CS done for placenta previa
7. History of sepsis in postpartum period after previous CS.

Vaginal Birth after CS—Conditions

1. Proper facilities and staff
2. Single vertex presentation with estimated weight < 4 kg
3. Previous CS done for nonrecurrent indications
4. No medical, surgical, obstructive contraindication for vaginal delivery
5. Obstetrician to tackle emergency CS and complications.

Scar Dehiscence—Amniotic Sac Intact

Disruption of part of the scar and fetal membranes remain intact. Visceral peritoneum is also intact. Bleeding is minimal.

Scar Rupture

1. Disruption of entire length of scar
2. Incomplete rupture—visceral peritoneum intact
3. Complete rupture—all broken.

Contraindications of Vaginal Birth after CS

1. Previous 2 CS
2. Previous classical CS
3. Previous inverted T or extension of uterine incision
4. Suspicion of CPD
5. History of postpartum fever or wound infection
6. Current obstetric factors—malpresentations, macrosomia, twins, thin lower segment
7. Short interval between CS and subsequent trial (< 2 years)
8. Uterine anomalies
9. Elderly patient.

Impending Signs of Scar Rupture

1. Increased maternal pulse
2. Scar tenderness
3. Blood stained urine
4. Edema +
5. Fetal tachycardia
6. Fresh bleeding PV
7. Bladder frequently filling (tenesmus)
8. All symptoms of fetal death.

Management of Previous Cesarean Section

During pregnancy

1. Previous LSCS-normal ANC
   Admit by 34–38 weeks or at term if normal
2. Previous classical CS—frequent ANC and admit at least by 34 weeks.

At term

1. If favorable factors for vaginal delivery are present, we can wait up to a max of 7 days with CTG monitoring on 5th day
2. Closely monitor mother and fetus
3. If any signs of impending uterine rupture or fetal distress arise immediately terminate by CS and CS done also when head is unengaged even after term.

At labor

First stage

1. Blood grouping and cross matching
2. IV line
3. Prophylactic antibiotics
4. Preparation for lower segment CS (LSCS) kept ready
5. Oxytocin may be used for augmentation in cases of inertia
6. Usual steps + maternal pulse every 15 min
7. Fetal heart sounds (FHS) every 15 min
8. Do not use prostaglandins for cervical ripening/induction
9. Watch for signs and symptoms of impending rupture
10. Epidural analgesia.

Second stage

1. Liberal episiotomy
2. Apply forceps to assist delivery of head.

Third stage

1. Active management is done
2. After delivery of baby check BP, pulse, blood loss
3. Placental delivery
4. If all are within normal limit (WNL) no need to explore uterus.

BAD OBSTETRIC HISTORY

Obstetric History

1. Gestational age at the time of pregnancy loss
2. Whether spontaneous or induced
3. Whether curettage was done after the spontaneous abortion
4. Whether the abortion was documented by histopathological examination
5. If the pregnancy loss was after the age of viability whether it was live birth or stillbirth
6. If it is live birth whether term or preterm
7. If it is stillbirth whether it is fresh or macerated
8. Congenital malformations, e.g. Neural tube defects.

Past History and Present History

1. History suggestive of uterine leiomyoma (1st trimester abortions)
2. History of maternal exposure to diethylstilbestrol
3. History suggestive of incompetent os—repeated second trimester abortion and preterm deliveries
4. History of trauma to cervix by dilatation, amputation or by traumatic forceps delivery
5. History of syphilis, chronic HTN (2nd trimester abortions)
6. History of chronic renal disease and diabetes mellitus, severe chronic respiratory disease
7. Low socioeconomic status

8. History of SLE, hydrops fetalis, neonatal jaundice
9. History of recurrent malpresentations
10. History of habituation to tobacco, alcohol
11. History of IUGR.

Examination (Pallor, Icterus, Cyanosis, Clubbing Lymph Nodes, Edema)

General examination—PICCLE

Vitals

Systemic Examination

Obstetric Examination

Diagnosis

Investigations

1. Complete hemogram
2. Urine R/E
3. RFT
4. LFT
5. Blood group
6. VDRL
7. TORCH titer
8. Thyroid function test (TFT)
9. LE cell preparation
10. Serum antinuclear antibody (ANA) and APLA
11. USG
12. GCT and GTT
13. Karyotyping of husband and wife
14. Hysteroscopy
15. Cervical culture for listeria monocytogenes, mycoplasma hominis, ureaplasma urealyticum from cervical discharge.

Definition

The term bad obstetric history is applied to a pregnant mother where her present obstetric outcome is likely to be affected adversely by the nature of previous obstetric disaster.

Abortion

Spontaneous termination of pregnancy before viability (22 weeks of gestation/weight < 500 g)
1. Incomplete abortion—abortion in which the part of product of conception have been passed but a part remains in uterus
2. Missed abortion—abortion in which fetus dies *in utero* but the products of conception is retained *in utero*.
3. Threatened abortion—crampy pains and slight show of blood that may or may not be followed by the expulsion of fetus during the first 20 weeks of pregnancy
4. Septic abortion—an infected abortion complicated by fever, endometritis and parametritis.

Causes of First Trimester Abortions

1. Chromosomal abnormality
2. Endocrinal—poorly controlled diabetes mellitus (DM); thyroid autoantibodies; inadequate luteal phase; polycystic ovarian syndrome
3. Infection
4. Immunological cause—autoimmunity, alloimmunity.

Causes of Second Trimester Abortions

1. Cervical incompetence—20%
2. Chronic maternal illness
3. Uterine synechiae
4. Uterine fibroid

5. Retroverted uterus
6. Infection
7. Defective Müllerian fusion—double uterus, septate uterus, bicornuate
8. Idiopathic.

APLA Syndrome Management

1. Low molecular weight heparin till termination
2. Low dose aspirin
3. Termination at 34 weeks.

ANEMIA COMPLICATING PREGNANCY

Symptoms

Cause of easy fatiguability, weakness, lassitude, palpitations, breathlessness on exertion.

History

1. History of excessive blood loss in the past—menorrhagia, polymenorrhagia, postpartum and postabortal hemorrhage in the past pregnancies, bleeding per rectum, melena, hematemesis, hookworm in stools, bleeding from any other site.
2. History of malnutrition, therapy for epilepsy, tapeworms in stools, bleeding per vaginum in present pregnancy.
3. History suggestive of malabsorption, hemolytic anemia, aplastic anemia, leukemia, malaria.

General Examination

Evidence of pallor, anemia, degree of anemia, nail changes, icterus, hepatosplenomegaly, edema feet.

Systemic Examination

Features of anemia—ejection systolic murmur at cardiac base, evidence of congestive cardiac failure such as raised JVP and basal crepitations. Evidence of some infection may be obtained.

Obstetric Examination

Number of fetuses, evidence of intrauterine growth restriction—fundal height and abdominal girthless than expected, small size of fetus, oligohydramnios.

Investigations

1. Establish the diagnosis of anemia
   a. Hemoglobin
   b. Packed cell volume
   c. RBC count.
2. Differentiate the type of anemia
   a. Mean corpuscular volume
   b. Mean corpuscular hemoglobin
   c. Mean corpuscular hemoglobin concentration
   d. Peripheral smear
   e. WBC count
   f. TC and DC
   g. Reticulocyte count
   h. Serum ferritin.
3. *In iron deficiency anemia*: Plasma iron and iron binding capacity, stool examination for stool occult blood, hookworms, test for malabsorption.
4. *Hemolytic anemia*: Peripheral smear for red blood cell morphology, (spherocytes, elliptocytes, sickle cells, red cells with Heinz bodies) osmotic fragility test, hemoglobin electrophoresis, acid elution or alkali denaturation test for hemoglobin F, assay for G6PD, blood smear for malarial parasite.
5. *Megaloblastic anemia*: Bone marrow examination, FIGLU test, serum folate and red blood cell folate estimation, serum vitamin B_{12} estimation, urinary methyl malonic acid excretion.

6. *To assess fetal growth*: Serial record of maternal weight, fundal height and abdominal girth, serial USG for fetal biparietal diameter, head/thoracic circumference ratio, femur length, amniotic fluid volume assessment.
7. *To assess fetal well being*: Nonstress test (NST), contraction stress test (CST), DFMC.

Complications

During Pregnancy

1. Pre-eclampsia
2. Infections
3. Heart failure or shock
4. Preterm labor.

During Labor

1. Postpartum hemorrhage
2. Cardiac failure
3. Shock
4. Uterine inertia.

During Puerperium

1. Sepsis/UTI/RTI
2. Subinvolution of uterus
3. Decreased lactation
4. Venous thrombosis/pulmonary embolism/heartfailure.

Fetal

1. Intrauterine hypoxia
2. IUGR
3. Increased perinatal death
4. Anemia in childhood.

Treatment

Prophylactic treatment

1. Avoid child birth for 2 years
2. Diet (iron rich foods)
3. Oral iron supplimentation 60 mg $FeSO_4$
4. Deworming.

Curative treatment

1. General measure
2. Specific measure—iron therapy (oral or parenteral), blood transfusion
   Oral iron tablets (sulfates, palmitate, carbonates of ferrous salts).

Parenteral Iron Therapy

Indications

1. Intolerance to oral iron
2. Severe anemia after 30 weeks
3. Severe malabsorption of oral iron.

Routes—IM/IV

Estimation of parenteral dose

1. 0.66 × % Hb deficit × weight in kg = mg of iron needed
2. This +50 % for iron stores are given.

Preparations

1. Iron dextran
2. Iron sorbitol citrate
3. Iron sucrose.

Intramuscular Route

Iron dextran/iron sorbitol citric acid complex contain 50 mg element. 2 mL given daily or alternate days in gluteal region by Z technique.

Intravenous Route

Iron dextran (1 mL = 50 mg elemental iron)

1. Advantages
   a. Definite correction of iron deficiency possible
   b. Not affected by other factors
2. Disadvantage
   a. Intramuscular injections are painful
   b. Costly
   c. Reactions/allergy
   d. Stains the skin
   e. Systemic disturbances.

Indications for blood transfusion
a. Refractory anemia
b. Anemia due to hemorrhage
c. Severe anemia after 36 weeks
d. Presence of infections.

Rh ISOIMMUNIZATION

History

1. Blood group of both partners
2. History of previous miscarriages/neonatal deaths/IUDs
3. History of injection of anti-D immunoglobulin
4. History of polyhydramnios, pre-eclampsia
5. History of previous neonatal jaundice.

Examination

1. Severe edema in maternal mirror syndrome
2. Polyhydramnios.

Indirect Coombs Test (ICT)

Rh negative woman with Rh positive partner—ICT at booking.

Procedure

1. Treat standard Rh positive RBCs with patient's serum
2. Treat these RBCs with Coombs reagent
3. RBCs will agglutinate if patient's serum has anti—Rh antibodies. Anti-Rh antibodies coat these RBCs and cause agglutination (Positive ICT)
4. RBCs will not agglutinate if patient's serum does not have anti-Rh antibody. (Negative ICT)

Management

Nonimmunized-Negative Indirect Coombs Test

1. Repeat ICT at
   a. 28 and 34 weeks in primigravida
   b. 28 and monthly there after in multigravida
2. ICT persistently negative proceed up to 40 weeks
3. Never allow to go beyond term.

Intrapartum

1. Early cord clamping
2. Sent Cord Blood for Hb, bilirubin and direct Coombs test.

Direct Coombs Test

1. Treat Baby's RBCs with Coombs reagent
2. Agglutination occurs if mother derived antibodies are present in baby's blood-positive Coombs test.

Postpartum

Anti-D prophylaxis: If baby is Rh positive Anti-D immunoglobulin must be given within 72 hours of delivery/abortion Anti-D immunoglobulin 300 microgram intramuscular is given—neutralize 15 mL of fetomaternal blood.

Indications for Anti-D Prophylaxis

First Trimester

1. Abortion
2. Ectopic pregnancy
3. Hydatidiform mole
4. Threatened abortion
5. MTP
6. Chorionic villous sampling.

Second and Third Trimester

1. Abortion
2. Amniocentesis
3. Fetal blood sampling
4. Antepartum hemorrhage
5. External cephalic version
6. Manual removal of placenta
7. Antepartum prophylaxis
8. Delivery.

Royal College of Obstetricians and Gynecologist

Before 20 weeks : 50 microgram
After 20 weeks : 100 microgram (for 4 mL fetomaternal blood)

Antepartum Prophylaxis

First dose at 28 weeks : 100 microgram
Second dose at 34 weeks : 100 microgram
Baby Rh positive : 100 microgram + Kleihauer

Immunized-Positive Indirect Coombs Test

1. ICT titer
2. Paternal blood group genotyping
3. Fetal blood group determination
4. Amniocentesis—amniotic fluid bilirubin evaluation—Liley's zones
5. Fetal blood sampling and intravascular transfusion
6. Ultrasound asessment—fetal hydrops (Buddha sign)/ascitis, liver/spleen enlargement and fetal MCA (middle cerebral artery) doppler
7. Antepartum steroids—betamethasone 12 mg 2 doses 24 hours apart for lung maturity
8. Delivery—mild cases at 38 weeks
9. Amniocentesis -> Lilley zone 3-> intravascular transfusion-> deliver at 34 weeks
10. Neonatal management.

Complications

Fetal Complications

1. Immune hydrops
2. Icterus gravis neonatorum
3. Congenital hemolytic anemia.

Maternal Complications

1. Pre-eclampsia
2. Polyhydramnios
3. Maternal mirror syndrome.

CONTRACTED PELVIS

History of Present Illness

Admitted for safe confinement—high-risk case; during antenatal checkup—short primigravida are found out and advise given regarding the complications.

Obstetric History

1. History of previous safe vaginal delivery of a average size baby
2. History of prolonged and tedious labor with instrumental delivery
3. History of difficult vaginal delivery ending in still born or early neonatal death (NND)
4. History of complete vaginal tear, vesicovaginal, rectovaginal fistula.

Past History

History of rickets, osteomalacia, tuberculosis of spine or pelvic joints, poliomyelitis.

General Examination

1. Height short stature < 140 cm
2. Abnormality of pelvic bone
3. Hip joints
4. Deformity of spine
5. Shortening of lower limb.

Abdominal Examination

1. Inspection—pendulous abdomen—in primi—inlet contraction
2. Palpation—look for malpresentations, mobile head at term
3. Bimanual examination.

Pelvic Examination

1. Cervix shrinking after amniotomy
2. Edema of the cervix
3. Head not well applied against the cervix
4. Head not engaged with leading point at 2 station
5. Caput formation
6. Molding (cranial bones overlapping)
7. Deflexion (anterior frontenelle easily palpable)
8. Asynclitism (sagittal suture is not in the middle of the pelvis).

Clinical Pelvimetric Findings Suggestive of Contracted Pelvis

1. Narrow subpubic arch
2. Biischial diameter less than 8 cm
3. Prominent ischial spines
4. Flat sacrum
5. Diagonal conjugate diameter less than 11.5 cm.

Diagnosed by

1. Clinical—abdominal method and abdominovaginal method (Münro-Kerr-Müller method)
2. X-ray pelvimetry
3. Cephalometry—X-ray and USG.

Clinical: Sacral promontory, measure diagonal conjugate, curve of sacrum, sacrosciatic notch, ischial spine, side wall, pubic angle, outlet measure.

X-ray: Lateral view (in standing position), helps to diagnose contracted pelvis (CPD) at 3 levels (inlet, midpelvic and outlet).

Cephalometry: Biparietal diameter measured by USG and its relation to pelvic diameter.

Management

Elective CS-2nd degree severe CPD, 1st degree CPD with maternal/fetal complications
1st degree CPD in a primi or multitrial labor.

Contraindications for Trial Labor

1. Elderly primi
2. IUGR
3. Postmaturity
4. Long history of infertility
5. Bad obstetric history
6. Severe PIH
7. Malpresentations
8. Post-CS
9. Heart disease complicating pregnancy.

Successful Trial

Undamaged baby born vaginally spontaneously or by forceps or ventouse with the mother in good condition.

Failure of Trial

Delivery by CS or delivery of a dead baby spontaneously or by craniotomy.

Classification

1. Nutritional and environmental
   a. Minor variation
   b. Major—rachitic or osteomyelitic.
2. Disease or injury to bones
   a. Pelvic—tumor, fracture pelvis, tubercular arthritis
   b. Spinal—kyphosis, scoliosis, spondylolisthesis
   c. Lower limb—congenital dislocation of hip.
3. Developmental defects
   a. Naegele's pelvis and Robert's pelvis
   b. High or low assimilation pelvis.

Differential Diagnosis of Mobile Head at Term

1. Mistaken date
2. Prematurity
3. Uterine anomaly
4. CPD due to contracted pelvis, large baby or both
5. Polyhydramnios
6. Retroverted gravid uterus
7. Occipitoposterior head/deflexed head
8. Low uterine fibroid
9. Hydrocephalus
10. Placenta previa.

Trial Labor

Keeping a lady with 1st degree CPD, thinking that good uterine contractions, dilatation of Cx, descent and moulding of the fetal skull, give away of the pelvis would result in the delivery of fetus with minimal injuries to fetus and mother.

Bishop's preinduction cervical scoring system

Factors	0	1	2	3
Cx dilatation	Closed	1–2	3–4	5+
Cervical length	>2	1–2	<1	Fully taken up
Consistency	Firm	Medium	Soft	
Position	Posterior	Midline	Anterior	
Head (station)	–3	–2	–1,0	+1, +2
Total score	13			
Favorable score	6–13			
Unfavorable score	0–5			

ANTEPARTUM FETAL SURVEILLANCE

Fetal Movement Count

Cardiff kick count—8 to 12 hours period must be chosen to record at least 10 fetal movements. Preferably, when fetus is most active.

Nonstress Test

1. Cardiotochography also known as admission test. Recording carried out for 20-60 minute baseline fetal heart rate, beat to beat variability, presence or absence of accelerations in response to movement and presence or absence of decelerations are looked for.
2. Reactive NST—presence of 2 or more fetal heart rate accelerations during 20 min with each acceleration of 15 beats or more per min lasting 15 or more second.
3. Nonreactive NST—in fetal hypoxia. Variable decelerations if nonrepetitive and brief are not significant. Repetitive or prolonged variable decelerations are considered abnormal.

Vibroacoustic Stimulation Test (VAST)

An acoustic stimulator placed over maternal abdomen and stimulus applied for one to two seconds.

Contraction Stress Test

Oxytocin challenge test.

Amniotic Fluid Volume

1. Amniotic fluid index (AFI)—sum of largest vertical pockets of liquor in four quadrants. Normal value 5-20 cm
2. Single deepest Pocket (SDP)—depth of single cord free pocket of liquor.

Biophysical Profile

Manning score

Component	Score 2	Score 0
NST	At least 2 accelerations, 15 bpm, 15s	0–1 acceleration
Fetal breathing	At least 1 FBM, lasting >30s	< 30s
Fetal movement	At least 3 discrete body/limb movement	< 3
Fetal tone	At least 1 episode of extension with flexion or opening or closing hand	No movements
Amniotic fluid volume	Single deepest pocket 2 cm or more	SDP < 2 cm
Maximum	10/10	
Normal	8–10/10	
Equivocal	6/10	
Abnormal	4/10	

Modified Biophysical Profile (Vintzileos Score)

Combination of NST + AFI

Doppler Velocimetry (Fig. 4.1)

Ratios

S/D : Systolic diastolic ratio (S/D ratio)
S-D/S : Resistance index
S-D/mean : Pulsatility index

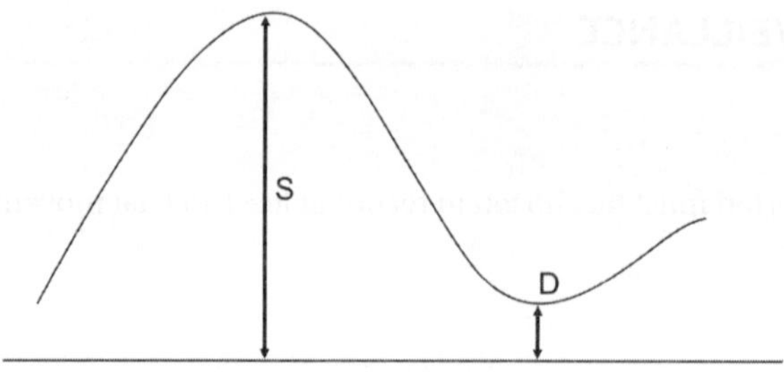

Fig. 4.1: Doppler velocimetry

1. Umbilical artery Doppler—placental Doppler. Flow patterns—reduced end diastolic flow, absent end diastolic flow (EDF), reversal of flow.
2. Middle cerebral vessels—once middle cerebral artery flow is abnormal delivery is indicated.
3. When there is fetal hypoxic stress fetus redistributes blood flow to brain and heart-brain sparing.
4. Venous doppler decreased flow suggestive of cardiac failure.

ULTRASONOGRAPHY IN OBSTETRICS

Methods

Transabdominal scanning (TAS) : Bladder should be full to act as a window.
Transvaginal scanning (TVS) : Bladder should be empty.

Timing

1. *Booking scan (10–14 weeks)*: Assessment of early pregnancy and fetal viability, dating of pregnanacy using CRL (Crown-Rump length), CRL between 9 weeks and 11 weeks—most accurate method of dating, ectopic pregnancy, multiple pregnancy, hydatidiform mole, evaluation of bleeding if present and evaluation of uterus and adnexa.
   Detection of some structural abnormalities and Nuchal translucency—screening for Down syndrome.
2. *Targeted anomaly scan (20 weeks)*: Fetal survey-anatomy, fetal number, viability, lie, placental location, liquor
   Fetal biometry—BPD, FL, AC and HC
   Fetal environment—placenta (R/o previa and retroplacental clots), Amniotic fluid (SDP and AFI)
   Pelvic anatomy—uterus, cervix, adnexa
   Targeted anomaly scan—head and neck, face, spine, thorax, abdomen, extremities and cord
3. *Third trimester scan*: For fetal growth and wellbeing (BPP, modified BPP, Doppler velocimetry) Localization of placenta, suspected IUD, confirmation of presentation, persistent cord around neck.

USG in Obstetrics

1. TAS—gestational sac—5th week
2. Fetal pole—6th week
3. Yolk sac—6th week
4. Cardiac pulsation—7th week
5. Embryonic movements—8th week
6. TVS—one week earlier.

Reliable Parameters to Predict Fetal Maturity

1. 1st trimester—CRL
2. 2nd trimester—BPD
3. 3rd trimester—FL
4. IUGR—AC (abdominal circumference).

POSTPARTUM HEMORRHAGE

1. Primary—hemorrhage occurs within 24 hours
2. Secondary—hemorrhage occurs beyond 24 hours up to 6 weeks postpartum
3. Blood loss is more than 500 mL.

Primary PPH—Causes

1. Atonic uterus—grand multipara, overdistention, malnutrition and anemia, APH, prolonged labor, anesthesia, malformation of the uterus, uterine fibroid, mismanaged 3rd stage, constriction ring, precipitate labor.
2. Traumatic
3. Combined
4. Blood coagulation disorders
   Management—uterus flabby—massage the uterus, injection methergine, oxytocin drip, to examine the expelled placenta, to catheterize the bladder—exploration of the uterus—blood transfusion and continue oxytocin drip—injection PGF2a (IM or intramyometrial)—bimanual compression—intrauterine packing—uterine artery ligation—internal iliac ligation—hysterectomy.

Secondary PPH—Causes

1. Retained placenta and membranes (the most common)
2. Infection
3. Subinvolution
4. Secondary hemorrhage from CS wound
5. Withdrawal bleeding following estrogen therapy to suppress the lactation
6. Rare causes—chorion epithelioma, CA cervix, placental polyp, infected fibroid, puerperal inversion.

Postpartum Hemorrhage—Management (Hemostasis Algorithm)

1. General medical management:
   H-Ask for Help
   A-**A**ssess (vital parameters, blood loss) and resuscitate
   E-Establish etiology, ecbolics, ensure availability of blood:
   i. **E**stablish etiology—4 Ts—tone, tissue, trauma, thrombin
   ii. **E**cbolics (syntometrine, ergometrine, bolus syntocinin)
   iii. **E**nsure availability of blood and blood products
   M-**M**assage the uterus
   O-**O**xytocin infusion, prostaglandins (intravenous, rectal, intramuscular, intramyometrial)
2. *Specific surgical treatment*:
   S : **S**hift to operation theater; bimanual compression; antishock garment especially if transfer is required
   T : **T**issue and **t**rauma to be excluded and proceed to **T**amponade using Sengstaken tube or condom, uterine packing
   A : **A**pply compression sutures
   S : **S**ystematic pelvic devascularization (uterine, ovarian, internal iliac)
   I : **I**nterventional radiology, uterine artery embolization
   S : **S**ubtotal or total hysterectomy.

Prevention of PPH

1. Correct anemia antenatally
2. High-risk pregnanacies should be managed at tertiary centers
3. Arrange adequate blood
4. Active management of 3rd stage.

Active Management of Third Stage

1. Early cord clamping
2. Prophylactic oxytocics
3. Deliver placenta by controlled cord traction (Brandt-Andrew's method)
4. Uterine massage.

ECTOPIC PREGNANCY

Triad

1. Amenorrhea, abdominal pain, vaginal bleeding
2. The most common site—ampulla and the most common cause—pelvic inflammatory disease (PID).

Criteria

1. Studdiford criteria—primary abdominal pregnancy
2. Spiegelberg criteria—ovarian pregnancy
3. Paalman and Mc Elin criteria (Rubin's)—cervical pregnancy.

Treatment of Ectopic Pregnancy

Drugs: Methotrexate, KCL, hyperosmolar glucose, Ru-486.
Surgery: Linear salpingostomy, linear salpingotomy, salpingectomy, milking of tube.

Indication of Methotrexate in Ectopic Pregnancy

1. Patient hemodynamically stable
2. Tubal diameter < 4 cm without cardiac activities
3. Beta hCG level < 10,000.

Tubal Rupture

Most common Isthmus	:	6–8 weeks
Ampulla	:	8–12 weeks
Interstitial (very late)	:	16 weeks.

MNEMONICS

Abdominal Pain: Causes during Pregnancy LARACROFT

1. **L**abor
2. **A**bruption of placenta
3. **R**upture (e.g. ectopic/uterus)
4. **A**bortion
5. **C**holestasis
6. **R**ectus sheath hematoma
7. **O**varian tumor
8. **F**ibroids
9. **T**orsion of uterus.

Alpha-fetoprotein: Causes for Increased Maternal Serum AFP during Pregnancy

Increased **m**aternal **s**erum **a**lpha **f**eto**p**rotein:
1. **I**ntestinal obstruction
2. **M**ultiple gestation/Miscalculation of gestational age/myeloschisis
3. **S**pina bifida cystica
4. **A**nencephaly/abdominal wall defect
5. **F**etal death
6. **P**lacental abruption.

Postpartum Hemorrhage Risk Factors

PARTUM

1. **P**rolonged labor/**p**olyhydramnios/**p**revious cesarean
2. **A**PH
3. **R**ecent history of bleeding
4. **T**wins (Multiple pregnancy)
5. **U**terine fibroids
6. **M**ultiparity.

Multiple Pregnancy: Complications

HI, PAPA

1. **H**ydramnios
2. **I**UGR
3. **P**reterm labor
4. **A**ntepartum hemorrhage
5. **P**re-eclampsia
6. **A**bortion.

Biophysical Profile: Constituents

Monitor **f**etus **t**o **c**onfirm **v**iability:

1. **M**ovement of fetal body
2. **F**etal respiratory movements
3. **T**one of the fetus
4. **C**TG monitoring of fetal heart rate (Nonstress test)
5. **V**olume of amniotic fluid (Amniotic fluid index).

Shapes of Female Pelvis

GAP

1. **G**ynecoid
2. **A**ndroid
3. **P**latypelloid.

Endometrial Carcinoma: Risk Factors

ENDOMET

1. **E**lderly
2. **N**ulliparity
3. **D**iabetes mellitus
4. **O**besity
5. **M**enstrual irregularity
6. **E**strogen therapy
7. Hyper**T**ension.

Endometriosis: Symptoms

5 'Ds

1. **D**ysmenorrhea
2. **D**isorders of menstruation
3. **D**yspareunia
4. **D**yschezia
5. **D**ull ache of abdomen.

5
CHAPTER

Gynecology

DYSFUNCTIONAL UTERINE BLEEDING

Symptoms

Cause of menorrhagia, polymenorrhea, polymenorrhagia, metrorrhagia, postcoital bleeding per vaginum, pre- or postmenstrual spotting.

History of Past Illness

1. History of dysmenorrhea, whitish discharge per vagina (p/v), passage of clots, spontaneous abortion prior to the present illness and whether curettage was done after abortion
2. History of D and C, sterilization, intrauterine contraceptive device (IUCD) insertion, sex steroid therapy for any reason
3. History of response to sex steroid therapy
4. History of bleeding disorders in past or in the family
5. History of administration of anticoagulants for any reason
6. History of tuberculosis (TB) or contact with TB, history of diabetes mellitus (DM)
7. History suggestive of hypo- or hyperthyroidism.

General Examination

Pallor, goiter, clinical evidence of hypo- or hyperthyroidism and bleeding disorders.

Systemic Examination

Refer supplementary book (SYNAPZ: The Complete Final MBBS Manual).

Abdominal Examination

Refer supplementary book (SYNAPZ: The Complete Final MBBS Manual).

Bimanual Pelvic Examination

1. **Uterus:** Size, shape, consistency, contour and mobility
2. **Ovarian tumors:** Granulosa cell tumor, theca cell tumor
3. **Ovarian enlargement:** Polycystic ovarian disease, corpus luteum cyst
4. Adnexal thickening, tenderness, tubo-ovarian masses
5. Carcinoma of cervix.

Speculum Examination

1. Cervical score, bleeding from uterine cavity, cervical erosion, ulcer, carcinoma
2. Cervical polyp, uterine polyp projecting through the cervix.

Per Rectum Examination

To stage cervical carcinoma.

Investigations

1. Hemogram including platelet count
2. Coagulation profile, thyroid function test (TFT)
3. Abdominopelvic ultrasonography (USG)
4. Exfoliative cytology—smear from cervix and posterior fornix of vagina
5. Endometrial cytology
6. Hysteroscopy with biopsy from suspicious area
7. Hysterography
8. *Endometrial histopathology*: Vibra aspirator, D and C

Dysfunctional uterine bleeding (DUB): Abnormal uterine bleeding occurring not associated with any organic cause present in the pelvis.

Treatment

1. Conservative
   a. Oral iron therapy
   b. Systemic iron therapy and blood transfusion
   c. Hormone therapy—oral contraceptive pills (OCPs)
   d. Progestrogens
   e. Progesterone impregnated intrauterine contraceptive devices (Mirena)
   f. Danazol (contraindicated in young women)
   g. Nonsteroidal anti-inflammatory drugs (NSAIDs) mefanamic acid
   h. Antifibrinolytic (tranexamic acid)
   i. Clomiphene citrate for anovulatory cycles
   j. Ethamsylate—efficacy not proven by studies
   k. Gonadotropin-releasing hormone (GnRH) analogs
2. Surgical
   a. D and C
   b. Hysterectomy
3. Minimal invasive surgery
   a. Hysteroscopic endometrial ablation by Nd:YAG
   b. Radiofrequency induced thermal endometrial ablation
   c. Balloon therapy
   d. Microwave endometrial ablation.

Classification

Anovulatory	Ovulatory
Threshold bleeding of puberty menorrhagia	Irregular ripening
Metropathia hemorrhagica	Irregular shedding
Premenopausal DUB	IUCD insertion

DUB-Spasmodic Dysmenorrhea (Primary)

1. No identifiable pelvic pathology
2. Mostly confined to adolescents
3. Almost always confined to ovulatory cycle
4. Pain usually cured following pregnancy and delivery
5. Appears within 2 years of menarche
6. Affluent society
7. Pain appears on 1st day of menstrual period
8. Pain usually lasts for 12 hours
9. Never persists beyond 48 hours.

Congestive Dysmenorrhea (Secondary)

1. Pain in presence of pelvic pathology
2. Patient is usually of thirties and often parous
3. For example, pelvic inflammatory disease (PID), endometriosis, adenomyosis, uterine fibroid, endometrial polyp, IUCD.

Definitions

1. Menorrhagia—bleeding either excessive (> 80 mL) or duration or both
2. Epimenorrhea (polymenorrhea)—cycle is reduced to 21 days or less
3. Epimenorrhagia—frequent cycles with excessive and prolonged bleeding
4. Metrorrhagia—irregular acyclic bleeding
5. Oligomenorrhea—bleeding occurs more than 35 days apart
6. Hypomenorrhea—bleeding lasts for less than 2 days.

Diagnostic Criteria for Menopause

1. Cessation of menstruation for consecutive 6 months during climacteric
2. Appearance of menopausal symptom
3. Vaginal cytology—10/85/5
4. Serum estradiol < 20 pg/mL
5. Serum FSH and LH > 40 mIU/mL.

GENITAL PROLAPSE

Symptoms

Cause of mass coming down from vaginum, difficulty in passing urine.

History

1. History of chronic (c/c) cough, constipation, lifting heavy weights, straining for micturition
2. History of dysuria, frequency of micturition, urgency, inability to pass urine until the prolapse has been reduced
3. Abdominal pain—dull aching, backache, worse towards the end of the day
4. History of urinary stress incontinence
5. History of leukorrhea, metrorrhagia, postcoital spotting (suggestive of decubitus ulcer on the cervix)
6. History of irreducibility (due to edema and congestion, retension of urine, bladder stone, pregnancy, impacted feces)
7. History of use of pessary
8. History suggestive of neurological disorder (nulliparous prolapse)
9. History suggestive of renal dysfunction
10. History of past attempts at repair of prolapse
11. History of hysterectomy in the past suggestive of posthysterectomy vault prolapse or vaginal wall prolapse.

Obstetric History

1. Home deliveries
2. Unattended deliveries
3. Forceps or vacuum deliveries and birth weight of babies
4. Resumption of household work soon after delivery
5. Interval between deliveries.

Menstrual History

Menopause attained or not, desire to retain menstrual status, desire to preserve the reproductive function and sexual function.

Examination

1. General condition, vitals and systemic examination (respiratory system for evidence of chronic obstructive pulmonary disease (COPD) or chronic infection) weight, spine for spina bifida (nulliparous prolapse)
2. Abdominal wall muscle tone is checked if abdominal suspensory operation is planned
3. Bimanual palpation of kidney to detect hydronephrosis, liver, spleen and kidney are palpated in case of nulliparous prolapse.

Local Examination

1. *Inspection*: Vulva; genital hiatus (urethral orifice to posterior fourchette); leading part (mostly cervix).
2. *Palpation*: Presence of pigmentation, ulceration, rugosity, erosion, discharge; describe the mass and tone of levator ani.

Speculum Examination

1. Degree of uterine prolapse
2. Degree of rectocele, cystocele, enterocele, urethrocele
3. *Condition of the perineum*: Lax with intact skin but torn perineal body
4. Urinary stress incontinence
5. Decubitus ulcer on cervix—site, size, shape, base, discharge, tenderness
6. Condition of cervix—hypertrophic, eroded, infected, keratinized uterocervical length, supravaginal elongation of cervix
7. Condition of vaginal mucosa—healthy, infected, atrophic.

Vaginal Examination

1. Uterine size, shape, consistency and mobility
2. Presence of pelvic masses
3. Tone and activity of levator ani and bulbospongiosus
4. Integrity of the perineal body.

Rectal Examination

To judge the strength of the uterosacral and cardinal ligaments.

Investigations

1. Hemogram, urinalysis, urine culture, colony count and antibiotic sensitivity
2. Blood urea nitrogen, serum creatinine
3. Chest radiograph—posteroanterior (PA) view
4. Excretory urography; viscerogram, cervical exfoliative cytology.

Diagnosis

Investigation

Lab findings: Hemoglobin, urine routine examination, blood urea, blood sugar, urine culture, high vaginal swab, chest X-ray, electrocardiogram (ECG).

Treatment

Conservative

Pessary-indicated

1. Before/during/after pregnancy
2. Preoperative period
3. In those people unfit for surgery.

Disadvantages of pessary

1. Only palliative not curative
2. Can cause vaginitis and dyspareunia
3. Must be changed every 3 months
4. Cannot be retained in patulous vagina
5. Does not cure stress incontinence.

Operative

1. Anterior colporrhaphy—repair cystocele and cystourethrocele
2. Kelly's plication—bladder incontinence
3. Posterior colporrhaphy and colpoperineorrhaphy—correct rectocele and repair deficient perineum

4. Fothergill's operation
   a. Preliminary D and C
   b. Amputation of cervix
   c. Sturmdorf suture
   d. Plication of Mackenrodt's ligament (Fothergill's stitch)
   e. Anterior colporrhaphy
   f. Colpoperineorrhaphy
5. Shirodkar's procedure—same as Fothergill's but cervix is not amputated this is to preserve child bearing function.

Treatment of Prolapse

Anterior colporrhaphy, posterior colporrhaphy and colpoperineorrhaphy with pelvic floor repair.

Vaginal Hysterectomy

Clamps
1. Pedicles containing Mackenrodt's and uterosacral ligament close to cervix
2. Uterine vessels
3. Upper portion of broad ligament holding the uterus containing round and ovarian ligament and fallopian tube.

Vaginal hysterectomy (VH) with pelvic floor repair (PFR) indications
1. UV prolapse in postmenopausal women
2. Genital prolapse in perimenopausal age group with dysfunctional uterine bleeding, unhealthy cervix or small fibroid
3. As an alternative to abdominal cyst or Fothergill operation or laparoscopically assisted vaginal hysterectomy (LAVH).

Complications

1. Hemorrhage
2. Anesthetic complications
3. Trauma to bladder and rectum
4. Sepsis
5. Urinary tract infection (UTI)
6. Vault prolapse.

Other Operative Procedures

Abdominal sling operations
1. Abdominocervicopexy Shirodkar's abdominal sling operation
2. Khanna's abdominal sling operation Moschcowitz's repair for enterocele
3. Le Fort's operation—old age with procidentia when the patient is unfit for longer duration of surgery.

Treatment for Vault Prolapse

1. Right transvaginal sacrospinous colpopexy
2. Colpocleisis sacral colpopexy
3. Laparoscopic colpopexy
4. Transabdominal
5. Ring pessary.

Treatment for Decubitus Ulcer

1. Cytology and biopsy from the site to rule out carcinoma cervix (Ca/Cx)
2. Clean the edge and the ulcer heals on reposition and vaginal packing.

Differential diagnosis of prolapse uterus
1. Congenital elongation of cervix
2. Cervical fibroid polyp
3. Cyst of anterior vaginal wall
4. Urethral diverticula.

Uterine descent (Grading of prolapse)
1°-descent of cervix into vagina
2°-descent of cervix up to introitus
3°-descent of cervix outside introitus
Procidentia—all of the uterus outside the introitus.

Sulci in Vaginal Wall

Submeatal sulcus, bladder sulcus, transverse sulcus of anterior vaginal wall.

Causes of Prolapse

1. Atonicity and asthenia—follow menopause due to estrogen deficiency
2. Birth injury
3. Peripheral nerve injury
4. Home delivery
5. Heavy work soon after delivery
6. Unmarried or nulliparous women
7. Ventouse extraction of fetus before the cervix is fully dilated
8. Delivery of big baby
9. Rapid succession of pregnancies
10. Raised intra-abdominal pressure
11. Postoperative like abdominoperineal excision of rectum
12. Radical vulvectomy.

Classification of Prolapse

Anterior vaginal wall

1. *Upper 2/3rd*: Cystocele
2. *Lower 1/3rd*: Urethrocele.

Posterior vaginal wall

1. *Upper 1/3rd*: Enterocele
2. *Lower 2/3rd*: Rectocele.

FIBROID OR OVARIAN TUMOR

Symptoms

1. Cause of lump in the lower abdomen
2. History of menstrual disturbances—menorrhagia (fibroids, endometrial carcinoma (Ca), feminizing tumors of ovary) amenorrhea (masculinizing tumors of ovary), metrorrhagia-submucous fibroid
3. History of infertility (uterine fibroids)
4. History of pain in the lower abdomen—acute (torsion of the ovarian tumor or subserous pedunculated uterine leiomyoma, hemorrhage into or from the tumor, acute pelvic infection, red degeneration) aching (malignant ovarian tumors), backache and sacral root pain (infilteration by malignant ovarian tumors)
5. Symptoms related to anemia
6. Loss of weight and appetite
7. History suggestive of pelvic inflammatory disease
8. History of defeminization, masculinization (virilizing ovarian tumors)
9. History of Ca breast in the past
10. History of female genital tract malignancy in the family/family history of fibroid
11. *History of pressure effects*: Frequency of micturition, retention of urine, edema of feet and vulva, varicose vein.
12. History suggestive of intestinal obstruction

Menstrual History

Obstetric History

History of OCP use/Cu-T/history of sterilization.

Treatment History

Examination

1. General condition, vital parameters, pallor, pedal edema, varicose vein, defeminization, virilization, supraclavicular lymph nodes and features of hermaphroditism.
2. Respiratory system (for evidence of TB or secondaries from pelvic malignancy).

Abdominal Examination

1. Degree of abdominal distention
2. *Umbilicus*: Distance from pubic symphysis and xiphisternum, shape (transversely stretched in ascitis and vertical in ovarian tumor)
3. Tenderness over lump or elsewhere (inflammation, hemorrhage, torsion, red degeneration)
4. Site, size, shape, surface, consistency and mobility of lump (lower border of pelvi-abdominal lump cannot be reached)
5. Hepatomegaly (metastases)
6. Percussion—dull note in central and lower abdomen tympanic in flanks—lump
7. Dull note in flanks, tympanic in center, shifting dullness—ascites
8. Para-aortic lymph nodes.

Bimanual Pelvic Examination

1. Catheterize bladder
2. Size of lump
3. Transmitted mobility
4. Position of lump with respect to uterus is noted.

Fixation of Tumor Indicates

Malignancy, endometriosis, intraligamentous growth, simultaneous inflammatory process, adhesion secondary to necrosis, impaction.

Investigations

1. Hemogram—Hemoglobin (Hb) (low in malignancy especially associated with bleeding PV), blood group
2. White blood cell (WBC) count (increased in infections, inflammation, red degeneration)
3. Ultrasonography—to differentiate between uterine and extrauterine masses/benign and malignant conditions and presence of ascitis
4. Electrocardiogram, liver function test, RFT-preoperative and prechemotherapy
5. Laparoscopy—adnexal mass of size small to moderate
6. Computed tomography (CT) scan for evaluation of ovarian Ca and metastasis
7. Nuclear magnetic resonance
8. Hysterography
9. X-ray chest posteroanterior (PA) view for metastasis
10. X-ray abdomen and pelvis anteroposterior (AP) view
11. Intravenous pyelography—in large abdominal mass and broad ligament fibroid
12. Abdominal paracentesis—biochemistry and exfoliative cytology
13. Tumor markers for ovarian tumors—β hCG, α FP carcinoembryonic antigen, Ca-125
14. Radionuclide imaging with I-125 labeled monoclonal antibody
15. Fine-needle aspiration cytology (FNAC) of pelvic mass
16. Exploratory laparotomy and frozen section.

Fibroid Uterine and Extrauterine

Uterine types	Degenerations
Intramural or interstitial	Hyaline
Submucous	Cystic
Subserous	Fatty
Submucous myxomatous polyp	Calcareous
	Red
	Leiomyosarcoma

Complications

1. Torsion
2. Capsular hemorrhage
3. Associated endometrial carcinoma
4. Inversion
5. Infection.

Differential Diagnosis (Varies according to Age and Marital Status)

1. Pregnancy
2. Adenomyosis
3. Endometriosis
4. Chronic PID
5. Malignant ovarian tumor
6. Myxomatous polyp
7. Pelvic kidney
8. Hematometra
9. Bicornuate uterus
10. Ectopic pregnancy
11. Benign ovarian tumor
12. Endometrial cancer
13. Chronic inversion.

Investigations

1. Hemoglobin
2. Ultrasonography (USG)
3. Hysteroscopy
4. Laparoscopy
5. CT scan
6. Blood group
7. Hysterosalpingography
8. D and C
9. Radiography.

Treatment

Medical	Surgical treatment
Iron therapy	Myomectomy
Mifepristone	Vaginal myomectomy
GnRH analogs	Hysteroscopic myomectomy
	Laparoscopic myomectomy
	Vaginal hysterectomy
	Laparoscopic hysterectomy
	Uterine artery embolization

Fibroid

1. Wandering or parasitic fibroid—subserous
2. Pseudocervical fibroid—fibroid polyp
3. Maximum symptoms—submucous
4. Lantern on dome of St Paul's—cervical fibroid.

Indications for Emergency Surgery in Fibroid

1. Torsion of subserous pedunculated fibroid
2. Massive intraperitoneal hemorrhage
3. Uncontrolled infected fibroid
4. Uncontrolled bleeding fibroid.

Indications for Surgery in Asymptomatic Fibroid

1. Size > 12 weeks
2. Diagnosis uncertain
3. Subserous pedunculated fibroid
4. Unexplained infertility
5. Unexplained recurrent abortion
6. Situated in lower part and likely to complicate delivery.

Ovarian Tumor

Investigations

1. Ultrasonography (USG)
2. Computed tomography (CT)
3. FNAC of solid tumors—nature of tumor
4. Magnetic resonance imaging (MRI)
5. Color flow Doppler
6. Ascitic tap for histopathological examination
7. Tumor markers—Ca-125 BRCA-1 AFP CEA, hCG, placental ALP, LDH
8. Staging laparotomy (overstaging of the disease so that proper treatment and better prognosis).

Management

1. Young girl 20 years—conservative ovariotomy; if peritoneal wash -ve no postoperative chemotherapy and if peritoneal wash +ve postoperative chemotherapy.
2. Perimenopausal women. Total abdominal hysterectomy (TAH) with bilateral salpingo-oophorectomy (BSO) with omentectomy.
3. Advanced cases—debulking surgery and removal of tumor [Postoperative chemotherapy (cisplatin, cyclophosphamide, vinblastin, paclitaxel) and radiotherapy depend on staging and type of tumor].

Clamps in Ovariotomy

1. Laterally—infandibulopelvic ligament
2. Middle—meso-ovarium
3. Medially—fallopian tube and ovarian ligament.

Benign Ovarian Tumors

Rx-unilateral ovariotomy/ovarian cystectomy/laparoscopic cystectomy/ovariotomy/laparoscopy/USG guided aspiration of cyst/abdominal hysterectomy and bilateral salpingo-oophorectomy (BSO).

Spread of Malignancy

1. Blood
2. Local
3. Lymphatic
4. Transcoelomic.

Complications

1. Axial rotation or torsion
2. Pseudomyoma of peritoneum
3. Extraperitoneal development
4. Rupture
5. Infection.

Ovarian Tumor

Findings	Benign	Malignant
Clinical	Size <10 cm Unilateral	Size >10 cm Bilateral
Consistency	Soft, cystic Mobile	Hard Fixed
Ascites	Absent	Present
Sec mass	Absent	Present/nodules in POD
Lymph node	Absent	Present
Ultrasonography (USG)	Thin-walled tumor Thin septa uniloculated	Thick wall Thick septa
Appearance	Black (liquid)	White (solid)
Volume	< 8 mL	> 8 mL
Cyst size	< 5 mm^3	> 5 mm^3
Doppler	Decreased blood flow	Increased blood flow

Prognostic factors in ovarian malignancy:

1. Stage—most important factor for survival
2. Histological grade
3. Volume of residual tumor should be < 1.5 to 2 cm
4. Ploidy status
5. Performance status
6. Age.

Krukenberg Tumor

1. Secondaries in ovary
2. Almost bilateral
3. Smooth freely mobile—no adhesion/infiltration
4. Retains shape of the ovary
5. Solid waxy consistency
6. Signet ring cells
7. Primary—stomach (70%), large bowel (15%), breast (6%).

Age Groups of Ovarian Tumors

1. Malignant epithelial tumors—40-60 years
2. Benign cystic teratoma—10-20 years
3. Dysgerminoma—< 20 years
4. Endodermal sinus tumor—15-20 years
5. Granulosa cell tumor—postmenopausal
6. Sertoli-Leydig cell tumor—20-30 years
7. Thecoma—postmenopausal.

1. Schiller-Duval bodies—endodermal sinus tumor
2. Signet ring cells—Krukenberg tumor
3. Coffee bean cells—granulosa cell tumor
4. Sertoli and Leydig cells—arrhenoblastoma
5. Psammoma bodies—papillary serous cystadenoma of ovary
6. Rokitansky's protuberance—dermoid cyst
7. Reinke's crystal—hilus cell tumor.

Staging of Ovarian Cancer

Stage 1: Limited to ovaries
  a. Growth limited to 1 ovary. No ascites, capsule intact.
  b. Growth limited to both ovaries. No ascites, capsule intact .
  c. Tumor either stage 1a or 1b with capsule rupture, ascites present with malignant cells or peritoneal washings positive.

Stage 2: Involving one or both ovaries with pelvic extension
  a. Extension or metastasis to uterus and tubes
  b. Extension to other pelvic tissues
  c. Tumor either 2a or 2b with capsule rupture, ascites present with malignant cells or peritoneal washings positive.

Stage 3: Tumor involving one or both ovaries with peritoneal implants outside the pelvis or positive retroperitoneal or inguinal lymph nodes. Superficial liver metastasis equals stage 3. Tumor is limited to true pelvis but with histologically proven malignant extension to small bowel or omentum.
  a. Tumor grossly limited to true pelvis with negative nodes but histologically confirmed microscopic seeding of abdominal peritoneal surfaces.
  b. Tumor involving one or both ovaries with histologically confirmed implants of abdominal peritoneal surfaces with none exceeding 2 cm in diameter. Nodes are negative.
  c. Abdominal implants > 2 cm in diameter or positive retroperitoneal or inguinal nodes.

Stage 4: Growth involving one or both ovaries with distant metastasis. If pleural effusion is present, there must be positive cytology to allot a case of stage 4. Parenchymal liver metastasis equals stage 4.

CARCINOMA OF CERVIX

History and Examination

1. History of present illness—complains of (C/o) irregular menses, menometrorrhagia, continuous bleeding, leukorrhea, blood stained discharge or offensive discharge, postcoital bleeding. C/o growth which bleeds on touch or ulcer—squamous cell cancer of ectocervix.
2. Menstrual history—irregular menses, menometrorrhagia.
3. Marital history—coitus before the age of 18 years; use of combined oral contraceptive pills and progestrogens over long periods can cause adenocarcinoma of cervix; multiple sex partners; exposure to smegma from uncircumcised partner.
4. Obstetric history—delivery of 1st baby before the age of 20 years; multiparity with poor birth spacing.
5. Past history—history of sexually transmitted diseases (STD), HIV infection, human papillomavirus (HPV) infection, herpes simplex infection. History of preinvasive lesions.

6. Personal history—poor personal hygiene.
7. Socioeconomic status—low.
8. Treatment history—history of transplant surgery for immunocompromised individual; history of irregular health check-ups and Pap smear.
9. Per vaginal examination—cervix reveals a growth or ulcer which bleeds on touch.

Investigations

1. *For diagnosis*: Pap smear, DNA study, colposcopy, cervicography, cone biopsy
2. *For staging*: Liver function test, renal function test, X-ray chest, IVP, cystoscopy, proctoscopy
3. *If operable preoperative work-up*: Blood group, hemogram, coagulation profile.

Differential Diagnosis

Cervical growth and ulcer (tubercular and syphilitic) fibroid polypus, sarcoma of cervix.

Staging

1. Carcinoma strictly confined to cervix
   a. Microinvasive ca1 a1 and ca1 a 2
2. Carcinoma spreads beyond Cx but not pelvic wall or lower 3rd of vagina
   a. Tumor without parametrial invasion
   b. Tumor with parametrial invasion
3. Tumor extends to lateral pelvic wall involves lower 3rd of vagina and/or functioning kidney
   a. Lower 3rd of vagina
   b. Extends to pelvic wall and involves kidney (hydronephrosis)
4. Metastasis
   a. Bladder/rectum/beyond the pelvis
   b. Widespread, distant metastasis.

Treatment

Carcinoma Cervix—Treatment

1. Stage 1a1—cone/simple hysterectomy—life long follow-up
2. Stage 1a2, 1b and 2a—radical hysterectomy with b/l pelvic lymphadenopathy, radiotherapy or combined therapy
3. Stage 2b—preoperative RT + surgery+ postoperative RT or only RT
4. Stage 3 and 4—only radiotherapy
5. Recurrent/persistant disease—RT in case initial treatment was surgery and surgery in case initial treatment was RT.

Radical Hysterectomy

1. *Wertheim's hysterectomy*: Exploration of abdomen, para-aortic lymph node biopsy, removal of entire uterus, both adnexae-pelvic lymph nodes, medial 1/3rd of parametrium upper 1/3rd of vagina.
2. *Extended vaginal hysterectomy*: Schuata's operation, Mitra's operation.

Carcinoma Cervix and Pregnancy

1. Incidence 1 in 2500 pregnancy
2. Most common malignancy in pregnancy
3. Cone biopsy may be necessary for confirmation
4. Microinvasive cancer—followed up to term
5. Advanced case—early pregnancy—treatment same as nonpregnant state
6. Late pregnancy—fetus is delivered by classical cesarean section + radical surgery or RT.

CARCINOMA OF ENDOMETRIUM

Symptoms

Menometrorrhagia in perimenopausal women, postmenopausal bleeding, bulky mass in abdomen

1. *Menstrual history*: Menometrorrhagia, postmenopausal bleeding
2. *Marital history*: Oral contraceptive pill has protective effect
3. *Obstetric history*: Infertile women or those with fewer children; PCOD patients are susceptible
4. *Past history*: History of hypertension and diabetes in 30% of cases, corpus cancer syndrome (obesity, hypertension, diabetes mellitus)
5. *Family history*: History of carcinoma due to genetic or dietetic habits. Lynch syndrome
6. *Treatment history*: Tamoxifen given to women with breast Ca are more prone to develop endometrial hyperplasia or cancer; unsupervised HRT with estrogen alone; Rx for cervical dysplasia by CO_2 laser or conization
7. *Abdominal examination*: Bulky uterus may be palpable due to fibroid or pyometra
8. Investigations:
   a. Pap smear—50–67%
   b. Endometrial aspiration cytology
   c. Fractional curettage
   d. Hysteroscopy
   e. Ultrasonography
   f. Cystoscopy—snow hill pattern, von Brunn's epithelial isles
   g. Others—CT, MRI, carcinoembryonic antigen (CEA), cytoplasmic steroid receptor, DNA ploidy.

Differential Diagnosis

1. Senile endometritis
2. Tubercular endometritis
3. Atypical endometrial hyperplasia
4. Lesions of the lower genital tract.

Treatment

1. *Prognostic factors*:
   a. Age at diagnosis
   b. Stage of tumor
   c. Grade of tumor
   d. Histological subtype
   e. Myometrial penetration
   f. Lymph node metastasis
   g. Peritoneal cytology.
2. *Treatment of Ca endometrium*:
   a. Stage 0 (endometrial hyperplasia) and stage 1a-abdominal hysterectomy with or without removal of ovaries
   b. All stages if possible — total abdominal hysterectomy + bilateral salpingo-oophorectomy, peritoneal washings, omental biopsy node sampling
   c. Stage 1b and 1c—add postoperative radiation
   d. Stage 2—surgery followed by postoperative radiotherapy (RT)
   e. Stage 3—if surgery possible (TAH+BSO+LN sampling + postoperative RT) if surgery not possible (radiotherapy) and stage 3c—whole body radiation
   f. Stage 4—(palliative therapy)—radiotherapy, chemotherapy, hormone therapy (large doses of progesterone).

VESICULAR MOLE (HYDATIDIFORM MOLE)

Symptoms

1. Amenorrhea, bleeding per vaginum, abdominal pain, hyperemesis
2. PIH < 24 weeks, passage of vesicles—rare
3. *Examination*: Uterine size more than period of amenorrhea
4. *Local examination*: Look for urethral nodule. Theca lutein cyst-P/V.

Investigations

1. Ultrasonography—snow storm appearance
2. Serum β-hCG—very high
3. *Chest X-ray*: To rule out lung metastasis
4. CT-brain and liver metastasis if suspected.

Classification

1. Benign
   a. GTD (Gestational trophoblastic disease)
   b. Hydatidiform mole—complete and partial.
2. Nonmetastatic malignant GTD
   a. Persistant GTD invasive mole
   b. Local choriocarcinoma.
3. Metastatic malignant GTD
   a. Good prognosis
      i. Duration of disease from termination of pregnancy to initiation of chemotherapy less than 4 months
      ii. Pretreatment urine hCG level less than 1000 IU/24 hours or serum β hCG < 40000 to 50000 mIU/mL
      iii. Metastatic disease limited to pelvis or lungs
      iv. No significant prior chemotherapy.
   b. Poor prognosis
      i. Duration of disease from termination of pregnancy to initiation of chemotherapy more than 6 months
      ii. High serum hCG levels > 50000 mIU/mL
      iii. Brain liver metastasis
      iv. Metastatic choriocarcinoma following a term pregnancy.

FIGO Anatomical Staging

1. *Stage 1*: Disease confined to uterus
2. *Stage 2*: Disease outside of uterus but limited to the genital structures
3. *Stage 3*: Disease extends to the lungs with or without known genital tract involvement
4. *Stage 4*: All other metastatic sites.

FIGO Prognostic Score

	0	1	2	4
Age (years)	< = 39	> 39		
Antecedent pregnancy	Hydatidiform mole	Abortion	Term pregnancy	
Interval from index pregnancy	< 4	4–6	7–12	> 12
Pre-treatment hCG	< 1000	1000–10,000	> 10,000–1,00,000	> 1,00,000
Largest tumor size + uterus	3–4 cm	5 cm		
Site of mets		Spleen, kidney	GI tract	Brain, liver
Previous failed chemotherapy			Single drug	2 or more drugs

Low-Risk Treatment Regime

1. Methotrexate/folinic acid—cycle repeated every 14 days
2. Methotrexate—50 mg by intramuscular injection repeated every 48 hours for a total of 4 doses
3. Folinic acid—15 mg orally 30 hours after each injection of methotrexate
4. Typical side effects—stomatitis, conjunctivitis, abdomen and chest pain.

High-Risk Treatment Regime

1. *Week 1, days 1 to 2*: Etoposide/actinomycin D/methotrexate + folinic acid rescue
2. *Week 2, day 8*: Vincristine/cyclophosphamide
3. *Typical side effects*: Myelosuppression (granulocyte colony stimulating factor used to prevent neutropenia and maintain dose intensity), nausea/vomiting , mucositis, reversible alopecia, neuropathy.

High-Risk Cases

1. Higher in eastern countries than in west
2. Blood group A
3. Young women and > 40-year-old women
4. Repeated incidence is 2%.

Prophylactic Chemotherapy in High-Risk Cases

1. Initial β-hCG > 1 lakh
2. Uterus > 24 weeks
3. Theca lutein cyst > 6 cm
4. Age > 40
5. Irregular follow-up.

Persistent Trophoblastic Disease

1. Serum hCG > 2 lakh IU after 4 weeks
2. Value double that of previous weeks
3. Plateauing, i.e. less than 10% fall in 3 consecutive weeks
4. Ultrasonography evidence of invasive mole
5. Uterus size or the theca lutein cyst not regressing
6. Histological evidence of invasive mole or choriocarcinoma
7. Persistence of β-hCG even at 12 weeks after evacuation
8. Metastasis to the lung or vagina.

Follow-up (For 2 Years)

1. Weekly β-hCG till 3 consecutive values are negative
2. Once a month for 3 months
3. Once in 3 months for next 9 months
4. Once in 6 months for next 1 year.

Indications for Hysterectomy

1. Advanced age (> 40 years) who have completed their family
2. Recurrent vesicular mole
3. Perforation/Life-threatening hemorrhage
4. Patient who may not come for follow-up.

Indications for Chemotherapy in GTD

1. Histological evidence of choriocarcinoma
2. Evidence of metastasis in brain, liver or GIT or radiological opacities > 2 cm on chest X-ray
3. Pulmonary, vulval or vaginal metastasis unless hCG falling
4. Heavy vaginal bleeding or evidence of GI or intraperitoneal hemorrhage
5. Rising hCG after evacuation
6. Serum hCG > 20,000 IU/L more than 4 weeks after evacuation because of risk of uterine perforation
7. Elevated hCG 6 months after evacuation even if still falling.

Chemotherapy

1. Methotrexate 1 mg/kg on days 1, 3, 5, 7 along with folinic acid 0.1 mg/kg on days 2, 4, 6, 8
2. Ideally values should fall by > 10%
3. Course may be repeated every 2 weeks. But do complete blood count (CBC), LFT, RFT in between
4. *Other drugs*: Actinomycin D 10–12 microgram/kg/day.

Pelvic Inflammatory Disease (PID)

Triad

1. Lower abdominal or pelvic pain (most common symptom)
2. Fever
3. Leukocytosis.

Criteria for Diagnosis of PID

1. Minimum criteria
   a. Lower abdominal tenderness
   b. Adnexial tenderness
   c. Cervical motion tenderness
2. Routine criteria
   a. Abnormal cervical or vaginal discharge
   b. ESR > 15 mm/hr
   c. Leukocytosis > 10,000 per mm^3
   d. Elevated C reactive protein
   e. Decreased or absent amylases in peritoneal fluid.

3. Elaborate criteria
   a. Histopathologic evidence of endometritis on endometrial biopsy
   b. Tubo-ovarian abscess on sonography or other radiographic test
   c. Laparoscopic abnormalities consistent with PID.

Criteria for Hospitalization of Patient with Acute Pelvic Inflammatory Disease (PID)

1. Suspected pelvic abscess
2. Severe illness, temperature > 38°C
3. Uncertain diagnosis
4. Unresponsive to outpatient therapy for 48 hours
5. Intolerance to oral antibiotics
6. Co-existing pregnancy
7. Patient known to have HIV infection
8. Patient is an adolescent.

Inpatient Antibiotic Therapy

1. Cefoxitin 2 g IV 6th hourly or cefotetan 2 g IV 12th hourly + doxycycline 100 mg orally or IV 12th hourly
2. Clindamycin 900 mg IV 8th hourly + gentamicin + metronidazole.

Indications for Surgery

1. Generalized peritonitis
2. Pelvic abscess
3. Tubo-ovarian abscess which does not respond to antibiotic therapy (48–72 hours).

OPERATIVE PROCEDURES

Lower Segment Cesarean Section

Preoperative Preparation

1. Get informed consent
2. Nil per orally after 10 pm
3. Tab rantac 150 mg at 7 am
4. Tab reglan 10 mg (metoclopramide) at 7 am
5. Tab alprax 0.5 mg hora somni (HS) (at bed time) (optional)
6. Inj pethidine 40 to 60 mg/inj morphine 8 mg intramuscular (IM) 1 hour prior to surgery
7. Inj phenergan 12.5 mg intramuscular (IM)
8. Inj cephazolin 1 g IV stat at 7 am
9. Prepare the patient (shaving).

On Table

1. IV line set-up with 16 G cannula
2. Anesthesia—subarachnoid block (spinal anesthesia) at L3-L4
3. Dorsal position
4. Catheterize the bladder
5. Drape the abdomen with betadine
6. Incision—pfannenstiel (suprapubic transverse incision)
7. Incision deepened, cut through subcutaneous fat, rectus sheath, rectus muscles separated
8. Doyen's retractor introduced to retract the bladder
9. Lower segment of uterus identified by white shiny uterovesical fold of peritoneum
10. Cut the peritoneum over the lower segment
11. Curvilinear incision put over the lower segment (max of 10 cm)
12. Cut through amniotic sac along with suction of amniotic fluid
13. Baby delivered by hooking the head between fingers
14. Secretions are suctioned only then rest of the baby is delivered
15. Cord is clamped and baby handed over

16. Wait for spontaneous separation of placenta
17. Before closing the uterus put finger to check the internal os if opened (should be opened for flow of blood)
18. Uterus closed in single layers continuous with vicryl (1-0)
19. Approximate the muscles by putting 1 or 2 interrupted cat gut sutures
20. Verify no of instruments and mops
21. Rectus sheath sutured with nonabsorbable prolene. The last knot should be buried deep in the muscle
22. Approximate the subcutaneous tissue (cat gut)
23. Skin sutured with interrupted mattress sutures (black silk)
24. Vaginal toileting done and note for any bleeding
25. Check the catheterized urine.

Postoperative Orders

1. 4th hourly temperature charting
2. BP, pulse ½ hourly
3. Catheterization of the bladder continued for 24 hours
4. Inj cefazolin 1 g BD IV for 5 days
5. IV fluids—1 pint RL, 2 pint NS and 2 pint 5% D
6. Inj phenergan 12.5 mg HS and si opus sit (SOS) (when required)
7. Early ambulation
8. Inj metrogyl 500 mg IV Q8H
9. Inj pethidine 40 mg HS and SOS
10. Early breastfeeding
11. Educate about sterilization.

Vaginal Hysterectomy

Indications

1. 3° prolapse
2. Only when patient insists for correction
3. Fibroids < 14 weeks size.

Preoperative Preparations

Same as in cesarean section.

On Table

1. Lithotomy position
2. Subarachnoid block (SAB)
3. Drape the area with betadine
4. Drain the bladder (catheterize)
5. Catch hold of the anterior lip of Cx—pull it down
6. Put an inverted T shaped incision on bladder sulcus
7. Reflect the anterior vaginal wall by dissecting through vesicovaginal space (bloodless space)
8. Cut the vesicocervical ligament (or fascia) and then push the bladder up
9. Extend the incision all around (make it circular)
10. Cut through the posterior vaginal wall and reflect it
11. Cut through the posterior rectovaginal peritoneum and enter the pouch of Douglas (take care not to injure the enterocele)
12. Insinuate the fingers through this and extend it till anterior peritoneal covering of uterus and then cut the uterovesical peritoneum
13. Put 3 clamps
    a. 1st clamp at Mackenrodt's and uterocervical ligament
    b. 2nd clamp—uterine artery
    c. 3rd clamp—round ligament, tube, ovarian ligament
14. Cut and ligate all these clamps bilateral.

Correction of Enterocele

1. Excise the redundant part of pouch of Douglas and suture it (purse string suture)
2. Approximate and suture the medial portion of uterosacral ligament.

Correction of Rectocele

1. Excise the lax vagina over the rectocele and rectovaginal fascia tightened after pushing the rectocele
2. Vagina sutured.

Colpoperineorrhaphy

Approximation and suturing of medial fibers of levator ani.

Anterior Colporrhaphy

Vesicovaginal fascia tightened and excess vaginal wall excised to correct laxity. vaginal wall sutured.

Stress Incontinence—Kelly's Suture

1. Vault repair—approximate the vault with uterosacral and Mackenrodt's ligament
2. Urine drained—catheter put
3. Vaginal pack kept.

Postoperative Orders

Same as in cesarean section.

Episiotomy

Structures Cut during Episiotomy

1. Posterior vaginal wall
2. Superficial and deep transverse perineal muscles
3. Bulbospongiosus
4. Part of levator ani
5. Fascia covering those muscles
6. Transverse perineal branches of pudendal vessels and nerves
7. Subcutaneous tissue and skin.

OBJECTIVE STRUCTURED CLINICAL EXAMINATION QUESTIONS

Drugs

1. Misoprostol—uses, side effects, complications
2. $MgSO_4$—indications, complications, mechanism of action, methods to assess toxicity
3. Oxytocin—indications and contraindications
4. OCP—ingredients, advantages, contraindications
5. Methergine—dose, route of administration, contraindications
6. Alpha methyl dopa—uses
7. Nifedipine—uses
8. Iron tablets—dosage, duration
9. Folic acid—dose in first trimester, late pregnancy, uses
10. Calcium supplements—dose, requirement
11. Methotrexate—uses, contraindications.

Instruments

1. Uterine sound—uses, complications
2. Dilators (Hegar)—uses, complications
3. Speculum-Sims—uses, advantages, disadvantages
4. Forceps—criteria to be satisfied, adverse effects, side identification
5. Menstrual regulation syringe with Karman cannula—identify, uses, complications

6. Vacuum cup—identify, uses, criteria to be satisfied
7. Cu T—copper T and other intrauterine devices (IUDs), contraindications, complications, advantages of medicated IUCDs over others, mechanism of insertion, noncontraceptive uses
8. Vulsellum—uses
9. Uterine curette—uses, complications
10. Punch biopsy forceps—uses; 2 other methods for screening the disease
11. Episiotomy scissors—identify, structures cut during episiotomy
12. Ovum forceps—identify, uses
13. Leech Wilkinson cannula—identify, uses.

Specimens

1. Ovarian cyst—complications
2. Endometrial carcinoma—method of diagnosis
3. Submucous fibroid—identify, complications; treatment-4 methods
4. Total abdominal hysterectomy (TAH) specimen with vesicular mole *in situ*—identify; confirmation of diagnosis; 2 tests or follow-up; 2 complications; 2 indications for hysterectomy
5. TAH with BSO specimen fibroid (all 3 types)—age group of patient; complications
6. TAH + BSO with papillary cystadenoma of ovary—identify; differentiate between benign and malignant; complications
7. TAH showing ruptured uterus—signs and symptoms of this condition; causes.

Charts

Cardiotocography (CTG)

1. Baseline heart rate—range of commonly repeated heart values within 6 to 7 beats
2. Beat-to-beat variability—expressed as (positive/negative) if the baseline is concentrated around 2 or 3 values only
3. Acceleration—increase by 15 beats or more from the current value (or lower value in baseline) on fetal movement or by artificial stimulation using VAST (instrument causing vibratory stress)
4. Expressed as acceleration present (up to beats/min)
5. Deceleration expressed as present or absent.

Partogram

1. Graphical record of progress of labor
2. Details, advantages, alert line, action line
3. WHO partogram.

INFERTILITY

1. Definition : Failure to conceive after one year of unprotected coitus
2. Primary infertility : Couples have never conceived
3. Secondary infertility : Conceived at least once in past.

Etiology

Male Factor

1. *Defective spermatogenesis*: Chromosomal (Klinefelter syndrome), cryptorchidism, hypogonadotropic hypogonadism, endocrine, infections (mumps orchitis), gonadotoxic factors (exposure to excessive heat, alcohol, smoking, anabolic steroids, cytotoxic drugs, nitrofurantoin), sertoli cell only syndrome, germ cell failure, testicular trauma, torsion, varicocele.
2. *Impaired sperm transport*: Obstructive azoospermia, impaired sperm motility (congenital/acquired).
3. *Sexual dysfunction*: Anatomical (hypospadias), ejaculatory abnormalities (retrograde ejaculation, premature ejaculation), impotence (psychogenic/organic), drugs (antidepressants, tranquilizers).

Female Factor

1. *Tubal factor*: Blocked tube due to PID, TB, endometriosis, adhesions
2. *Ovarian factor*: PCOS, dysgenesis/agenesis of ovary, luteal phase defect, luteinized unruptured follicle, hyperprolactinemia, premature ovarian failure
3. *Cervical factor*: Stenosis, cervicitis, hostile cervical mucous, immunological
4. *Uterine factor*: Tuberculosis, fibroids, intrauterine adhesions, anomalies, hypoplasia
5. *Systemic factor*: Diabetes, hypopituitarism, thyroid dysfunction.

Case Taking

Female Partner

History

1. Duration of infertility
2. Menstrual history—age at menarche, interval, duration, quantity and regularity
3. Symptoms of ovulation—premenstrual symptom, midcycle pain, spotting, increased discharge and dysmenorrhea
4. Contraceptive history
5. Sexual history—technique of coitus, use of artificial lubricant, postcoital douche, dyspareunia
6. Past obstetric history—Medical termination of pregnancy (MTP), abortion, delivery with complications
7. History regarding galactorrhea, hirsutism
8. Past medical history—PID, tuberculosis, diabetes, thyroid dysfunction
9. Past surgical history—pelvic surgery, appendicectomy, vaginal operations.

Examination

1. *General examination*: Body habitus (obese, anorexia), endocrine abnormalities, hirsutism and breast for galactorrhea
2. *Pelvic examination*: Inspection-pubic hair distribution, size of clitoris:
   a. P/S examination—cervix for pinhole os, infection, erosion, laceration and mucous quality
   b. Bimanual examination—uterus-size, shape, position and tenderness, ovaries, parametrial thickening and masses in adnexa
   c. Rectal examination—for endometriosis.

Investigations

1. *Routine*: Complete blood count (CBC), erythrocyte sedimentation rate, URE, Venereal Disease Research Laboratory and investigations for TB
2. *Ovarian factor*: Ultrasonogram, basal body temperature (BBT), endometrial biopsy, D and C
3. *Tubal factor*: Hysterosalpingogram, laparoscopy
4. *Cervical factor*: Cervical mucous, postcoital test, immunological testing
5. *Uterine factor*: Hysterosalpingogram (HSG), ultrasonography (USG), laparoscopy, D and C, hysteroscopy.

Male Partner

History

1. Duration of infertility
2. *Sexual history*: Technique, frequency of coitus, sexual dysfunction
3. Exposure to heat—hot baths, tight underwears, occupational
4. *Past history*: Tuberculosis, diabetes, liver disease, mumps, sexually transmitted diseases (STDs)
5. *Treatment history*:
   a. Drugs—nitrofurantoin, cimetidine, ketoconazole, betablockers, antihypertensives, phenytoin, imipramine, irradiation
   b. Surgery on gonads, inguinoscrotal operations (hernia, hydrocele)
6. *Personal history*: Alcohol, smoking, exposure to toxins
7. Past marital status.

Examination

1. *General examination*: Height, weight, BP, secondary sexual characters (body habitus, gynecomastia, hair pattern)
2. *Urological*:
   a. Testis size and consistency
   b. Epididymis and vas
   c. Penis size, urethral meatus.

Investigations

1. *Routine*: Hemoglobin, total count (TC), differential count (DC), ESR, urine routine examination, postprandial blood sugar (PPBS), VDRL
2. *Semen examination*: Produced preferably by masturbation collected in a wide mouthed clean glass bottle
3. *Hormonal assay*: Follicle-stimulating hormone (FSH), luteinizing hormone (LH), testosterone
4. Testicular biopsy
5. Scrotal Doppler
6. Antisperm antibody testing
7. Semen penetration assay.

Normal Semen Study

1. Volume 2 to 5 mL
2. pH Alkaline (7.2–8)
3. Liquification Within 30 min
4. Sperm conc > 20 million/mL
5. Total sperm count ≥ 40 million/ejaculate
6. Motility > 50% progressively motile
7. Morphology > 30% normal
8. Viability > 70% live
9. WBC < 1 million/mL
10. Fructose > 120 mg%

No significant sperm agglutination.

Management

Female Partner

1. *Anovulation*: Clomiphene citrate, letrozole, gonadotropins
2. *Tubal factor*: Laparoscopic surgery, microsurgery (adhesionolysis, end-to-end anastomosis, implantation, fimbrioplasty), hysteroscopic canulation for corneal block, medical Rx for TB and endometriosis
3. *Uterine factor*: Hysteroscopic adhesionolysis, myomectomy, polypectomy, septum resection, metroplasty operation in bicornuate uterus
4. *Cervical factor*: Medical treatment for cervicitis, IUI
5. Improving general health of patient, treatment of systemic illness.

Male Partner

Treatment of identifiable causes

1. Avoid gonadotoxic factors—exposure to heat, harmful drugs, chemical toxins, alcohol intake and smoking
2. Treatment of genital tract infections, diabetes, thyroid disease and hypoprolactinemia
3. Management of varicocele
4. Ejaculatory disturbances—sympathomimetic drugs, electroejaculation
5. Immunological—intermittent steroids
6. Obstructive azoospermia—microsurgical reconstructive surgery.

Medical Therapy

1. Clomiphene citrate
2. Androgens
3. Gonadotropins
4. Sperm vitalizing therapy.

Assisted Reproductive Technology

1. *In vitro* fertilization (IVF) and embryo transfer (ET)
2. Zygote intrafallopian transfer (ZIFT)
3. Gamete intrafallopian transfer (GIFT)
4. Intracytoplasmic sperm injection (ICSI)
5. Intrauterine insemination (IUI).

6 CHAPTER Pediatrics

CARDIOVASCULAR SYSTEM

Congenital Heart Disease

History of Present Illness

Left to right

1. Frequent chest infection
2. Effort intolerance
3. Palpitation
4. Dyspnea—older children
5. Increased head sweating
6. Feeding difficulty (Inability to suck continuously)
7. Rapid labored breathing
8. Excessive cry
9. Chest pain
10. Visible precordial pulsation
11. Growth failure (due to interrupted feeding and more calories for breathing)
12. Facial puffiness.

Right to left

1. Bluish discoloration of skin, lips, palm
2. Cyanotic spell (convulsion, loss of consciousness)
3. Squatting episodes
4. Swelling of fingertips (clubbing).

History suggestive of infective endocarditis

1. History of fever with chills
2. Petechial hemorrhages
3. Hematuria
4. Hemoptysis
5. Dental procedures or surgery.

History suggestive of congestive cardiac failure (CCF)

1. Orthopnea relieved by putting on shoulder
2. History of breathlessness/cyanosis
3. Excessive perspiration over head on feeding (↓ Cardiac output → Sympathetic stimulation)
4. History of suck—rest—suck cycle
5. History of decreased intake during feeds
6. Edema over legs or body
7. History of repeated respiratory tract infection (RTI)
8. Failure to thrive
9. History of abdominal distention/pain.

Past History

1. Diagnosed soon after birth
2. Exact time of detection.

Antenatal/natal/postnatal

1. Diabetes mellitus
2. Alcoholism
3. Fever with rash in intrauterine period
4. Drug intake (Phenytoin, Valproate) and alcohol
5. Metabolic factor—hypercalcemia
6. Birth at high altitude
7. History of cyanosis.

Development

1. Developmental delay
2. Gross motor delayed
3. Regression during CCF episodes.

Dietetic

Feeding difficulty, deficiency may be present.

Family History

1. **Whether normal at birth:** History of consanguinity
2. **History of treatment:** History of genetic disease like Marfan, Ehlers Danlos Syndrome, Hurler
3. History of chronic illness in the sibling
4. History of sudden death
5. History of rheumatic fever.

Socioeconomic status

1. *Place of living*: High altitude
2. *Diabetic mother*: Assymetrical septal defect.

Examination

Left to right	Right to left
Cleft lip/palate	Polycythemia
Precordial bulge	Cyanosis
	Clubbing

Examination

Head to Foot

1. Look for feature of chromosomal anomalies (Downs)
2. All pulses better palpable in PDA
3. Feature of infective endocarditis
4. Collapsing pulse in PDA
5. High volume pulse in patent ductus arteriosus (PDA)/ventricular septal defect (VSD)
6. Hepatomegaly (CCF)
7. Dysmorphic features—microcephaly, cataract (rubella)
8. Dentition and oral hygiene—infective endocarditis.

Examination of cardiovascular system: Refer to supplementary book (SYNAPZ: The Complete Final MBBS Manual—Format Book).

Examination of gastrointestinal tract (GIT): Liver, spleen, ascites.

Examination of respiratory system: Basal creps.

Rheumatic Fever

Complaints

Fever—high-grade or low-grade.

Joint pain and swelling

1. Whether sudden or insidious
2. History of trauma
3. Whether pain and swelling confined to the joint or migratory
4. Joints affected small or large
5. Number of joints affected
6. Symmetry
7. Limitation of movements
8. Redness and swelling over the joint
9. Local rise of temperature
10. Subsidence with drugs
11. Whether any early morning stiffness
12. Whether pain increased after inactivity and relieved by activity (degenerative disease).

Chest pain, palpitation, edema

1. Abnormal movements of the limbs (chorea)
2. "Teacher scolds for bad handwriting"
3. "Grandma scolds for making faces"
4. "Mom scolds for breaking glasses".

Past History

1. History of sore throat with fever 10 days to 2 weeks prior
2. History of drug prophylaxis
3. Similar attacks in the past.

To rule out differential diagnosis

1. History of bleeding disorders (hemarthrosis)
2. History of urinary or enteric infections (reactive arthritis)
3. History of sickle cell disease/leukemia/tuberculosis (TB)/Systemic lupus erythematosus (SLE).

Rheumatic Fever

1. It is an immunological disorder initiated by group A beta hemolytic streptococci
2. Acute nonsuppurative inflammation affecting mainly connective tissues of joints, blood vessels and myocardium due to antigen antibody reaction to group A beta hemolytic streptococci
3. Age group is 5–15 years
4. Mitral valve is most commonly and severely affected.

Guidelines for the Diagnosis of Initial Attack of Rheumatic Fever (Jones Criteria, Updated 1992)

Major Manifestations

1. Carditis
2. Polyarthritis
3. Erythema marginatum
4. Subcutaneous nodules
5. Chorea.

Minor Manifestations

Clinical features

1. Arthralgia
2. Fever.

Laboratory features

1. Elevated acute phase reactants
2. Erythrocyte sedimentation rate
3. C-reactive protein
4. Prolonged PR interval.

Supporting Evidence of Antecedent Group A Streptococcal Infection

1. Positive throat culture or rapid streptococcal antigen test
2. Elevated or increasing streptococcal antibody titer.

Pathological hallmarks in rheumatic fever—Aschoff nodules and Anitschkow cells

During acute rheumatic fever, widely disseminated but focal inflammatory lesions are found in various sites. They are most distinctive within the heart where they are called Aschoff bodies. They constitute foci of fibrinoid degeneration surrounded by lymphocytes (primarily T cells), occasional plasma cells, and plump macrophages called Anitschkow cells (pathognomonic for rheumatic fever).

Treatment

Bed rest and monitored closely for evidence of carditis. Patients with carditis require longer periods of bed rest.

Antibiotic Therapy

The patient should receive 10 days of orally administered penicillin or erythromycin, or a single intramuscular injection of benzathine penicillin to eradicate GAS (Group A Streptococci) from the upper respiratory tract. After this initial course of antibiotic therapy, the patient should be started on long-term antibiotic prophylaxis.

Anti-inflammatory Therapy

Patients with typical migratory polyarthritis and those with carditis without cardiomegaly or congestive heart failure should be treated with aspirin at a dose of 100 mg/kg/day in 4 divided doses per orally (PO) for 3 to 5 days, followed by 75 mg/kg/day in 4 divided doses PO for 4 weeks.

Patients with carditis and cardiomegaly or congestive heart failure should receive corticosteroids. The usual dose of prednisone is 2 mg/kg/day in 4 divided doses for 2 to 3 weeks followed by a tapering of the dose that reduces the dose by 5 mg/24 hours every 2–3 days. At the beginning of the tapering of the prednisone dose, aspirin should be started at 75 mg/kg/day in 4 divided doses for 6 weeks.

Supportive therapy for moderate to severe carditis—digoxin, fluid and salt restriction, diuretics and O_2.

Sydenham Chorea

Phenobarbitone (16–32 mg every 6–8 hours PO) is the drug of choice.
If phenobarbitone is ineffective, haloperidol (0.01–0.03 mg/kg/24 hours divided bid PO) or chlorpromazine (0.5 mg/kg every 4–6 hours PO) should be initiated.

Prevention

Primodial prevention

1. Primary prevention
2. Secondary prevention.

The regimen of choice for secondary prevention is a single intramuscular injection of benzathine penicillin G (1.2 million IU) every 4 weeks.

Drug	Dose	Route
Penicillin G benzathine	1.2 million U, every 4 weeks	Intramuscular
OR		
Penicillin V	250 mg, twice a day	Oral
OR		
Sulfadiazine or sulfisoxazole	0.5 g, once a day for ≤ 27 kg	Oral
	1.0 g, once a day for > 27 kg	
For people who are allergic to penicillin and sulfonamide drugs		
Erythromycin	250 mg, twice a day	Oral

Fetal Circulation

1. Normal 4 chambered heart by 6 weeks of intrauterine life
2. *Ductus venosus*—bypass between the portal vein and inferior vena cava (IVC)
3. *Foramen ovale*—bypass between right atrium and left atrium
4. *Ductus arteriosus*—bypass between pulmonary artery and descending aorta.

Circulatory adjustments at birth

1. Flow through ductus venosus disappears by 7th day of postnatal life
2. Functional closure of foramen ovale soon after birth
3. In full term neonates ductus arteriosus closes within 10–21 days.

Congenital Heart Diseases—Classification

Acyanotic

1. Left to right shunt
2. Lesions resulting in increased volume load—atrial septal defect (ASD), ventricular septal defect (VSD), patent ductus arteriosus (PDA)
3. Lesions resulting in increased pressure load—valvular pulmonic stenosis, valvular aortic stenosis, and coarctation of the aorta CCF present, precordial bulge
4. Frequent chest infections, hyperemic or plethoric lung field.

Cyanotic

1. Right to left shunt
2. Lesions with decreased pulmonary blood flow
3. Lesions with increased pulmonary blood flow
4. Eisenmenger syndrome, clubbing present, CCF absent.

Obstructive lesions

1. Right side—PS
2. Left side—AS coarctation of aorta
3. No cyanosis and no frequent chest infections
4. No precordial bulge and heaving apex.

Nada's Criteria

1. Assessment of a child for the presence of heart disease
2. One major or two minor are essential.

Major

1. Systolic murmur with grade 3 or more in intensity
2. Diastolic murmur
3. Central cyanosis after excluding lung disease
4. CCF.

Minor

1. Systolic murmur with less than grade 3 intensity
2. Abnormal second sound
3. Abnormal electrocardiogram (ECG)
4. Abnormal X-ray.

Atrial Septal Defect

1. Abnormal communication between two atria.
2. Ostium secundum located at fossa ovalis—most common.
3. Ostium primum situated inferior to fossa ovalis and is associated with cleft in anterior mitral valve leaflet with or without a cleft in septal tricuspid leaflet.
4. A sinus venosus ASD is situated in the upper part of the atrial septum in close relation to the entry of the superior vena cava.

Clinical Features

1. General asymptomatic
2. Parasternal impulse
3. Mild-to-moderate cardiomegaly (marked cardiomegaly + mitral valve obstruction—Lutenbacher syndrome
4. S1 is normal may be accentuated due to a loud tricuspid component of S1
5. S2 is widely split and fixed with P2 being accentuated and widely transmitted along left sternal border and up to apex
6. Ejection systolic murmur (ESM) at second and third left interspace and is widely transmitted all over chest
7. Delay diastolic murmur at lower left sternal border (tricuspid area).

Investigation

1. *ECG*: *ASD (ostium secundum)*: Characterized by right axis deviation and right ventricular hypertrophy.
2. *X-ray chest*: Mild-to-moderate cardiomegaly
   a. Right atrial and right ventricular enlargement
   b. Prominent main pulmonary artery plethoric lung fields.

Complications

Pulmonary arterial hypertension.

Treatment

1. *Medical*: Supportive care
2. Treating chest infection
3. *Surgical*: Definitive surgical or transcatheter device closure is advised for all symptomatic patients and also for asymptomatic patients with a Qp : Qs ratio (the ratio of pulmonary to systemic blood flow) of at least 2:1.
   The timing for elective closure is usually after the 1st year and before entry into school.

Ventricular Septal Defect

1. Communication between two ventricles
2. Most common congenital cardiac lesion

3. *Common site*: Membranous part of septum—posteroinferior position, anterior to the septal leaflet of the tricuspid valve
4. *Other sites*: Muscular part of septum—midportion or apical region of the ventricular septum, supracristal—superior to the crista supraventricularis—are less common
5. VSDs between the crista supraventricularis and the papillary muscle of the conus may be associated with pulmonary stenosis and other manifestations of the tetralogy of Fallot
6. VSDs in the are muscular in type and may be single or multiple (Swiss cheese septum).

Clinical Features

Symptoms

1. Palpitation
2. Dyspnea on exertion
3. Frequent chest infection.

Signs

1. Wide pulse pressure
2. Hyperkinetic precordium with systolic thrill at left sternal border
3. Moderate cardiomegaly (LVH)
4. S1 and S2 masked by a PSM at left sternal border
5. Widely split and variable S2 with accentuated P2
6. S3 at apex may be audible
7. ESM at pulmonary wall (flow murmur)
8. Delayed diastolic murmur (DDM) at apex (mitral valve) (flow murmur).

Investigations

1. ECG-LVH
2. X-ray chest:
   a. Pulmonary plethora
   b. Left atrial enlargement
   c. Membraneous VSD
   d. Supracristal VSD
   e. Muscular VSD
   f. Swiss cheese VSD.

Types

1. *Very small VSD*: ESM, most common cause of functional systolic murmur in children
2. *Small VSD*: PSM (Maladie de Roger—loud murmur), S2 normal split, P2 normal
3. *Large VSD*: ESM
4. *VSD with P2*: Soft P2
5. *VSD with pulmonary hypertension*: Loud P2
6. *Obstructive*: Thrill absent, ESM, S2 closely split no mitral murmur
7. *Hyperkinetic*: Thrill present PSM, wide and variable S2 split, mitral DDM. In 90% of patients spontaneous closure of VSD occurs at the age of 3 years.

Complications

1. Pulmonary stenosis
2. Pulmonary arterial hypertension
3. Aortic regurgitation
4. CCF
5. Infective endocarditis.

Treatment

1. *Medical*: Control of CCF
   a. Treatment of chest infection
   b. Prevention and treatment of anemia and infective endocarditis
2. *Surgical*
   a. Indication
      i. CCF
      ii. Large left to right shunt
      iii. VSD associated with pulmonary stenosis, pulmonary arterial hypertension, aortic regurgitation.

b. *Procedure*: Closure with Dacron patch
c. *Complications of surgery*:
   i. Complete heart block
   ii. Bifascicular block
   iii. Reopened or residual VSD.

Patent Ductus Arteriosus

1. Communication between pulmonary artery and aorta
2. Functional closure 3 hours to 3 days
3. Anatomical closure 3 weeks to 3 months.

Clinical Features

Symptoms
1. Effort intolerance
2. Palpitation
3. Frequent chest infections.

Signs
1. Wide pulse pressure
2. Prominent carotid pulsations
3. Hyperkinetic apical impulse
4. Systolic/continuous thrill/2nd left interspace and also heard well below left clavicle
5. Loud S1
6. Paradoxical split of S2 in large left to right shunt
7. Third sound at apex followed by DDM in large shunt.

Shunt murmur : Continuous/machinery/Gibson/train in tunnel murmur in 2nd left intercostal space

Flow murmur : Mitral—DDM
Aortic—ESM

Investigations

1. ECG-LVH, volume overloading of left ventricle
2. X-ray chest—cardiomegaly directly proportional to left to right shunt size
3. Asceding aorta and aortic knuckle are prominent
4. Pulmonary plethora present.

Complications

Pulmonary hypertension.

Differential diagnosis of continuous murmur
1. Coronary arteriovenous (AV) fistula
2. Ruptured sinus of Valsalva fistulae into right side
3. Aorticopulmonary septal defect
4. Systemic AV fistula over chest
5. Bronchial collateral murmur
6. Pulmonary AV fistula
7. Peripheral pulmonic stenosis
8. Small ASD with mitral stenosis.

Treatment

Indomethacin—if diagnosis made within first 2 weeks.

Tetralogy of Fallot (TOF)

Most common congenital cyanotic heart disease in children above the age of 2 years.

Tetralogy (VARP)

1. Ventricular septal defect
2. Aorta—overriding of aorta
3. Right ventricular hypertrophy (RVH)
4. Pulmonary stenosis.

Severity of cyanosis directly proportional to severity of pulmonary stenosis.
ESM is inversely proportional to severity of pulmonary stenosis
Congestive cardiac failure occurs in TOF when it is associated with:

1. Anemia
2. Infective endocarditis
3. Systemic hypertension
4. Unrelated myocarditis complicating TOF
5. Aortic/pulmonary valve regurgitation.

Clinical Features

Symptoms

1. Dyspnea on exertion
2. Exercise intolerance
3. Sitting posture—squatting when they get dyspneic
4. Paroxysmal attacks of dyspnea.

Signs

1. Cyanosis
2. Clubbing
3. Normal sized heart
4. Mild parasternal impulse
5. Systolic thrill
6. Flow murmur—ESM at pulmonary area.

Investigations

1. **ECG**
   - Right axis deviation
   - Right ventricular hypertrophy
2. **X-ray chest**
   - Normal sized heart with upturned apex suggestive of right ventricular hypertrophy (RVH)
   - Cor En Sabot/wooden shoe-shaped heart
   - Unilateral rib notching
   - Oligemic lung fields
3. **Echocardiography**
   - Large overriding aorta
   - RVH
   - Aortic—mitral valve continuity is maintained.

Complications

1. Cardiac enlargement
2. Congestive cardiac failure
3. Infective endocarditis
4. Hemiplegia
5. Paradoxical embolism
6. Venous thrombosis
7. Brain abscess.

Treatment

Medical

1. Management of complications
2. Correction of anemia
3. Management of anoxic spells.

Surgical

1. Palliative systemic anastomosis to pulmonary artery
   Blalock-Taussig shunt: Subclavian to pulmonary artery
   Pott's shunt: Descending aorta to pulmonary artery
   Waterson's shunt: Ascending aorta to right pulmonary artery
2. *Definitive*: Closing VSD and resecting infundibular obstruction.

Fallot's trilogy: PS + RVH + reversed interatrial shunt
Fallot's pentalogy: tetralogy + ASD
Acyanotic (pink) Fallot's: Where right ventricular outflow tract obstruction is mild.

Management of Anoxic Spells

1. Knee-chest position
2. Humidified oxygen
3. Subcutaneous morphine
4. Correct acidosis with sodium bicarbonate IV

5. Propranolol
6. Vasopressors—methoxamine IM/IV
7. Correct anemia
8. Consider operation.

Congestive Cardiac Failure

Inability of heart to maintain an output, at rest or during stress, necessary for the metabolic needs of the body (systolic failure) and inability to receive blood into the ventricular cavities at low pressure during diastole (diastolic failure).

Causes

Infants

1. Congenital heart disease
2. Myocarditis and primary myocardial disease
3. Paroxysmal tachycardia
4. Anemia.

Children

1. Rheumatic fever and rheumatic heart disease
2. Hypertension
3. Congenital heart disease complicated by anemia/infection
4. Upper respiratory obstruction.

Signs of congestive cardiac failure in infants

Left sided failure	Failure of either side	Right sided failure
Tachypnea	Cardiac enlargement	Hepatomegaly
Tachycardia	Gallop rhythm(S3)	Facial edema
Cough	Peripheral cyanosis	Jugular venous engorgement
Wheezing	Small volume pulse	Edema on feet
Rales in chest	Absence of weight gain	

Stepwise Management of CCF

Step 1 : Frusemide with amiloride or triamterene
Step 2 : Adding digoxin
Step 3 : ACE inhibitors and stop potassium sparing diuretics
Step 4 : Adding isosorbide nitrate
Step 5 : Intermitent dobutamine or dopamine with dobutamine
Step 6 : Adding immunosuppressives with steroids or beta blocker
Step 7 : Cardiac transplantation.

Dosage of Digoxin

Premature/neonate	0.04 mg/kg
1 month–1 year	0.08 mg/kg
1–3 years	0.06 mg/kg
> 3 years	0.04 mg/kg.

Steps of Digitalization

1. Obtain baseline ECG—rhythm and PR interval
2. Serum electrolytes-K^+, Ca^{++}
3. Calculate total digitalizing dose
4. Give half stat, one-fourth after 8 hours and one-fourth after next 8 hours
5. Obtain repeat ECG
6. Maintenance dose after 24 hours of final dose.

Manifestations of Infective Endocarditis

History

1. Prior congenital or rheumatic heart disease
2. Preceding dental, urinary tract, or intestinal procedure
3. Intravenous drug use
4. Central venous catheter
5. Prosthetic heart valve.

Symptoms

1. Fever
2. Chills
3. Chest and abdominal pain
4. Arthralgia, myalgia
5. Dyspnea
6. Malaise
7. Night sweats
8. Weight loss
9. CNS manifestations (stroke, seizures, headache).

Signs

1. Elevated temperature
2. Tachycardia
3. Embolic phenomena (Roth spots, petechiae, splinter nail bed hemorrhages, Osler nodes, CNS or ocular lesions)
4. Janeway lesions
5. New or changing murmur
6. Splenomegaly
7. Arthritis
8. Heart failure
9. Arrhythmias
10. Metastatic infection (arthritis, meningitis, mycotic arterial aneurysm, pericarditis, abscesses, septic pulmonary emboli)
11. Clubbing.

Laboratory

1. Positive blood culture
2. Elevated erythrocyte sedimentation rate; may be low with heart or renal failure
3. Elevated C-reactive protein
4. Anemia
5. Leukocytosis
6. Immune complexes
7. Hypergammaglobulinemia
8. Hypocomplementemia
9. Cryoglobulinemia
10. Rheumatoid factor
11. Hematuria
12. *Renal failure*: Azotemia, high creatinine (glomerulonephritis)
13. *Chest radiograph*: Bilateral infiltrates, nodules, pleural effusions
14. Echocardiographic evidence of valve vegetations, prosthetic valve dysfunction or leak, myocardial abscess, new-onset valve insufficiency.

The Duke Criteria—Nelson

Major criteria

1. Positive blood cultures (two separate cultures for a usual pathogen, two or more for less typical pathogens).
2. Evidence of endocarditis on echocardiography (intracardiac mass on a valve or other site, regurgitant flow near a prosthesis, abscess, partial dehiscence of prosthetic valves, or new valve regurgitant flow).

Minor criteria

1. Predisposing conditions
2. Fever

3. Embolic-vascular signs
4. Immune complex phenomena (glomerulonephritis, arthritis, rheumatoid factor, Osler nodes, Roth spots)
5. A single positive blood culture or serologic evidence of infection
6. Echocardiographic signs not meeting the major criteria

Two major criteria, one major and three minor, or five minor criteria suggest definite endocarditis.

A modification of the Duke criteria may increase sensitivity while maintaining specificity. The following minor criteria are added to those already listed:

1. The presence of newly diagnosed clubbing, splenomegaly, splinter hemorrhages, and petechiae
2. A high erythrocyte sedimentation rate
3. A high C-reactive protein level
4. The presence of central nonfeeding lines, peripheral lines, and microscopic hematuria.

Diagnosis of Infective Endocarditis (Modified Duke Criteria)—Davidson

Major criteria

Positive blood culture

1. Typical organism from two cultures
2. Persistent positive blood cultures taken > 12 hours apart
3. Three or more positive cultures taken over more than 1 hour.

Endocardial involvement

1. Positive echocardiographic findings of vegetations
2. New valvular regurgitation.

Minor criteria

1. Predisposing valvular or cardiac abnormality
2. Intravenous drug misuse
3. Pyrexia $\geq$ 38°C
4. Embolic phenomenon
5. Vasculitic phenomenon
6. Blood cultures suggestive—organism grown but not achieving major criteria
7. Suggestive echocardiographic findings.

Definite endocarditis: Two major, or one major and three minor, or five minor
Possible endocarditis: One major and one minor, or three minor.

RESPIRATORY SYSTEM

History

1. Difficulty in breathing
2. Fever with chills and rigor
3. Cough with sputum
4. Difficulty in feeding
5. Nasopharyngeal infection
6. Pyoderma
7. Anorexia
8. Bluish discoloration of skin, lips, palm
9. History of allergy
10. Weather change
11. Nasal discharge
12. Incessant crying
13. Aggravating factors—exercise, at night.

Past History

1. Similar illness history of bronchial asthma, PTB
2. Treatment history.

Family History

History of consanguinity history of similar illness.

Socioeconomic Status

Place of living—high altitude.

Development

Head to foot

1. Febrile, irritable, crying and dyspneic
2. Movement of accessory respiratory muscles
3. Nasal discharge grunting respiration
4. Cyanosis intercostal indrawing
5. Bronchophony crepitation
6. Bronchial breathing evident suprasternal notch
7. Retraction of lower intercoastal spaces.

Case Discussion

Common Causes of Wheezing

1. Wheeze associated with LRTI
2. Tropical eosinophilia
3. Hypersensitivity pneumonitis
4. External compression
5. Bronchiolitis and bronchial asthma
6. Loeffler's syndrome
7. Inhaled foreign bodies
8. Cystic fibrosis.

First episode of wheezing before 6 months of age is usually bronchiolitits.

Distinguishing between stridor due to supraglottic and tracheal obstruction

Clinical features	Supraglottic obstruction	Tracheal obstruction
Stridor	Inspiratory and often less serious	Usually expiratory and more serious
Cry	Muffled	Normal
Dyspnea	Less severe	More marked
Cough	Less marked	Deep barking or brassy

Pneumonia

Acute Respiratory Infection (ARI)

Acute infection of respiratory tract including ear, nose, throat, paranasal sinus and pleura of less than 30 days duration (14 days in case of ear).

Classification of ARI

	No pneumonia	Pneumonia	Severe pneumonia	Very severe pneumonia
Fever, cough and breathlessness	Present	Present	Present	Present
Tachypnea	Absent	Present	Present	Present
Chest indrawing	Absent	Absent	Present	Present
Danger signs	Absent	Absent	Absent	Present
Treatment	1. Steam inhalation 2. Saline nasal drops 3. Antipyretics 4. Look for danger signs	1. Cotrimoxazole is the drug of choice 2. Antipyretics 3. Reassess after 2 days 4. If worse Advice hospitalization	1. Benzyl penicillin/ ampicillin 3 days and switch to oral penicillin 2. Reassess after 48 hours if worse switch to chloramphenicol	1. Chloramphenicol/ benzyl penicillin + Gentamycin for 2 days then switch to oral 2. Reassess after 48 hours if worse Cloxacillin + Gentamycin

Danger Signs

1. Not feeding/drinking
2. Abnormally drowsy/difficulty to wake up
3. Grunting, stridor
4. Unconsciousness/convulsions
5. Cyanosis, apneic spells
6. Abdominal distention and malnutrition.

Pneumonia Age Groups

1st 2 months	: *Klebsiella*, *E. coli*, pneumococci, staphylococci
3 months to 3 years	: Pneumococci, *H. influenzae*, staphylococci
After 3 years	: Pneumococci, staphylococci.

Pneumococcal Pneumonia

Symptoms

1. High fever with chills
2. Cough with thick rusty sputum
3. Difficulty in feeding
4. Headache
5. Rapid respiration.

Signs

1. Cyanosis
2. Impaired percussion
3. Diminished air entry
4. Bronchophony
5. Bronchial breathing
6. Crepitations
7. Whispering pectoriloquy.

Diagnosis

1. History
2. Physical examination
3. Blood routine examination leukocytosis
4. X-ray–lobar consolidation
5. Sputum gram staining and culture
6. Blood culture.

Treatment

1. Penicillin G 50,000 units/kg/day IV or IM in divided doses for a week to 10 days
2. Procaine penicillin 6,00,000 units IM/day
3. Penicillin V may be used orally
4. If cyanosis and respiratory distress present give O_2.

Staphylococcal Pneumonia

Clinical features

1. URTI
2 Fever
3. Listlessness
4. Pyoderma
5. Anorexia
6. Irritable
7. Distended abdomen.

Sign

Grunting respiration cyanosis may be present.

Diagnosis

1. X-ray
2. Blood culture.

Treatment

1. Immediate hospitalization and isolation
2. Antipyretics and hydration for control of fever
3. Oxygen administration for dyspnea and cyanosis
4. Empyema is aspirated and pus is sent for culture and sensitivity
5. Vigorous antibiotic therapy—penicillin G, erythromycin, cloxacillin, cephalosporin
6. In resistant cases—vancomycin/teicoplanin.

Complications

1. Respiratory distress
2. Pleural thickening
3. Pyopneumothorax
4. Metastatic abscess
5. Empyema.

Hemophilus Influenzae Pneumonia

Clinical features

1. Nasopharyngeal infection
2. Dyspnea
3. Retraction of lower intercostal spaces
4. Fever
5. Grunting respiration.

Complication

1. Bacteremia
2. Empyema
3. Polyarthritis
4. Pericarditis
5. Meningitis.

Treatment

1. Ampicillin a dose of 100–150 mg/kg/day and chloramphenicol 50 mg/kg/day in four divided doses
2. *Other alternative*: Cefotaxime (100 mg/kg/day) or ceftriaxone (50–75 mg/kg/day).

Streptococcal Pneumonia

Clinical features

1. Fever with chills
2. Dyspnea rapid respiration
3. Cough
4. Ill looking
5. Blood streaked sputum
6. Extreme prostration.

Complications

1. Serosanguineous or purulent empyema
2. Pulmonary suppuration
3. Bacteremia.

Diagnosis

1. X-ray—interstitial pneumonia segmental involvement diffuse peribronchial densities or an effusion
2. Complete blood count—increased neutrophil.

Treatment

1. Penicillin G in dose of 50,000 to 100,000 units/kg of body weight daily in divided doses for a fortnight
2. Empyema—aspiration of pus.

Acute Bronchiolitis

1. **Common organism:** Respiratory syncytial virus (RSV)
2. **Other agents:** Parainfluenza, adenovirus, *Mycoplasma*, and, occasionally, other viruses. Human metapneumovirus co-infection with RSV
3. Common age group 1 to 6 months (affect up to 2 years).

Clinical features

1. Symptoms
   a. Upper respiratory tract infection
   b. Retraction of lower intercostals spaces
   c. Cyanosis may present
   d. Fast breathing respiratory distress
   e. Evident suprasternal notch.
2. Signs
   a. Hyper resonance on percussion
   b. Increased anteroposterior diameter of chest
   c. Fine rales and rhonchi on auscultation.

Investigations

1. X-ray chest - Hyperinflation and infiltrate
   - Diaphragm is pushed down
2. Monoclonal antibody test can detect RSV from nasal swab.

Treatment

1. Oxygen inhalation
2. Maintain fluid and electrolyte-balance
3. Nebulized adrenaline preferred over Salbutamol/Ipratropium
4. Antiviral agent—Ribavirin as aerosolized mist
5. No role for antibiotics.

Monoclonal antibody used against RSV—Palivizumab.

Differential diagnosis

1. Bronchial asthma
2. Foreign body
3. Congestive heart failure.

Bronchial Asthma

Characterized by increased responsiveness of trachea and bronchi to various stimuli.

Triggers of Asthma

1. Allergy
2. Exercise
3. Emotional factors
4. Endocrine factors
5. Viral infection
6. Weather change
7. Role of food.

Clinical Features

1. Wheezing and dyspnea
2. Hyperinflation of chest
3. Nocturnal coughing and is nonproductive (early phase)
4. Child sweats profusely and looks fatigued
5. May develop cyanosis
6. Symptoms are aggravated by exercise and more at night.

Examination

1. Pulse—pulsus paradoxus
2. BP—hypotension
3. Respiration—tachypnea
4. Temperature—febrile
5. Head to foot—ill looking, dyspnea
6. Respiratory system:
   a. Bulging chest
   b. Moving nasal alae
   c. Hyperresonance
   d. Accessory muscle involvement
   e. Wheeze/Rhonchi.

Diagnosis

1. Chest X-ray
2. Pulmonary function test
3. Absolute eosinophil count
4. Allergy test—skin test and RAST (radioallergosorbent allergen specific IgE).

Differential Diagnosis

1. Bronchiolitis
2. Congenital malformations
3. Cystic fibrosis
4. Aspiration of foreign body
5. Extrinsic allergic malformations.

Grading and treatment of asthma

Clinical parameter	Mild	Moderate	Severe
Color	Normal	Normal	Pale
Sensorium	Normal	Anxious	Agitated
Respiratory rate	Increased	Increased	Increased
Dyspnea	Absent, can speak sentence	Moderate, can speak in phrases	Severe, difficulty in speech
Accessory muscles	Nil or minimal	Chest indrawing flaring up of ala nasae	Chest indrawing
Pulses paradoxus	< 10 mm	10–20 mm	> 20 mm
Rhonchi	Expiratory	Expiratory and inspiratory	Inspiratory, expiratory or absent
Peak expiratory flow rate (PEFR)	> 80%	60–80%	< 60%

Contd...

Contd...

SaO_2	> 95%	90–95%	< 90%
Rx	α_2 agonist by Nebulizer or MDI + Spacer with or without face mask—6 to 8 hours	1. Inhaled α_2 repeated every 20 minute for 1 hour 2. Oral prednisolone 3. O_2 inhalation	1. Immediate O_2 inhalation 2. Subcutaneous inj terbutaline for 1 hr: adrenaline 3. Inhalation of salbutamol/ipratropium bromide 4. IV hydrocortisone 5. Transfer to ICU

Danger signs in bronchial asthma

1. Altered sensorium
2. Bradycardia
3. Low volume pulse
4. Cyanosis even with oxygen therapy
5. Silent chest.

Chest signs of some common respiratory disorders of children

Disorder	Chest movement	Percussion	Auscultation
Bronchiolitis	Restricted, with hyperinflation, often tracheal tug and subcoastal recession	Hyperresonant	Widespread crepitations or wheezing
Pneumonia	Rapid, shallow respirations with audible grunt may be reduced on affected side	Dull or resonant	Localized bronchial breathing or crepitations. May have no abnormal signs
Asthma	Restricted with hyperinflation use of accessory muscles and subcostal retraction	Hyperresonant	Expiratory wheeze
Croup	Inspiratory stridor with subcostal recession	Normal	Inspiratory coarse crepitations (crackles)

Differences between bronchial asthma and bronchiolitis

Bronchial asthma	Bronchiolitis
Age > 18 months	< 6 months
Recurrent episodes	First episode
Positive family history	Negative
Responds to bronchodilators	Not much response

RENAL SYSTEM

Case Taking

Presenting Complaints

1. Pedal edema
2. Facial puffiness
3. Abdominal distention
4. Hematuria
5. Oliguria.

History of Present Illness

1. **Edema:** Onset, where appeared first, progress, relieving on rest, abdominal distension, scrotal swelling.
2. **Cola colored urine:** When color progress, dysuria, flank pain trauma, other bleeding manifestations.
3. Oliguria, hematuria, dysuria.

Causes of Edema

1. Dyspnea/orthopnea/paroxysmal nocturnal dyspnea (PND)—CCF
2. Jaundice/hematemesis/melena—liver
3. Alleric to food/drugs/insect bite—angioedema
4. Diarrhea/steatorrhea—protein energy malnutrition (PEM)
5. Abdominal pain, rash arthritis—Henoch-Schönlein purpura (HSP)
6. Abdominal pain/diarrhea—hemolytic uremic syndrome (HUS)
7. History of prior viral infection—IGA nephropathy.

For Complications of Acute Glomerulonephritis (AGN)

1. Altered sensorium, blurring of vision, headache, convulsions (HTN encephalopathy) cough, dyspnea (LVF)
2. Symptoms of acute renal failure (Anuria alteration of sensorium, acidotic breathing)
3. Rashes, joint pain (Vasculitis and collagen vascular disease)
4. Fever with chills
5. Abdominal pain.

Past History

1. Similar episodes and history of Rx-nephrotic syndrome
2. History of remissions/relapses
3. Sore throat, skin infections 1–4 weeks prior
4. History of mumps, measles, hepatitis B, IMN, malaria, infective endocarditis
5. History of GBS or steroid therapy
6. Any history of remission of relapse.

Dietetic History

Modification of diet advised—salt and fruit restriction.

Diet in NS

1. Salt < 2 gm/day
2. Protein 2 gm/kg/day
3. Avoid egg yolk
4. Increase vegetable fibers.

Examination

General examination

Anemia, pyoderma and scabies, LNE, BP, edema, ascites, hydrothorax, scrotum, abdominal wall and sacral edema.

1. CNS – Signs of encephalopathy
2. CVS – Signs of LV dysfunction/pulmonary edema
3. Renal – Renal angle tenderness
4. RESP – Basal creps, hydrothorax
5. GIT – Pharaynx and tonsils, ascites, abdominal tenderness.

Urine casts

1. Red cell cast—AGN
2. WBC cast—Pyelonephritis
3. Borad cast—CRF
4. Fatty cast—NS.

Heat and acetic acid test

Slight opalescence – Trace
Cloudiness – 1+ (fine print can be read–15–30 mg of protein/dL)
Coagulum – 2+
Floculum – 3+ (black lines are not visible—150–350 mg)
Precipitate – 4+ (acetic acid is added to dissolve phosphate)

Urine protein: Creatinine ratio
Massive proteinuria—40 mg/m^2/hr—1 g/m^2/24 hours

Acute Glomerular Nephritis

Characterized by hematuria, oliguria, hypertension and edema.

Common Causes

1. Postinfectious—Streptococci, staphylococci, hepatitis B and C, bacterial endocarditis
2. Systemic vasculitis—HSP, systemic lupus erythematosis (SLE), polyarteritis nodosa (PAN)
3. Membranoproliferative glomerular nephritis
4. IgA nephropathy
5. Familial nephropathy—Alport syndrome.

Clinical Features

1. **Typical:** Puffiness around the eyes and pedal edema, oliguria, cola colored urine, hypertension
2. **Atypical:** Convulsions—due to hypertensive encephalopathy
3. LVF and pulmonary edema—due to malignant HTN and hypervolemia
4. Acute renal failure.

Investigations

1. *Urine-1+ to 2+ proteinuria with red cells and granular casts*: Normocytic anemia due to hemodilution, ESR elevated
2. *Blood urea and creatine elevated—indicate degree of renal impairment*: Hyponatremia and hyperkalemia
3. Throat swab culture—shows beta hemolytic *Streptococcus*
4. ASO titer increased
5. Anti-DNase B is elevated in streptococcal skin infection
6. Serum C_3 level-Low
7. X-ray chest—shows prominent vascular markings, cardiomegaly.

Management

1. **Diet:** Intake of protein, Na and K restricted till blood urea value reduce and urine output increases. Absolute bed rest
2. **Weight:** Gain in weight necessitate reduce in fluid intake
3. **Diuretics:** Not indicated. Only indicated in presence of pulmonary edema—IV frusemide.
4. Hypertension
5. LVF.

Hypertension
1. Mild HTN controlled by salt restriction and water intake
2. Antihypertensive drugs—atenolol, hydralazine, nifedipine
3. In malignant hypertension treated with IV nitroprusside or labetalol
4. *LVF*: Venesection with removal of 100–200 mL of blood, control the hypertension with IV frusemide
5. Prolonged oliguria—dialysis.

Prognosis
1. Excellent prognosis in childhood
2. Significant proteinuria disappear within two weeks.

Differential diagnosis
1. Nephrotic syndrome
2. Hemolytic urine syndrome
3. Henoch-Schonlein purpura
4. Immune thrombocytopenic purpura
5. Ig A nephropathy.

Differentiating features between IgA nephropathy and Poststreptococcal glomerulonephritis

IgA nephropathy	Poststreptococcal glomerulonephritis
Onset of hematuria 2–4 days after URTI	Onset of hematuria 7–21 days following URTI and skin infection
Serum complement C3 level normal	Serum compliment C3 level decreased
Recurrence common	Recurrence rare, one attack confers life-long immunity
No elevation of antibody titer	Elevation of antistreptococcal antibody titer

Nephrotic Syndrome (NS)

Characterized by massive proteinuria (40 mg/m^2/hr), hypoalbuminemia and edema.

Clinical Features

1. Edema around eyes and pedal edema
2. Features of anasarca—generalized edema with ascites, hydrothorax and hydrocele.
3. 3+ to 4+ proteinuria
4. Low albumin level hypercholesterolemia
5. **Protein sensitivity:** The ratio of clearance of high molecular weight to low molecular weight proteins.

Investigations

1. **Blood:** Hb (low-CRF, hematuria—high-hypoalbuminemia), erythrocyte sedimentation rate (ESR)
2. **Urine:** Proteinuria, RBC, pus cells (urinary tract infection)
3. 24 hours urine protein
4. Renal function test (RFT)
5. Serum electrolytes—hyponatremia, low total serum calcium
6. USG abdomen KUB
7. Chest X-ray—pleural effusion—to rule out other causes of effussion
8. LFT-albumin-low
9. **Lipid profile:** Hyper lipidemia
10. **Others:** Serum C3, ANA ds-DNA, VDRL, HbsAg, Renal biopsy.

Indications of renal biopsy in nephrotic syndrome

1. Persistent gross hematuria
2. Persistent hypertension
3. Low C3
4. Persistent uremia
5. Age of onst < 2 years and > 10 years
6. Congenital nephrotic syndrome
7. Steroid resistant nephrotic syndrome
8. Frequent relapses.

Management

1. Initial episode
   a. Salt restricted and high protein diet
   b. Prednisolone 2 mg/kg/day in 2–3 divided doses for 6 weeks.
2. First 2 to 3 recurrence
   Prednisolone 2 mg/kg/day in 1–2 divided doses for 10–14 days.

Complications

1. Edema
2. Thrombotic complication
3. Steroid toxicity
4. Infection
5. ARF.

Steroid resistance: Failure to remission after 8 weeks of steroid therapy

Steroid dependance: Unable to discontinue steroid without experiencing relapse

Steroid responder: Disappearance of proteinuria within 8 weeks of starting steroids
Remission of NS: Urine protein negative for a period of at least 3 days
Relapse of NS: Proteinuria > 4 mg/m²/hr on 3 consecutive days within 7 days of stopping steroids
Frequent relapses: More than 2 episodes in 6 months/more than 3 episodes in 1 year.

Indications for dialysis in ARF (Acute renal failure/injury)

1. Volume overload with evidence of hypertension and/or pulmonary edema refractory to diuretic therapy
2. Persistent hyperkalemia
3. Severe metabolic acidosis unresponsive to medical management
4. Neurologic symptoms (altered mental status, seizures)
5. Blood urea nitrogen greater than 100–150 mg/dL (or lower if rapidly rising)
6. Calcium/phosphorus imbalance, with hypocalcemic tetany strong indications for RRT.

GASTROINTESTINAL SYSTEM

Viral Hepatitis

Presenting Complaints

Prodrome (1–2 weeks)

1. Moderate fever
2. Anorexia, nausea, vomiting
3. Abdominal pain.

Icteric phase

1. Discoloration of urine (staining the clothes)
2. Clay colored stools
3. Jaundice
4. Rarely may present as GBS, myocarditis.

History of Present Illness

1. Acute/insidious in onset
2. Associated
3. Chills, headache, nausea, vomiting
4. Abdominal pain, malaise, anorexia, loose stools
5. Yellow discoloration of urine and normal color of stools
6. Itching and symptoms of obstructive jaundice during the cholestatic phase
7. Rash and arthralgia
8. Bleeding tendencies.

Past History

History of contact, blood transfusion, drugs immunization dental extraction.

Antenatal, Natal and Postnatal

1. Jaundice in mother
2. Rh negative mother (Exchange transfusion)
3. Any instrumentation during delivery.

Immunization History

Hepatitis vaccination.

Socioeconomic

Details of drinking water and sanitation.

Family History

1. Similar illness in the family
2. History of neurological deficits in family (Wilson's disease)

3. History of surgery following jaundice (to rule out HS)
4. History of contact.

Head to foot examination

1. Jaundice
2. Cervical lymph nodes (Hepatitis B)
3. Signs of vitamin deficiency
4. Signs of liver failure.

Vital signs

Bradycardia.

GIT

1. Fetor hepaticus
2. Mild to moderate abdominal distension
3. Tenderness in right hypochondrium
4. Tender soft to firm liver
5. Splenomegaly — 10%
6. Ascites.

Respiratory system

Pleural effusion

CVS

Myocarditis, pericarditis.

Investigations

1. Blood : Relative lymphocytosis
2. LFT :
   - Plasma bilirubin reflects the degree of liver damage
   - Serum transaminases (ALT, AST) typically between 200 and 2000 U/L—ALT is liver specific
   - The alkaline phosphatase and GGT elevated in hepatitis A.
3. IgM HAV : Recent infection
4. HBsAg, HbcAg, HBeAg
5. IgM HCV
6. Prolongation of the prothrombin time in severe hepatitis.

Management

1. **Hepatitis A:** Bed rest, nutritious diet, fat restriction and normal salt
2. **Hepatitis B:** Alpha interferon, lamivudine
3. **Hepatitis C:** Alpha interferon
4. **Hepatitis E:** Alpha interferon, ribavirin.

Causes of viral hepatitis

Common

1. Hepatitis A
2. Hepatitis B ± hepatitis D
3. Hepatitis C
4. Hepatitis E.

Less common

1. Cytomegalovirus
2. Epstein-Barr virus.

Rare

1. Herpes simplex
2. Yellow fever.

Complications of Acute Viral Hepatitis

1. Fulminant hepatitis—development of hepatic failure and encephalopathy within 2 weeks
2. Subfulminant hepatitis—from 2 weeks to 3 months after onset of jaundice
3. Hepatocellular carcinoma—hepatitis B
4. Acute liver failure
5. Cholestatic hepatitis
6. Aplastic anemia
7. Chronic liver disease and cirrhosis (hepatitis B and C)
8. Relapsing hepatitis.

Hepatomegaly in Pediatrics

Infants

1. *Infections*: TORCH infection, neonatal hepatitis
2. *Biliary obstruction*: Extrahepatic biliary atresia (EHBA)
3. *Infiltration*: Erythroblastosis fetalis, histiocytosis, tumors
4. *Storage disorders*: Glycogen storage disease, hemochromatosis, galactosemia
5. *Congestion*: Congestive cardiac failure (CCF).

Older children

1. *Infections*: Acute (A/c) and chronic (C/c) hepatitis, liver abscess, infectious mononucleosis (IMN), hydatid cyst
2. *Storage disorders*: Glycogen storage disease, Wilson's disease
3. *Fatty infiltration*: Kwashiorkor, tuberculosis, cystic fibrosis
4. *Congestion*: CCF, Budd-Chiari syndrome, veno-occlusive disease of liver
5. *Infiltration*: Hepatic neoplasm, lymphoreticular malignancies, metastasis.

Diarrhea

Passage of liquid or watery stool more than 3 times a day.

1. *Persistent diarrhea*: Diarrhea of presumed infectious origin that begins acutely and lasts for 14 days or more and associated with rapid weight loss.
2. *Chronic diarrhea*: Associated with "abnormal stools" which continues or recurrently occurs over several months, dehydration is rare.

Presenting Complaint

Loose watery stools, blood in stools.

History of Present Illness

1. Loose stools—onset, number of episodes, consistency, blood stained/not, mucous, frothy
2. **Associated symptoms:** Vomiting, abdominal pain, fever
3. **Complications:** Urine output and thirst to assess dehydration, altered sensorium, seizures, irritability, abdominal distention, tears, eyes.
4. History of contact with similar illness
5. Food intake from outside
6. History of UTI, pharyngitis/pneumonia
7. Any ear discharge
8. **Any drugs:** Oral antibiotics.

Past History

1. History of infections TB, measles
2. Travel outside.

Antenatal, Natal, Postnatal History—LBW or Not

Dietetic History

1. Prelacteals, cow's milk, bottle feeding, artificial feeds
2. Weaning problems.

Immunization History

Rotavirus immunization (most common cause of diarrhea).

Family History

Similar illness.

Socioeconomic Status

1. Source of drinking water, boiled water
2. Cutting nails
3. Sanitary latrines present or not.

General Examination

Head to foot

1. Anterior fontanelle—depressed/not
2. Eyes—sunken/not, tears
3. Oral mucosa and tongue—dry/moist
4. Ears—discharge
5. Thirst
6. Abdomen—skin pinch, abdomen distended or not
7. Limbs—capillary filling time.

GIT

Respiratory system—pneumonia.

CVS

CNS—altered sensorium, meningitis.

Danger Signs of Diarrhea

1. Drowsiness
2. Watery stools
3. Repeated vomiting
4. Not able to drink and feed
5. Fever and abdominal distention
6. Decreased urine output
7. Blood in stools.

Nature of Stools

1. *Watery*: Rotavirus, ETEC, EVEC
2. *Rice water*: Cholera
3. *Pus, mucous, blood*: *Shigella, Campylobacter*
4. *Watery, blood, mucous*: *Salmonella.*

Causes of Abdominal Distention in Diarrhea

1. Hypokalemia
2. Necrotizing enterocolitis
3. Septicemia.

Cause of Convulsion in Diarrhea

1. Hyponatremia and hypernatremia
2. Hypokalemia
3. Reye's syndrome
4. Meningitis
5. Encephalitis (*Shigella*)
6. Cerebral venous/sagittal sinus thrombosis.

Features	No signs of dehydration	Some dehydration	Severe dehydration
Condition	Well, alert	Restless, irritable lethargic/unconscious	Floppy
Eyes	Normal	Sunken	Very sunken and dry
Tears	Present	Absent	Absent
Mouth and tongue	Moist	Dry	Very dry
Thirst	Drinks normally	Thirsty, drinks eagerly	Drinks poorly
Skin pinch	Goes back quickly	Slowly	Very slowly
Treatment	**Plan A** 1. Home available fluids± 2. ORS after each stool	**Plan B** 1. *Rehydration therapy*: 75 mL/kg of ORS in first 4 hours 2. *Maintenance fluid therapy*: 10–20 mL/kg body weight of ORS for each liquid stool 3. ORS administered till diarrhea stops	**Plan C** 1. *Start IV fluids*: RL or NS 2. ORS solution 5 mL/kg/hr 3. *Monitor*: PR, BP 4. If improving start plan B 5. Not improving continue 1 and 2

Dysentery

Presence of blood and pus in the stools, associated with abdominal cramps and fever.

Causes

Rotavirus, enterotoxigenic *E. coli, Cholerae, Salmonella, Shigella*, etc.

Management

1. Cotrimoxazole TMP—8 mg/kg (ampicillin if allergic to cotrimoxazole)
2. Reassess after 2 days if improvement continue for 3 more days
3. If no improvement change to nalidixic acid.

Reassess after 2 days if no improvement examine stool for *Entamoeba*—if present metronidazole.

Advise on Discharge of a Child with Diarrhea

1. Explain the condition of the disease to the mother
2. Explain about the preparation of oral rehydration solution (ORS)
3. Explain about quantity and frequency of giving ORS
   a. Boil and cool 1 liter of water (5 glasses)
   b. One packet dissolved in 5 glasses of water
   c. 2–3 tsp every 5–10 min after every bout of diarrhea
4. Explain about other home available solutions—sugar and salt solution, rice water with salt, *lassi* with salt, lemon water, coconut water
5. Tell about the complications
6. If complications arise, to get the child back to the hospital
7. Encourage breastfeeding and normal diet
8. If ORS is used up, return for more
9. Explain the importance of immunization.

Reduced osmolarity ORS

Reduced osmolarity ORS	Grams/liter
Sodium chloride	2.6
Glucose anhydrous	13.5
Potassium chloride	1.5
Trisodium citrate, dihydrate	2.9
Total weight	20.5

Reduced osmolarity ORS	mmol/liter
Sodium	75
Chloride	65
Glucose, anhydrous	75
Potassium	20
Citrate	10
Total osmolarity	245

Fluids

Crystalloids

1. **Isotonic fluids**

Normal saline : 0.9% NaCl Na^{+}-150, Cl^{-} 150 mEq/L
Ringer lactate : Na^{+}-131, K^{+}-5, Cl^{-} 111, Ca^{++}-4, lactate—29 mEq/L
NaCl : 0.6 g, NaOH-0.114 g, KCl-0.04 g, calcium chloride dihydrate—0.027 g, lactic acid—0.24 mL

2. **Hypotonic fluids**
   5D : 5% dextrose
   Osmolarity : 277 mOsmol/L
3. **Hypertonic**
   10 D : 10% dextrose
   Osmolarity : 556 mOsmol/L
   25 D : 25% dextrose
   Osmolarity : 1385 mOsmol/L
   DNS : 0.9% NaCl and 5% dextrose
   Na-150, Cl-150
   Total osmolarity 560 mOsmol/L
   NaCl—0.9 g, anhydrous dextrose—5 g
   3% saline

Colloids

Natural: Human albumin
Artificial: Hydroxyethyl starch, hemasil.

HEMATOLOGICAL DISORDERS

Bleeding Disorders

Case Taking

Presenting complaints
Bleeding from gums/bleeding spots/epistaxis/bleeding from vaccination sites/menorrhagia.

History of Present Illness

1. Age of onset
2. Bleeding episode—site, history of trauma/spontaneous, number of bleeds, history of hospital admission
3. History of mucosal bleeds, gum bleeds, petechiae, purpura—primary hemostatic defect
4. History of deep bleeds, muscle bleeds, hematuria, hematemesis—secondary hemostatic defect
5. History of trauma/drug intake
6. History of easy fatiguability and exertional dyspnea—CCF
7. History of recurrent fever, infections—aplastic anemia
8. History of abdominal pain, arthritis, edema, oliguria—HSP
9. History of rash/joint pain—SLE
10. History of abdominal swelling, bone pain, arthralgia—infiltrative disorder
11. History of left sided mass, pain—splenic sequestration
12. History of diarrhea, edema,convulsions—HUS
13. History of vomiting, seizures, altered sensorium, weakness—complications like intracranial hemorrhage.

Past History

1. History of similar episodes
2. History of viral infection—immune thrombocytopenic purpura (ITP)
3. Transfusions
4. History of bleeding—umbilicus, vaccination site, circumcision, tooth extraction, epistaxis
5. History of drug intake—anticoagulants, NSAIDs, anticonvulsants, quinine, sulfonamides
6. History of jaundice—liver disease
7. History of skin rash, arthralgia, edema—SLE
8. History of prosthetic valve—infective endocarditis
9. History of TB.

Antenatal History

1. History of drug intake during pregnancy
2. History of infections—neonatal thrombocytopenia—CMV, rubella
3. History of DIC.

Natal History

1. Low birth weight
2. Bleeding from umbilical cord.

Postnatal History

Passage of blood in stools—hemorrhagic disease of newborn.

Developmental History

Delay in mile stones in case of intracranial bleeds.

Immunization History

1. Bleeding from immunization sites
2. Hepatitis B immunization should be taken
3. Precautions—limit number of injections, avoid IM injections, use small diameter needles and use ice pack after injections.

Dietetic History

Adequate intake.

Family History

1. History of similar illness in family—trace 3 generations
2. History of menorrhagia
3. Abortion/stillbirth.

Socioeconomic Status

General Examination

1. Pallor, jaundice, lymphadenopathy, edema
2. Pulse, BP-shock, RR-tachypnea.

Head to Foot

1. Any bleeding spots—petechiae, purpura, ecchymosis
2. Head—subconjunctival hemorrhage
3. Face-malar rash—SLE
   a. Blebs in lips and oral cavity—immune thrombocytopenic purpura (ITP)
   b. Gum hypertrophy
   c. Oral thrush.
4. Chest—bone pain and sternal tenderness, petechiae
5. Abdomen—petechiae
6. Limbs—joint examination, petechiae, capillary filling time, rash and hyperpigmentation.

Joint Examination

1. **Inspection:** Contour, swelling, redness, deformity, muscle wasting
2. **Palpation:** Temperature and tenderness, patellar tap
3. Movements.

Systemic Examination

1. **CVS:** CCF, murmurs
2. **Abdomen:** HSM

3. **CNS:** Intracranial bleeds
4. **Respiratory system:** Recurrent infections, TB.

Immune Thrombocytopenic Purpura

Characterized by petechial hemorrhages, ecchymosis, thrombocytopenia, reduced platelet survival, presence of platelet antibodies and a normal or increased number of megakaryocytes in the bone marrow.

Classification

Acute ITP and chronic ITP.

Clinical Features

1. Age incidence 2–6 years
2. Subcutaneous hemorrhages—petechiae
3. Ecchymosis, mucosal bleed
4. Hematemesis, melena and brain hemorrhages
5. No hepatosplenomegaly and lymphadenopathy (in C/c ITP spleen may be palpable)
6. Easy bruisability.

Investigations

1. **Thrombocytopenia:** Below 100,000/mm^3
2. Prolonged BT while CT, PT and aPTT are normal
3. Platelet antibody positive
4. Peripheral smear—large platelet (reaches up to the size of RBC), megakaryocytic fragments
5. Bone marrow—normal or increased number of megakaryocytes.

Indication for bone marrow in ITP
1. Cutaneous ITP
2. Abnormal total count and differential count
3. Unexplained anemia
4. Findings suggestive of bone marrow disease.

Differential Diagnosis

1. Aplastic anemia
2. Henoch-Schönlein purpura
3. Leukemia
4. Thrombotic thrombocytopenic pupura
5. Hemolytic uremic syndrome (HUS).

Treatment

1. No need of therapy in asymptomatic children with platelet counts above 40,000/mm^3
2. Supportive care
   a. Restriction of physical activities
   b. Avoid IM injections.
3. Corticosteroids—prednisolone 1–2 mg/kg/day for 2–3 weeks
4. IV immunoglobulin (IVIG) 400 mg/kg/day for 5 days
5. Anti-Rh (D) therapy 25 micro gm/kg/day for 3 days
6. Splenectomy—indicated in:
   a. Chronic ITP
   b. Uncontrolled bleeding
   c. Not responding to steroids/IVIG.

Hemophilia (X-Linked Recessive)

Congenital deficiency of plasma coagulation factor VIII (hemophilia A) or factor IX (hemophilia B).

History

1. Mild and moderate cases—asymptomatic
2. History of prolonged bleeding during tooth extraction, trauma surgery, circumcision

3. History of muscle hematoma, hemarthrosis
4. Newborn—bleeding from umbilical cord, headache and vomiting due to intracranial bleed
5. History of blood transfusion, jaundice, fever.

Clinical Features

1. Prolonged bleeding, muscle hematoma
2. Joint bleeding (hemarthrosis), painful joint swelling along with restriction of movements.

Head to Foot Examination

1. Subconjunctival hemorrhage, oral bleed, epistaxis, ecchymosis, muscle hematoma
2. Joints—painful swelling of weight-bearing joints
3. Restriction of movements and ankylosis
4. Atrophy of muscles around the joint
5. Joint bleeding (hemarthrosis).

Investigations

1. Hb-anemia due to blood loss
2. Normal BT with prolonged CT and aPTT, platelet count is normal or elevated
3. X-ray—synovial hypertrophy, hemosiderin deposition, fibrosis, damage to cartilage.

Differential Diagnosis

1. Von Willebrand disease
2. DIC
3. Vitamin K deficiency
4. Immune thrombocytopenic purpura
5. Leukemia
6. Aplastic anemia.

Treatment

Principle

To control and prevention of bleeding disorder, treatment of complications and rehabilitation.

Replacement therapy

1. Fresh frozen plasma—contains factor VIII and IX
2. Cryoprecipitate—contains factor VIII.

Hemarthrosis-Rx

1. Administration of factor VIII
2. Check aPTT
3. Immobilization of joint for 48 hours
4. Start ambulation and muscle strengthening exercises
5. Paracetamol, pethidine and diazepam used for pain relief.

Drug therapy for bleeding manifestation

1. Epsilon aminocaproic acid
2. Tranexamic acid
3. Desmopressin acetate
4. Fibrin glue—to seal the bleeding sites.

Prevention: Perinatal diagnosis by chorionic villus sampling, analysis of fetal blood or amniocentesis.

Henoch-Schönlein Purpura (HSP)

It characterized by the presence of nonthrombocytopenia palpable purpura, transient arthralgia and abdominal symptoms.

1. The most common nonthrombocytopenic purpura in children
2. The most common leukocytoclastic vasculitis in children.

Clinical Features

1. Purpuric rashes over extensor aspects of lower extremities and buttocks
2. Abdominal pain—intermittent, colicky, periumbilical abdominal pain
3. Glomerulonephritis—hematuria, hypertension.

Investigations

1. Total serum IgA level increased
2. Microscopic hematuria and proteinuria
3. Deposits of IgA and C3 in skin and renal biopsies.

Diagnostic Criteria for HSP

Criteria for diagnosis of HSP:
1. Palpable purpura
2. Age less than 20 years at first onset of symptoms
3. Bowel angina
4. Wall granulocytes on biopsy of arterioles or venules (at least 2 criteria for diagnosis).

Treatment

1. Maintenance of hydration
2. Drugs for pain relief
3. Avoid trauma
4. Prednisolone in GI bleed or CNS involvement.

Classification of Platelet Dysfunction

Quantitative Disorders

1. Decreased production
2. Increased production.

Qualitative Disorders

Inherited disorders
1. Glanzmann's thrombasthenia
2. Bernard-Soulier syndrome
3. Gray-Platelet syndrome
4. Wiskott-Aldrich syndrome.

Acquired disorders
1. Medications
2. Chronic renal failure
3. Cardiopulmonary bypass.

Comparison of bleeding disorders

Disorder	APTT	Thrombin time	Platelet count	Bleeding time
ITP	N	N	↓	↑
DIC	↑	↑	↓	↑
Liver disease	↑	N/↑	N/↑	↑/N
Platelet function disorder	N	N	N	↑
Hemophilia	↑	N	N	N
Von Willebrand	↑	N	N	↑

Anemia

1. *Hb < 11 gm/dL*: 6 months to 6 years
2. *Hb < 12 gm/dL*: Above 6 years
3. *Hb 5–10 gm/dL*: Moderate anemia
4. *Hb < 5 gm/dL*: Severe anemia.

Case Taking

Presenting complaints
1. Pallor
2. Breathlessness
3. Easy fatiguability
4. Jaundice
5. Fever.

History of Present Illness

1. History of hematemesis, melena, hemoptysis
2. History of bone pain, epistaxis, gum bleeds, skin discoloration—leukemia, aplastic anemia
3. History of jaundice, abdominal distention, abdominal pain, leg ulcers—hemolytic anemia
4. History of edema, oliguria—chronic renal disease.

Past History

1. Age of onset
2. Frequency of blood transfusion
3. History of splenectomy
4. History of chemotherapy
5. History of drug intake
6. History of jaundice, recurrent fever, bleeds.

Neonatal History

1. Neonatal jaundice
2. History of sepsis
3. Exchange transfusion.

Developmental History

Developmental delay.

Dietetic History

History of intake of iron rich food.

Immunization History

1. Hepatitis B—repeated blood transfusions
2. Pneumococcal, meningococcal—in case of splenectomy.

Family History

1. History of similar illness
2. Consanguinity
3. Major abdominal surgery—splenectomy.

General Examination

1. Pallor, jaundice, clubbing, edema, lymph nodes
2. Pulse, BP, RR, JVP
3. Hemolytic facies
4. Hyperpigmentation—vitamin B_{12} deficiency, Fanconi anemia
5. Mucocutaneous bleed
6. Skeletal deformity
7. Skin infection, leg ulcers
8. Abdominal distention
9. Signs of liver failure.

Anthropometry

1. Increased HC
2. Decreased height.

Abdomen

1. *Oral cavity*: Hyperpigmentation, tonsils, pharyngitis, gum hypertrophy
2. Abdominal distention
3. Hepatosplenomegaly.

CVS

ESM pulmonary area.

Diagnosis

1. Type of anemia
2. With/without complications—CCF
3. With/without blood transfusion, hypersplenism, PEM, developmental delay, signs of overload.

Microcytic Hypochromic Anemia

1. Iron deficiency anemia
2. Thalassemia
3. Lead poisoning.

Macrocytic Anemia

1. Vitamin B_{12} deficiency
2. Folate deficiency
3. Kwashiorkor
4. Drugs—phenytoin, primidone
5. Cirrhosis of liver.

Normocytic Normochromic Anemia

1. Physiological anemia of infancy
2. Hypothyroidism
3. Aplastic anemia
4. Hemolytic anemia
5. Leukemia.

Iron Deficiency Anemia

1. Common cause of nutritional anemia
2. Common age group—6 months to 2 years
3. Daily requirement of elemental iron—1st year (5–7 mg); childhood (10 mg); adult (15–20 mg)
4. Site of absorption of iron—duodenum and upper part of jejunum
5. Lactose, ascorbic acid, lysine, cysteine, histidine enhance iron absorption
6. Phosphates, phytates, carbonates, oxalate, milk and egg inhibit iron absorption
7. Principal supply of iron is reticuloendothelial system
8. Storage forms of iron—ferritin and hemosiderin.
   a. *Symptoms*: Pallor, easy fatiguability, koilonychia, atrophied tongue, pica
   b. *Signs*: Cardiac enlargement, systolic, diastolic flow murmurs.

Laboratory Investigations

Sequence of events in iron deficiency:
1. Decreased hemosiderin (Absence of hemosiderin by prussian blue staining)
2. Decreased serum ferritin level
3. Increased TIBC
4. Increased free erythrocyte protoporphyrin level
5. Decreased activity of iron containing enzymes
6. Reticulocyte count is decreased
7. Peripheral smear shows anisocytes and poikilocytes
8. MCH, MCV, MCHC are low.

Treatment

Deworming of patient.

Oral Iron Therapy

1. Iron preparations (anhydrous ferrous sulfate, ferrous fumarate, ferrous succinate, ferrous carbonate)
2. Optimal dose of elemental iron is 3–6 mg/kg of body weight given orally in 3 divided doses—Hb level rise by about 0.4 gm/dL/day
3. Oral iron therapy should be continued for at least 6–8 weeks after the Hg has reached normal levels to replete the iron stores
4. **Parenteral iron therapy:** Iron dextran, iron sucrose, iron sorbitol citrate
5. **Iron requirement:** Iron (mg) = weight (kg) × Hb deficit (gm/dL) × 4
6. *Blood transfusion* in severe anemia.

Source of Iron

1. Meat
2. Pulses
3. Liver
4. Kidney
5. Green vegetables
6. Fruits
7. Egg yolk.

Hemolytic Anemia

It is defined as anemia due to increased red cell destruction coupled with increased erythropoiesis.

Causes

1. Intracorpuscular defects
   a. **Hereditary red cell enzyme deficiency:** G6PD deficiency, Pyruvate kinase deficiency, Hexokinase deficiency
   b. **Hereditary defects of red cell membrane:** Hereditary spherocytosis, Hereditary elliptocytosis
   c. **Ineffective erythropoiesis:** Thalassemia (α or β)
   d. **Hemoglobinopathies:** Sickle cell and Hb C, D, E disease
   e. Paroxysmal nocturnal hemoglobinuria.
2. Extra corpuscular defects
   a. **Immune hemolytic anemia:** Isoimmunization
   b. **Infections:** Malaria, kala-azar
   c. **Schistocytic:** Disseminated intravascular coagulation (DIC), HUS.

Thalassemia

It is a heterogeneous group of hereditary disorders of reduced Hb synthesis.
Types: Alpha, beta and delta beta.
Beta thalassemia: Mutation on short arm of chromosome 11.

Clinical Features

1. Pallor, mild icterus and growth retardation
2. HSM due to extramedullary hemopoiesis.

Hemolytic Facies

1. Prominent frontal and parietal eminence, bossing of skull, with flattened vault, straight forehead, hypertrophy of maxilla, prominent malar eminence, depressed bridge of nose and puffy eyes
2. Fractures of long bones in untreated cases
3. Death may due to severe anemia, cardiac or liver failure.

Laboratory Investigation

1. Hb is reduced. Hb F is increased while HbA_2 is normal
2. Low total erythrocyte counts
3. Low hematocrit, MCV and MCH or MCHC
4. Bone marrow—erythroid hyperplasia
5. Osmotic fragility is decreased
6. Serum bilirubin moderately elevated
7. Fecal stercobilinogen is markedly elevated
8. Serum iron levels are high
9. **X-ray skull:** Hair on end appearance.

Treatment

1. Blood transfusion—maintain Hb level between 10 g/dL and 12 g/dL
2. Neocyte transfusion (younger cells with longer life span)
3. Chelation therapy
4. Desferrioxamine
5. Deferiprone
6. Splenectomy
7. New therapeutic approaches
8. Bone marrow transplantation
9. Gene manipulation
10. Gene therapy.

Leukemia

Most common form of childhood malignancy.

Subtypes

1. Acute lymphoblastic leukemia (ALL)
2. Acute myeloid leukemia (AML)
3. Chronic myeloid leukemia (rare).

ALL

1. *L1*: Scanty cytoplasm and inconspicuous nucleoli
2. *L2*: Abundant cytoplasm and large nucleoli
3. *L3*: Abundant cytoplasm and prominent nucleoli.

Clinical features

Pallor, fatigue, petechiae, purpura and bleeding, fever and infection, lymphadenopathy, HSM, bone tenderness.

Differential diagnosis

1. ITP, aplastic anemia, juvenile rheumatoid arthritis, IMN
2. Treatment—4 phases
   a. *Induction of remission*: Vincristine + Prednisolone + L asparaginase/Anthracycline (4–6 weeks)
   b. *Intensification (consolidation)*: Methotrexate + L asparaginase + Cyclophosphamide + Cytarabine + Epidophylotoxin
   c. *CNS prophylaxis*: Intrathecal methotrexate + Hydrocortisone + Cytarabine ± Cranial irradiation
   d. *Maintenance therapy*: 6 mercaptopurine + Methotrexate ± Vincristin + Prednisolone.

AML

1. *M1*: A/C Myeloblastic leukemia with minimal maturation
2. *M2*: A/C Myeloblastic leukemia with maturation
3. *M3*: A/C Promyelocytic leukemia (Associated with DIC)
4. *M4*: A/C Myelomonocytic leukemia
5. *M5*: A/C Monoblastic leukemia
6. *M6*: Erythroblastic leukemia
7. *M7*: A/C Megakaryoblastic leukemia (Associated with Down syndrome).

Clinical features

Pallor, fatigue, bleeding, fever.

Investigations

1. Low Hb, thrombocytopenia, high WBC counts
2. Peripheral smear—blast cells
3. Bone marrow aspiration—plenty of blast cells
4. In ALL lymphoblast are PAS positive but myeloperoxidase and Sudan black negative (code: ALL PAS).

Treatment

1. Induction therapy
2. Cytocine arabinoside + anthracycline
3. Postremission therapy (consolidation therapy)
4. Cytocine arabinoside + etoposide or bone marrow transplantation
5. Treatment of AML M3—by all trans retinoic acid (single agent therapy).

NERVOUS SYSTEM

Acute Flaccid Paralysis

Approach

Polio

1. Fever along with onset of paralysis in history
2. Affects muscle group, i.e. asymmetric
3. No sensory involvement
4. Cranial nerve involved is bulbar and bulbo spinal nerves.

Guillain-Barré Syndrome (GBS)

1. Affecting cranial nerves 7, 9, 10, 11, 12
2. History of fever, diarrhea, injections weeks or days prior to onset of weakness
3. Symmetric, ascending, plantar—flexor or no response. No or minimal distal subjective sensory symptoms
4. Bladder involvement nil or transient (only 20%).

Transverse Myelitis

1. Sensory, motor and reflex Level +
2. Plantars upgoing
3. Bladder involvement present DTR +++ after shock state.

Pseudoparalysis

1. Joint pathologies, fractures, scurvy to be ruled out in history and examination
2. Traumatic neuritis
3. History.

Surveillance

1. Report on Mondays even if nil report
2. Nodal officer reports to district immunization officer (DIO)
3. DIO reaches the site within 48 hours.

Clinical features of conditions causing acute flaccid paralysis

Site	Clinical features	Conditions
Muscles	Neck, limb girdle, proximal muscles affected, possible cardiomyopathy, occasional respiratory muscle involvement	Myoglobinuric myopathy, hypokalemic paralysis, toxic paralysis, myopathy of intensive care
Neuromuscular junction	Cranial, limb girdle and proximal muscles, may affect respiratory muscles, autonomic signs (presynaptic), fatiguability (post-synaptic)	Myasthenia gravis, botulism, hypermagnesemia
Peripheral nerve	*Weakness*: Distal, symmetrical, sensory, may have associated autonomic signs, may involve cranial nerves, deep tendon reflexes reduced/ lost early	Guillain–Barré syndrome, diphtheric neuropathy, porphyria, lead neuropathy, hypophosphatemia, cobalamine deficiency
Anterior horn cells	Predominantly motor signs, hyporeflexia, sensory symptoms uncommon, often asymmetric	Poliomyelitis, other enteroviruses

Number of collection of stool—8 g or thumb size 2 samples within 24–48 hours.
Sample send to Coonoor by reverse cold chain follow-up on the 60th day.
Outbreak response immunization: 500 children below the age of 5 years around the index case are immunized.
Polio will be considered eradicated if no case of polio is reported for 3 years.

Cerebral Palsy

Nonprogressive neurological disorder of tone, posture and movement due to defect/lesion in developing brain and often associated with mental retardation, epilepsy and special sense defects such as speech, vision, etc.

Presenting Complaints

1. Developmental delay
2. Abnormal movements
3. Aspiration causing respiratory infections
4. Seizures
5. Feeding problems
6. Difficulty in changing diapers
7. Scissoring at lower limbs.

History of Present Illness

Child known to have a development delay from the age of...., now presents with .... (if already diagnosed) and elaborate the presenting complaint, then to the following:

Developmental Delay

1. When noticed?
2. Consulted for what?
3. Which all developmental spheres affected?
4. Progress of development.

Higher Functions

1. Intelligence, speech, hand preference
2. Cranial nerve symptoms from 1 to 12
3. Motor, bulk—thinning of limb
4. Power—weakness, hand preference, bottom shuffling
5. Tone—spasticity, difficulty in changing diapers
6. Coordination—gait, day to day activities
7. Abnormal movements
8. Seizures—when noticed first, describe the pattern of seizure cleary, i.e. duration, stages, frequency of seizuers, Rx for chorea, athetosis, failure to thrive?

Past History

History of seizures, jaundice, tuberculosis.

Mother's Past Obstetric History

History of stillbirth, abortion.

Antenatal

1. Maternal age > 35
2. History of fever with rash
3. History of radiation
4. Drugs, trauma, UTI
5. Delayed quickening
6. History of diabetes mellitus (DM), hypertension (HTN)—macrosomia, difficult labor
7. Maternal sepsis
8. History of chorioamnionitis.

Natal

1. Preterm/term
2. Vaginal/Cesarean/Forceps/Vacuum-indication—Vertex/Breech
3. Hospital/home—increased risk of infection
4. Birth weight-GDM/Big head—toxoplasma
5. History of prolonged labor
6. Birth injuries
7. History of meconium stained amniotic fluid (MSAF)
8. Leaking/bleeding per vaginum.

Postnatal

1. Cried soon after birth/not
2. Fever, seizures
3. Jaundice—kernicterus
4. History of blood transfusion/exchange transfusion/phototherapy
5. Feeding problems

6. Umbilical sepsis
7. Any perinatal complications
8. Hospital admission.

Development History

1. Gross motor-neck steadyness applied or not
2. Fine motor
3. Language
4. Social
5. Loss of attained milestones
6. Deviated development.

Dietetic History

Feeding difficulties.

Immunization History

1. All vaccines can be give as per NIP
2. Pertussis vaccine can be given in CP as it is a nonprogressive neurological disorder.

Family History

1. History of similar illness
2. History of mental retardation
3. History of developmental delay
4. Seizures
5. Consanguinity.

Examination

General Examination

1. Bed ridden, conscious and cooperative
2. Abnormal movements
3. Edema—PEM
4. Vitals—aspiration pneumonia.

Head to Foot

1. Skull—microcephaly/macrocephaly, fontanelle, over-riding of sutures, flat occiput
2. Face—facial dysmorphism
3. Hair—PEM features
4. Eyes—pallor, jaundice, nystagmus, squint, cataract (intrauterine infections), bitot spots, gaze palsy.
5. Ears—discharge, deformities, hearing
6. Oral cavity—hygiene, dental caries, drooling, angular stomatitis, palate
7. Neck—shortening
8. Chest—skeletal deformities—pectus carinatum, rickety rosery, harrison sulcus, kyphoscoliosis.
9. Abdomen—PEM features
10. Spine-deformities—spinal, presacral edema
11. Limbs—posture and attitude, wasting, abnormal movements
12. Skin—neurocutaneous markers.

Anthropometry

Higher Functions

Motor system

1. *Bulk*: Inspection, palpation, measurements.
2. *Power*: Test muscle groups—observation and stimuli
3. *Tone*: Muscle groups
4. *Reflexes*: Superficial reflexes may be preserved in CP, deep reflexes, neonatal reflexes, abnormal movements
5. *Coordination*: Gait and activities.

Systemic Examination

Diagnosis

Topographical

Spastic quadriplegia/Spastic diplegia/Flacid diplegia.

Etiological

Birth asphyxia/Kernicterus/Preterm insult.

Functional

Associated deficits.

Mental retardation/Speech/Seizures/Vision/Hearing.

Early Markers of Cerebral Palsy

1. High pitch crying
2. Persistent primitive reflexes
3. Assymetrical movements and abnormal movements
4. Exaggerated deep tendon reflexes
5. Head circumference not adequate
6. Hand preference at an age < 1 year
7. Feeding problems
8. Hypertonicity/hypotonicity.

Neonatal reflexes

Reflex	Age of appearance	Age of disappearance
Rooting	Birth	3 months
Moro	Birth	5–6 months
Palmar grasp	Birth	6 months
Tonic neck	Birth	9–10 months
Landau	10 months	2 years
Parachute	8–9 months	Persists throughout life

Management

1. Treatment and management are directed at assisting the child to attain maximal physical functioning and potential physical, occupational, and speech therapy
2. Occupational therapy
3. Special education assistance
4. Orthopedic monitoring and support
5. Social and emotional support
6. Rehabilitation and vocational guidance
7. Medications for spasticity—baclofen, diazepam, dantrolene sodium and seizures
8. General support of the parents and family with counseling, educational programs, and support groups.

Apgar Scoring System

Criteria	0	1	2
Breathing	Nil	Slow gasping	Crying
Heart rate/min	Nil	Up to 100	> 100
Muscle tone	Flaccid	In between	Flexed
Reflex response	Nil	Grimace	Cry
Color	Pale/ blue	Peripheral cyanosis	Pink
7–10	Good		
3–6	Moderate CNS depression		
0–2	Severe CNS depression		

Types of Cerebral Palsy

1. Spastic—diplegia, quadriplegia and hemiplegia
2. Hypotonic/Atonic
3. Extrapyramidal.

Classification of cerebral palsy and major causes

Motor syndrome	Neuropathology	Major causes
Spastic diplegia	Periventricular leukomalacia (PVL)	Prematurity, infection, ischemia and endocrine/ metabolic (e.g. thyroid)
Spastic quadriplegia	PVL, malformations and multicystic encephalomalacia	Ischemia, infection Endocrine/metabolic, genetic/ developmental
Spastic hemiplegia	*Stroke*: *In utero* or neonatal	Thrombophilic disorders, infection, genetic/ developmental and periventricular hemorrhagic infarction
Extrapyramidal (athetoid, dyskinetic)	*Pathology*: Putamen, globus pallidus, thalamus, basal ganglia	Asphyxia, kernicterus, mitochondrial and genetic/metabolic

Down Syndrome

Trisomy 21

Presenting complaints

1. Abnormal facies
2. Mental retardation
3. Delayed milestones
4. Difficulty in feeding.

Prenatal, natal and postnatal history

1. Age of conception
2. Any exposure to radiation or drugs
3. Any spontaneous abortions
4. Delay in passage of meconium
5. Prolongation of physiological jaundice.

Developmental history

Developmental delay.

Head to Foot Examination

General Attitude

Playful, cooperative, fond of music.

Head and Face

1. *Head*: Flat occiput, microcephaly, brachycephaly, low posterior hair line, wide opened anterior fontanelle,
2. *Neck*: Short and broad with abundant neck skin
3. *Face*: Round moon face, flat facies, small nose with depressed nasal bridge, narrow short high arched palate with furrowed protruding tongue, pseudo-macroglossia, grimace in crying
4. *Teeth*: Small teeth, delayed dentition, malocclusion, caries teeth
5. *Eye*: Cataract, nystagmus, squint, abnormalities of visual acuity, epicanthal folds, mongoloid slant of eyes, hypertelorism, norrow palpebral fissures, keratoconus, Brushfield spot
6. *Ear*: Small and dysplastic low set ears, conductive hearing loss, serous otitis media.

Limbs

1. *Hand*: Short and broad small fingers clinodactyly (hypoplasia of middle phalanx with a single flexion crease of fifth finger) simian crease (single transverse palmar crease) and Sydney crease.
   More ulnar loops in finger tips
   Distal migration of proximal triradiate

2. *Feet*: Sandle gap (wider gap between first and second toe), subhallucial pad of fat, single longitudinal and deep crease on sole (Kennedy crease).
   Joints: Hypotonia, hyperflexibility of joints, poor Moro reflex.

Other Systems

CVS: PDA, VSD, ASD (ostium primum type)—endocardial cushion defects
RS: Recurrent infections, sleep apnea, pulmonary hypoplasia
GIT: Umbilical hernia, duodenal stenosis, duodenal webs, duodenal, ileal and jejunal atresia, Hirschsprung's disease, annular pancreas, imperforate anus, tracheoesophageal fistula and atresia, Meckel's diverticulum
Duodenal atresia—most common
External genitalia—undescended testes, hypospadiasis, micro penis and scrotum
CNS: Hypotonia, neonatal reflex, poor Moro's reflex
Blood: Acute leukemia most common—AML-M7, juvenile CML.

Screening in Down Syndrome

1. First trimester ultrasound screening by nuchal translucency—at 10–14 weeks. Maximum thickness of subcutaneous translucent area between the skin and soft tissue that overlies the fetal spine in sagittal plane is measured
2. *Second trimester ultrasound*: Duodenal atresia, nuchal thickness
3. *Second trimester serum screening*: Triple test—high beta hCG, low MSAFP, low unconjugated serum estriol
   Quadruple test—Triple test + Inhibin A (increases).

GROWTH AND DEVELOPMENT

Growth

Increase in size or mass of tissue.

Development

Maturation of functions.

Period of Growth

1. Postnatal period
   a. Newborn first 4 weeks after birth
   b. Infancy first year
   c. Toddler 1–3 years
   d. Preschool child 3–6 years.
2. Prenatal period
   a. Ovum 0–14 days
   b. Embryo 14 days to 9 weeks
   c. Fetus 9 weeks–birth.
   Perinatal period 22 weeks of gestation—7 days after birth
3. School age child 6–10 years (girls)
   6–12 years (boys)
4. Adolescence 10–19 years.

Failure to Thrive

It is a term given to infants whose rate of weight gain is sluggish. Length of the child may or may not be affected.

Causes

1. Intrinsic causes
   a. Defect in absorption
   b. Persistent vomiting
   c. Metabolic disorders
   d. Chronic disease of heart, lungs, kidney or liver.

2. Extrinsic causes
   a. Inadequate nutritional intake
   b. Social and environmental deprivation
   c. Or combination of both.

NUTRITION

It is the process by which organisms utilize foods. Carbohydrates, fats and proteins are termed as proximate principles.

Net protein utilization (NPU) = Digestibility coefficient × Biological value/100
= Nitrogen retained by body/Nitrogen intake

This gives us a more complete expression of protein value than amino acid score.

Amino acid score is a measure of concentration of each essential amino acid in the test protein expressed as a percentage of that amino acid in the reference protein.

= No. of miligram (mg) of essential amino acid per gm of protein/No of miligram of that amino acid in the egg protein

Biological value = Retained nitrogen (N_2) in the body × 100/Absorbed nitrogen (N_2)

Protein energy ratio (PE Ratio) = Energy from protein × 100/Total energy of food, i.e. the % of total energy of the food that is obtained from proteins.

Carbohydrates and proteins provide an energy of 4 kcal/g, whereas fats (long chain fatty acids) give 9 kcal/g short chain fatty acids give 5.3 kcal/g and medium chain fatty acids give 8.3 kcal/g.

Exclusive Breastfeeding

Only breast milk is given, no other food or drink, not even water is given. Medicines, vitamins or mineral drops are permitted if indicated.

Advantages of Breast Milk for the Baby, Mother and the Family

1. Nutritive value and digestibility
2. Protects from allergy
3. Emotional bonding
4. Low risk of infection
5. Physiological adaptation
6. Other benefits—babies have a higher IQ
7. Maternal advantages—lactational amenorrhea, economical factors, emotional bonding.

True contraindication for breastfeeding is when mother is on anti-cancer drugs, galactosemia and phenylketonuria.

Complimentary Feeding

Giving the child other nutritious food in addition to breast milk.

Criteria for Complimentary Food

1. Culturally acceptable
2. Physiologically suitable
3. Easily prepared at home with the existing facilities
4. Locally available and inexpensive
5. Easily digestible and nourishing
6. Adequate to provide all nutritional requirement of the infant with respect to energy, protein, vitamins and minerals.

Age independent anthropometric indices

Method	Name of index	Normal (severely malnourished)
Weight in kg/(height in cm)1.6 ×100	Dugdale's	0.88–0.97 (< 0.79)
Weight in kg/(height in cm)^2×100	Rao's	0.15–0.16 (< 0.14)
MAC (cm)/HC(cm)	Kanawati	0.32–0.33 (≤ 0.25)
MAC (between the age of 1–5 years)		> 13.5 cm (< 12.5 cm)

National Nutritional Programs

1. Mid-Day Meal Program
2. Balwadi Nutrition Program
3. National Vitamin A Prophylaxis Program
4. National Anemia Control Program.

Aim of the Programs

1. To improve general health and quality of the population
2. To control the infections
3. To provide nutritional supplementation.

Integrated Child Development Services (ICDS)

For children below 6 years, pregnant and lactating woman and other woman in the age group of 15–44 years.

Objectives

1. Improve the nutritional and health status of children in the age group 0–6 years
2. Laid the foundation for proper psychological, physical and social development of the child
3. Reduce the incidence of mortality, morbidity, malnutrition and school drop out
4. Achieve effective co-ordination of policy and implementation amongst the various departments promoting child development
5. Enhance the capability of mother to look after the normal health and nutrition needs through proper nutrition and health education.

Overweight
BMI exceeds the 85th percentage for that age and sex.
Obesity
BMI exceeds 95th percentage for that age and sex.
Cereals
(Cereals are poor in vitamin A, D, C, Ca and Fe)

i. *Rice*: 100 g gives 350 kcal, 7 g proteins. It is deficient in *lysine*. Polished rice causes *beri beri*
ii. *Wheat*: 100 g gives 350 kcal, 11 g proteins. It is deficient in *lysine* and *threonine*
iii. *Ragi*: 100 g gives 350 kcal, 7 g proteins, 3.14 mg Ca, 3.9 mg Fe and iodine. It is a weaning food
iv. *Maize*: It has high leucine content. It interferes with the absorption of niacin, vitamin B_2: causes *Pellagra* (Diarrhea, dermatitis, dementia).

Consequences of Delayed Weaning

1. Fe deficiency anemia
2. Triple M complex (Malnutrition, morbidity, mortality).

Pulses

1. Deficient in methionine
2. Combined in the ratio of 1:4 with cereals

Green gram (cherupayar)	350 kcal	24 g protein
Red gram (unakkapayar)	350 kcal	20 g protein
Black gram (uzhunnu)	350 kcal	24 g protein
Bengal gram (kadalai)	350 kcal	17 g protein
Soybean	350 kcal	43 g protein

Chemical score = mg of amino acid per 1 gm of protein
Essential amino acids are leucine, isoleucine, lysine, methionine, phenylalanine, threonine, tryptophan and valine.
Histidine is essential for infants.
Arginine, cysteine, taurine are essential for **LBW** babies.
Pulses lack vitamin A and C, but germinated pulses contain vitamin C.
Egg (reference protein): High quality, easily available, can be stored, contain all amino acid, easily absorbed. Human milk is very close to reference protein standard.
Deficient in **carbohydrates** and **vitamin C**.
Biological value 100 (BV of fish, milk-75; meat-80; rice-67)
Shell-12%; white-58%; yolk-30%
60 g egg contains 80 kcal energy 6 g fat 30 mg calcium
6 g protein 1.5 mg Iron 250 mg cholesterol
(Duck egg has increased amount of avidin which decreases the availability of biotin).

Milk

1. Deficient in vitamin C and iron
2. 100 mL of cows milk gives 70 kcal and 3.5 g protein
3. 100 mL of human milk gives 70 kcal and l.5 g protein.

Fiber

Complex unabsorbed carbohydrate seen in cereals vegetables, fruits and dried beans.

Types

1. Soluble-gums, pectins—decreases the absorption of glucose and cholesterol
2. Nonsoluble-cellulose—decreases the GI transit time.

Advantages

1. Increases bulk
2. Prevents constipation
3. Increases GI transit time
4. Limit glucose absorption
5. Decrease absorption of cholesterol
6. Prevents carcinoma colon
7. Decrease absorption of cholesterol.

Disadvantages

Decreases absorption of fat soluble vitamins and minerals.

Vitamin D—Rickets Features

1. Craniotabes
2. Rachitic rosary
3. Delayed dentition
4. Bow legs
5. Frontal bossing
6. Pigeon chest
7. Umbilical hernia
8. Kyphosis
9. Delayed closure of AF
10. Harrisons sulcus
11. Wrist broadening
12. Scoliosis.

X-ray

1. Mainly in the lower end of radius and ulna
2. Saucer like depression seen at the lower end of bone
3. Epiphyseal plate appears widened due to uncalcified osteoid
4. Splaying and flaring of ends
5. Osteoporosis.

Rx

1. Six lakh units of vitamin D orally or IM
2. Look for the healing line in the X-ray
3. If no healing line repeat the dose after 4 weeks
4. After this give vitamin D at a dose of 400 IU/day.

Vitamin E is given in preterms in order to prevent hemolytic anemia and as a prophylaxis against retrolental fibroplasia.

Vitamin A Deficiency

1. < 6 months : 50,000 IU/day till recovery.
2. 6 months - 1 year : 1 lakh IU
3. > 1 year : 2 lakh IU

In keratomalacia give 5000 IU/g/day × 5 days (Mega vitamin A therapy) followed by 25,000 IU /day till recovery.
Vitamin A prophylaxis program—given along with measles 1 lakh IU.
At 18 months along with DPT booster 2 1akh IU
Then every 6 months 2 lakh IU till 3 years.
Riboflavin deficiency:

1. Magenta tongue
2. Dermatitis
3. Angular stomatitis
4. Glossitis
5. Cheilitis.

Pyridoxin dependent syndromes

1. Dependent seizures
2. Responsive anemia
3. Homocystinuria.

For refractory neonatal seizures—therapeutic trial of 100 nanogram (ng) pyridoxin is given IM.

World Health Organization Classification (WHO) of Xerophthalmia

	Primary signs	Secondary signs
X1A	Conjunctival xerosis	XN night blindness
X1B	Bitot's spots	XF fundal changes
X2	Corneal xerosis	XS corneal scarring
X3A	Corneal ulceration (less than 1/3rd of cornea)	
X3B	Corneal ulceration (more than 1/3rd of cornea)	

Vitamin C (Seen in Citrus Fruits)

1. Scurvy
2. Pseudoparalysis
3. Skin and conjunctival bleeds
4. Gum bleeds
5. Scorbutic rosary
6. Delayed wound healing.

X-ray: Lower end of femur, upper end of humerus, ground glass appearance of bones is seen.
White line of Frenkel—metaphyseal line of calcified cartilage.
Wimburgers sign—epiphyseal centers of ossification surrounded by white ring.

Oral Rehydration Solution (ORS)

One packet mixed in 1 liter of boiled and cooled water (5 glasses). Use within 24 hours. It is ineffective in:

1. Persistant vomiting
2. High stool purge
3. Severe dehydration
4. Incorrect preparation.

Each packet contains

NaCl	3.5 g	Na^+	90 mEq
KCl	1.5 g	K^+	20 mEq
Na Citrate	2.9 g	Cl	80 mEq
Glucose	20 g	Citrate	10 mEq
Water 1 liter		Glucose	111 mEq
			311 mEq

Improved ORS Solution

1. Glucose replaced by starch based cereal powder 50 g/L such as cooked rice powder
2. Glucose polymers like maltodextrins or AA are either combined with or replaced with glucose. AA and dipeptides can promote water and salt absorption by mechanisms distinct from that of glucose
3. Low osmolality ORS—by reducing glucose and sodium.

Advantages

1. Reduce severity and duration of diarrhea
2. Reduce need for IV fluids.

Groundnut

100 g contains 540 kcal and 24 g protein.

1. It is rich in fat, carbohydrate (CHO), protein, vitamin A, B complex and some minerals.
2. Ten groundnuts contain 20 kcal and 1 g protein.

Tubers

1. Carrots—beta carotene
2. 1 unit vitamin A= 0.3 ug of retinol = 0.6 ug of β carotene = 1.2 ug of other carotenoids
3. Potato contains carbohydrates and vitamin C.

Green Leafy Vegetables

1. Rich in vitamin A, B Complex, calcium and iron.
2. Requirement 50 g/day.
3. Drumstick leaves contain increased amounts of Ca and Fe.
4. Amaranthin (cheera) is rich in carotenoids—100 g contains 20 kcal and 4 g proteins
5. Tomatoes are rich in vitamin C. 100 g contains 20 kcal and 1 g protein
6. Dates and dried fruits are rich in Fe.

Fish

1. It is rich in calcium and protein
2. 100 g contains 70 kcal and 20 g protein
3. It is also rich in PUFA both ω_6 (linoleic acid, arachidonic acid) and ω_3 (linolenic, eicosapentaenoic acid, docosahexaenoic acid).

Fats

1. Concentrated source of energy—its deficiency causes phrynoderma
2. It increases the palatability and acts as a vehicle for fat soluble vitamins. It causes satiety.

Antinutrients

1. Phytates—bind Fe, Zn, Ca-seen in cereals
2. Tannin—bind Fe-seen in tea
3. Oxalates—decreases Ca absorption
4. Goitrogens-isothiocyanates-cabbage—rich in vitamin C excess fiber binds trace elements
5. *Kesari dal*
6. Avidin-biotin
7. Aflatoxins.

Protein Energy Malnutrition

Clinical finding	Marasmus	Kwashiorkor
Occurrence	More common	Less common
Edema	Absent	Present
Activity	Active	Apathetic
Appetite	Good	Poor
Liver enlargement	Absent	Present
Mortality	Less than kwashiorkor	High in early stage
Recovery	Recover early	Long to recover
Infection	Less prone	More prone

Management of Severe Malnutrition

Hypoglycemia

1. Blood glucose level < 54 mg/dL or 3 mmol/L
2. If blood glucose cannot be measured, assume hypoglycemia
3. Hypoglycemia, hypothermia and infection occur as a triad.

Treatment

In asymptomatic hypoglycemia:
1. Give 50 mL of 10% glucose or sucrose solution orally or by nasogastric tube followed by first feed
2. Feed with starter F-75 every 2 hourly day and night.

In symptomatic hypoglycemia:
1. Give 10% dextrose intravenous (IV) 5 mL/kg
2. Follow with 50 mL of 10% dextrose or sucrose solution by nasogastric tube
3. Feed with starter F-75 every 2 hourly day and night
4. Start appropriate antibiotics.

Prevention

1. Feed 2 hourly starting immediately
2. Prevent hypothermia.

Hypothermia

1. Rectal temperature less than 35.5°C or 95.5°F or axillary temperature less than 35°C or 95°F
2. Always measure blood glucose and screen for infections in the presence of hypothermia.

Treatment

1. Clothe the child with warm clothes
2. Ensure that the head is also covered well with a scarf or a cap
3. Provide heat using radiation (overhead warmer), conduction (skin contact), convection (heat converter)
4. Avoid rapid rewarming as this may lead to disequilibrium
5. Feed the child immediately
6. Give appropriate antibiotics.

Prevention

1. Place the child's bed in a draught free area
2. Always keep the child well covered. Ensure that the head is also covered well

3. The child could also be put in the contact with the mother's bare chest or abdomen (skin to skin) as in the kangaroo mother care to provide warmth
4. Feed the child 2 hourly starting immediately after admission.

Dehydration

1. Difficult to estimate the dehydration status accurately in the severely malnourished child
2. Assume that all severely malnourished children with watery diarrhea have some dehydration
3. Low blood volume (hypovolemia) can co-exist with edema.

Treatment

1. Use reduced osmolarity ORS with potassium supplements for rehydration and maintenance
2. Amount depends upon how much the child wants, volume of stool loss and whether the child is vomiting
3. Initiate feeding within 2–3 hours of starting rehydration with F-75 formula on alternate hours with reduced osmolarity ORS
4. Be alert for signs of overhydration.

Prevention

1. Give reduced osmolarity ORS at 5–10 mL/kg after each watery stool, between feeds to replace the stool losses
2. If breastfed, continue breastfeeding
3. Initiate refeeding with starter F-75 formula.

NEWBORN INFANTS

1. Neonatal period—from birth to under four weeks
2. Early neonatal period—first week of life
3. Late neonatal period—extends from 7th to < 28th day
4. Postneonatal period—period of infancy from 28 days to < 365 days of life
5. Perinatal period—from 20th week of gestation to less than 7 days of life
6. Term neonate—any neonate born between 37 and < 42 weeks (259–293 days) of gestation irrespective of birth weight
7. Preterm neonate—any neonate born before 37 weeks (< 259 days) of gestation irrespective of birth weight
8. Post-term neonate—a neonate born at a gestation age of 42 weeks or more (294 days or more) gestation irrespective of birth weight
9. Low-birth weight neonate—any neonate weighing less than 2500 g at birth irrespective of the gestational age
10. Very low birth weight neonate—any neonate weighing less than 1500 g at birth irrespective of gestational age
11. Extremely low birth weight neonate—any neonate weighing less than 1000 g at birth irrespective of gestational age
12. Neonatal mortality rate—deaths of the infants under the first 28 days of life per 1000 live births.

Steps of Warm Chain

1. Warm delivery room
2. Warm resuscitation
3. Immediate drying
4. Skin to skin contact
5. Breastfeeding
6. Bathing postponed
7. Appropriate clothing
8. Mother and baby together
9. Professional alertness
10. Warm transportation.

Problems of Preterm Babies Versus Those in IUGR Babies

Problems in Preterm Babies

1. Hypothermia
2. Birth asphyxia
3. Respiratory (hyaline membrane disease, pulmonary hemorrhage, pneumothorax, bronchopulmonary dysplasia, pneumonia)

4. Apnea of prematurity
5. Metabolic (hypoglycemia, hypocalcemia)
6. Hematologic (anemia, hyperbilirubinemia)
7. Bacterial sepsis
8. Feeding problems and poor weight gain.

Problems in IUGR Babies

1. Perinatal asphyxia
2. Meconium aspiration
3. Hypothermia
4. Hypoglycemia
5. Feed intolerance
6. Polycythemia
7. Growth retardation.

Essential Criteria for Perinatal Asphyxia

1. Prolonged metabolic or mixed academia (pH < 7.0) on an umbilical arterial blood sample
2. Persistence of APGAR score of 0–3 for > 5 minutes
3. Neurological manifestations, e.g. seizures, coma, hypotonia or hypoxic ischemic encephalopathy in the immediate neonatal period
4. Evidence of multiorgan dysfunction in the immediate neonatal period.

Differences between caput succedaneum and cephalohematoma

Characteristics	Caput succedaneum	Cephalohematoma
Incidence	Very common	Less common
Location	Subcutaneous plane	Located over parietal bones, between skull and periosteum
Time of presentation	Maximum size and firmness at birth	Increasing size for 12–24 hours and then stable
Clinical time course	Softens progressively from birth and resolves within 2 or 3 days	Takes 3 to 6 weeks to resolve
Characteristic findings	Diffuse, crosses suture line	Does not cross the suture line, has distinct margins
Association	None	Linear fracture of skull bone in 5–25%; hyperbilirubinemia (due to break down of hemoglobin in the bleed)

PEDIATRIC SURGERY

Infantile Hypertrophic Pyloric Stenosis

The pylorus is thickened and elongated and its lumen is narrowed due to hypertrophy of circular muscle fibers of pylorus.

Clinical Features

1. Nonbilious vomiting at 3 to 6 weeks of age
2. Dehydration, failure to thrive, constipation
3. Visible peristalsis, palpable pyloric mass.

Investigations

1. X-ray barium meal-dilatation and hypertrophy of stomach, narrow pylorus (string sign)
2. Ultrasonography (USG) abdomen—dome shaped thickened pyloric sphincter.

Treatment

1. Correction of dehydration and dyselectrolytemia
2. Stomach wash with isotonic saline
3. Ramstedt's operation (pyloromyotomy).

Intussusception

Acute intestinal obstruction in infancy (around the age of 1 year).

Clinical Features

1. Episodic crying (due to severe colicky abdominal pain)
2. Blood stained stool (red current jelly)
3. Vomiting
4. Sausage shaped mass palpable in right quadrant of abdomen.

Investigation

1. X-ray barium enema—shows cupping, as it is obstructed by intussusception
2. USG abdomen.

Treatment

1. It is a surgical emergency
2. Shock is treated and rehydrated
3. Uncomplicated cases relieved by hydrostatic pressure of barium enema
4. Complicated cases managed surgically.

Wilm's Tumor

Most common malignant tumor of kidney under 5 years of age. Tumor usually unilateral or may be bilateral. Tumor gene has been identified at chromosome 11.

Clinical Features

1. Abdominal mass, pain
2. Hematuria, hypertension
3. Anorexia, vomiting.

Investigations

1. Complete blood cell and urine routine examination
2. X-ray chest for metastasis in lung
3. USG abdomen
4. CT scan.

Staging of Wilm's Tumor

Stage

1. Tumor concerned to kidney and completely excised
2. Tumor extends beyond kidney and completely excised
3. Tumor infiltrate renal fat, residual tumor after surgery, LN+ (hilar and para-aortic)
4. Metastasis in lung/liver, rarely bone and brain
5. Bilateral renal involvement.

Treatment

Surgery (Nephrectomy) + chemotherapy (actinomycin D and vincristine) + radiotherapy.

Posterior Urethral Valve

1. Most common cause of obstructive uropathy in children
2. Only boys affected
3. Can extend anywhere from prostatic urethra to external sphincter
4. Dilatation of proximal urethra with bladder hypertrophy-hydroureter-hydronephrosis-end stage renal disease (ESRD)
5. 50%—VUR and 30%—ESRD
6. Antenatal diagnosis
   a. Oligohydramnios/pulmonary hypoplasia
   b. B/L hydronephrosis/distended bladder.

7. *Antenatal treatment*: Vesicoamniotic shunt/Fetal surgery
8. Postnatal symptoms
   a. Poor urinary stream
   b. Palpable bladder.
   c. May present later as UTI/FTT/uremia.
9. Postnatal diagnosis
   a. Vesicoureteric reflux
   b. Perineal USG.
10. Postnatal management
    a. Catheterization with feeding tube and not balloon catheter
    b. Transurethral ablation
    c. If not possible or RFT abnormal, temporary vesicostomy and ablation later
    d. Irreversible renal damage—pyelostomy
    e. Correction of sepsis/uremia/electrolyte imbalance
    f. Antibiotic prophylaxis.
11. Good prognostic factors
    a. Normal prenatal USG from 18 to 24 weeks
    b. S creatinine < 1.0 mg% after bladder decompression
    c. Intact corticomedullary differentiation of the kidneys on USG.
12. Bad prognostic factors
    a. Oligohydramnios and pulmonary hypoplasia
    b. Diurnal incontinence beyond 5 years of age
    c. Cortical cysts in both kidneys.
13. Prenatally diagnosed PUV's especially by 2nd trimester have poorer prognosis
14. 15% of boys with PUV-U/L reflux into dysplastic kidney—VURD (valve, U/L reflux, dysplasia) syndrome.

Vesicoureteric Reflux

1. 80% are females and average age at diagnosis is 2–3 years
2. Diagnosed during evaluation of UTI
3. Graded 1–4 by voiding cystourethrogram (VCUG)
4. Leads to pyelonephritis/rennin induced hypertension/ESRD—reflux nephropathy
5. 50% duplication of upper UT has reflux
6. May present as prenatal hydronephrosis
7. Investigations
   a. Contrast VCUG
   b. Radionuclide VCUG
   c. Cystourethrosonogram.
8. Mean age of spontaneous resolution of reflux is 6 to 7 years
9. Chance of spontaneous resolution decreases with increasing age.

OBJECTIVE STRUCTURED CLINICAL EXAMINATION (PEDIATRICS)

General Points to Remember

1. Always ask for consent from the mother
2. Enquire about the name of the child
3. Establish a rapport
4. Explain briefly what is going to be done.

Do not Forget to Ask

1. The age of the child (precisely in months) (if the child is only of a few days age, ask the precise time of birth of the child)
2. For what reason the child has come
3. About the vaccination status
   a. While advising the mother, both the doctor and the other should be seated and facing each other
   b. After completing the objective structured clinical examination (OSCE), if time remains, keep talking and do not just sit mum
   c. Any examination done on a particular side is to be repeated on the other side too
   d. In case of giving advice after doing it, asks the mother if she has any doubts (Remember that the mother asking you any doubts is going to fetch you extra marks as it shows that you have gained the confidence of the mother)

e. Before palpating, or placing your hand on the child, remember to warm your hands
f. After completing the OSCE, return the child to the same state as before (dress him) or place the instrument as it was before (e.g. thermometer)
g. In case of neonates always remove the cap of the baby if he is wearing one (for instance there may be cephalhematoma) inspect after removing the diaper—there may be an undescended testis or abnormalities of the external genitalia.

History Taking and Advise

1. **Take a case history of diarrhea**
   a. When did the episodes started?
   b. Number of stools passed, frequency
   c. Is it bloody?
   d. Is there associated fever and vomiting?
   e. Urine passed or not, frequency
   f. Are the eyes sunken or normal?
   g. Are tears coming while crying?
   h. Is the child breastfeeding vigorously or not?
   i. Is there associated seizures?
   j. Is there abdominal distension?
   k. Is the child thirsty?
   l. Is there any recent change in food?
   m. Any previous history?
   n. Is the child fully immunized?
2. **Assessment of a case of diarrhea**
   Look for:
   a. Depressed anterior fontanelle
   b. Tears in eyes
   c. Sunken eyes
   d. Dry tongue
   e. Palpate with finger for dryness of buccal mucosa
   f. Pulse
   g. BP
   h. Skin pinch
   i. Edema
   j. Kussmaul's breathing
   k. Ask for urine output frequency
   l. Ask for a glass of water and bring it near the baby to assess the thirst of child.
3. **Advise on discharge of a child with diarrhea**
   a. Explain the condition of the disease to the mother
   b. Explain to her about the preparation of ORS
   c. Explain to her about quantity and frequency of giving ORS :
      i. Boil and cool 1 liter (5 glasses)
      ii. One packet dissolved in five glasses of water
      iii. Two to three tsp every 5 to 10 minutes after every bout of diarrhea.
   d. Explain about other home available solutions
   e. Tell about the complications
   f. If complications arise, to get the child back to the hospital
   g. Encourage breastfeeding and normal diet
   h. If ORS is used up, return for more
   i. Explain the importance of immunization.
4. **Advice on immunization**
   a. Ask the age of the child
   b. Explain the importance of immunization
   c. Ask about vaccination like BCG (injection on left arm at birth), OPV (oral drops), DPT (inj on lateral aspect of thigh)
   d. Tell her about optional vaccines
   e. Tell her that is available at her nearest PHC on all Wednesdays
   f. Even in case of slight fever, get the child for immunization
   g. It will not cause any harm to the child
   h. Explain the importance of pulse polio immunization
   i. Ask if she has any doubts.
5. **History in case of febrile seizures**
   a. Age of child
   b. Is this the first episode or recurrent?
   c. Whether occurred within 24 hours of fever
   d. Whether moving all his limbs or local (focal/gen)
   e. Any loss of consciousness

f. Any abnormal behavior in the postictal period
g. Duration of attacks
h. Any associated vomiting? (raised ICT)
i. Whether seizures in absence of fever
j. Whether seizures present before 6 months
k. Any family history of seizures.

6. **Advice on prophylaxis of febrile seizures**
   a. Explain the condition to the mother
   b. During febrile episodes explain her to decrease temperature by using
      i. Light clothing
      ii. Ventilated room
      iii. Tepid sponging
      iv. Tab paracetamol
      v. Diazepam (oral/suppository)
   c. Rush to doctor if temperature does not subside
   d. *In case of seizures*:
      i. Keep child away from dangers
      ii. Do not put anything in the mouth
      iii. Keep the head tilted to one side
   e. Explain on immunization.
7. **Immunization of an unimmunized child**

Visits	< 5 years	> 5 years
1st visit	BCG , DPT, OPV, HB	TT, DT. HiB
2nd visit (1 month later)	OPV, DPT, HB	TT/DT. HiB
3rd visit (1 month later)	OPV, DPT, MMR/measles	MMR, typhoid
4th visit (1 year later)	OPV, DPT, HB	HB
Every 3 years	Typhoid booster	Typhoid booster

8. **Mother of a 3-month-old child complains that the child is not feeding adequately. Weight of the child is 4.2 kg and the child has incessant cry during evenings**
   a. Ask for birth weight
   b. Reassure the mother that the child has adequate weight gain
   c. Ask whether the child is suckling properly (Drinks for 0–15 min and sleeps for about 2 hours each drink: 8–10 such feeds per day; passes urine 6–8 times/day)
   d. Explain about positioning of the child (tummy-to-tummy, chest-to-chest, child-to-breast, baby-to-mother)
   e. Feed alternatively from both breasts
   f. Ask whether she changes diapers as and when the child passes urine (reason for incessant cry—wet diapers)
   g. Ask for fevers (meningitis)
   h. Explain on immunization.
9. **Assessment of jaundice in a neonate**
   a. Age of the child in days (if possible in hours) (less than 30 hours indicate pathological jaundice)
   b. First apply pressure over the tip of the nose and look for yellowish discoloration in the blanched skin
   c. Apply the pressure over face, chest, abdomen below the level of the umbilicus, over the shin, over the foot, palms and soles in that order. (Kramers dermal zone)
   d. Urine and stool color
   e. Umbilical sepsis
   f. Activity
   g. Cephalhematomas
   h. Bleeding
   i. Comment on the level of jaundice.

10. **Advise on discharge of child with nephritic syndrome**
    a. Dietary advice—avoiding yolk, fatty foods and excess salt
    b. Explain the disease and prognosis (like say there are chances of relapse)
    c. Weekly BP monitoring
    d. Explain on administration of steroids and its side effects like appearance of moon face
    e. Educate mother on heat and acetic acid test, the procedure and interpretation. Take 3/4 of a test tube with clean urine heat it by tilting it over a flame; then add 8 drops of acetic acid (vinegar) and note the color.
11. **Keep it in front of the newspaper and try reading it**
    a. Can read small letters clearly nil
    b. Can read but unclear 1+
    c. Can read only headlines 2+
    d. Cannot read headlines but can see them as dark areas 3+
    e. Cannot see the paper at all 4+
    f. If the reading comes to 3+ or 4+ for 3 consecutive days then ask her to report to a doctor
    g. Early management of infections.
12. **Assess the developmental status**
    a. In order to save time do the assessment while taking history.
    b. Developmental history (age must)
       i. Gross motor
          - Ventral suspension (child < 16 weeks)
          - Prone
          - Supine
          - Pull to sit and sitting
          - Standing
       ii. Fine motor
          - Hand mouth coordination
          - Hand eye coordination
          - Grasp-palmar/pincer
          - Writing
       iii. Vision and hearing
       iv. Language, social and adaptive
       v. Bowel and bladder development can be assessed from the history.
13. **Assess the nutritional status**
    Dietetic history
    Head-to-foot examination
    a. Edema, ascites, hair and skin changes of PEM
    b. Pallor and other stigmatas of Fe deficiency anemia
    c. Eye changes of vitamin A deficiency.
    d. Vitamin D
       i. Delayed closure of AF
       ii. Craniotabes
       iii. Delayed dentition
       iv. Harrison's sulcus/rickety rosary (painless)
       v. Pectus carinatum and other bony abnormalities
       vi. Widening of wrist and malleoli
       vii. Heparin-surface-modified (HSM).
    e. Vitamin B complex
       i. Glossitis, cheilitis
       ii. Peripheral neuropathies (B_1, B_6, B_{12}), hyperdynamic circulation, cardiomegaly
       iii. Angular stomatitis, magenta tongue, circumcorneal vascularization
       iv. Diarrhea, dementia, dermatitis, pellagrous boot and glove, casals necklace.
    f. Vitamin C
       i. Perifollicular hemorrhage
       ii. Gum bleeding
       iii. Pseudoparalysis

iv. Scorbutic rosary (painful)
   - Anthropometry grading
   - Vital signs
   - Look for any foci of infection; skin, ear, lung

14. **Other neonatal spotters**
   a. Mongolian Blue Spot
   b. Cradle Cap (Seborrheic dermatitis)
   c. Erythema toxicum
   d. Umbilical hernia.

Clinical assessment of term and preterm

	Preterm	Term
Hair	Fuzzy, wooly	Normal
Ear	Cartilage deficient , poor recoil	Normal
Breast nodule	> 5 mm	< 5 mm
Genitalia		
Labia	Separate	Apposed
Testis	Not descended	Descended
Scrotal rugosity	Absent	Present
Soles superficial crease	Present	Absent
Neurological	Square window (+)ve	Absent
Tone		
Popliteal angle	Obtuse	Acute
Adductor angle		
Scarf sign	Present	Absent
Arm recoil	No recoil	Recoil
Moro reflex	Present	Absent
Arm to ear		

CASE CHARTS

1. A fully immunized 5-year-old boy comes with high fever, stridor and difficulty in swallowing. He is not able to talk and sits up learning forward with neck extended and saliva dribbling from his chin.
   a. What is the most probable diagnosis? (Ans: Acute epiglotitis)
   b. What is the causative organism?
   c. What is the radiological finding?
   d. What is the immediate management if stridor worsens?
   e. What is the drug of choice?
2. A 10-year-old boy presents with high fever jaundice; severe myalgia, headache, conjunctival congestion. Total Count—18000 with predominant neutrophils.
   a. What is the most probable diagnosis? (Leptospirosis)
   b. What is the etiological agent?
   c. Give 2 important complications (Also refer viral hepatitis and compare).
3. A 2-year-old girl presents with fever, vomiting and convulsions since 2 days. CSF examination shows. Sugar—15 mg/dL, Protein—100 mg/dL, Cells—500/mm^3 (polymorphs).
   a. What is your diagnosis? (Bacterial meningitis)
   b. Duration of treatment in a child less than 1 month.
   c. Mention 3 complications.
   d. What are the clinical signs you will elicit? (Also refer TB meningitis and viral meningitis and compare).
4. A 3-year-old boy presents with fever and one episode of convulsions lasting for 5 minutes. Blood picture: TC-14,000, lymphocytes-8000 CSF shows: Pressure-75 cm of CSF, Cells-5 lymphocytes/mm^3, Sugar-70 mg/dL, Protein-30 mg/dL.
   a. What is the most probable diagnosis? (Febrile seizures)
   b. Comment on the blood and CSF values.
   c. How will you manage this case?

5. A 5-day-old girl presents with yellowish discoloration of skin up to the umbilicus since 1 day. Total serum bilirubin-10 mg/dL, Direct bilirubin-1.2 mg/dL.
   a. What is your diagnosis? (Physiological jaundice)
   b. How will you manage if the bilirubin level rises?
   c. What are the possibilities if the jaundice developed on the first day?
   d. What are the complications you can anticipate? (Also refer extrahepatic biliary atresia (EHBA) and Rh incompatibility and compare).
6. A 4-week-old male child presents with nonbilious vomiting since 5 days.
   a. What is the electrolyte and acid base balance abnormality expected?
   b. Which is the IV fluid of choice?
   c. What is the definitive management?
   d. Mention 2 causes of bilious vomiting in a child.
7. A 6-month-old girl presented with acute watery diarrhea since 2 days and was treated with ORS solution for 2 days. Now she develops abnormal consciousness and on examining skin has a doughy feel. Serum electrolytes-K^+4.5 mEq/L, Na^{+}-165 mEq/L.
   a. What is the diagnosis? (Hypernatremia)
   b. What is the dreaded complication if a child with TOF develop diarrhea?
   c. Give 3 possibilities if a child with diarrhea develops seizures.
   d. What are the improved ORS solution?
8. A 2-month-old infant presents with yellowish discoloration of sclera with normal colored urine and pallor.
   a. What is the most probable diagnosis? (Hereditary spherocytosis)
   b. What are the peripheral smear findings?
   c. What is the confirmatory test you will do?
   d. What is the pattern of inheritance? (Also refer thalassemia and sickle cell anemia and compare).
9. A 1-year-old Sandeep presents with 2 episodes of epistaxis and gum bleeding. On examination multiple ecchymotic patches are seen. Abdomen was normal.
   a. Bleeding time—12 minutes APTT—1 minutes
   b. Clotting time—16 minutes PTT—12 seconds
   c. Platelet — 3 lakh/mm^3
      i. What is your diagnosis? (Von Willebrands disease)
      ii. What are the confirmatory tests you will do?
      iii. What are the drugs used?
      iv. What is the pathogenesis? (Also refer ITP, Hemophilia and acute lymphocytic leukemia (ALL) and compare).
10. A 14-day-old baby of Sangeetha presents with prolonged jaundice, delayed passage of meconium, poor cry, floppiness and poor sucking.
    a. What is your diagnosis? (Congenital hypothyroidism)
    b. What is the radiological investigation you will do?
    c. What is the most important screening test?
    d. What is the drug used and for how long?
11. A 2-year-old boy develops fever with cough with a respiratory rate of 50/min. He is grunting with retraction of the chest wall.
    a. What is the diagnosis? (Severe pneumonia) (according to ARI control programme)
    b. What is the drug of choice?
    c. What will you do if the child develops cyanosis and is unable to feed?
    d. What are the other danger signs?
12. A 7-year-old boy comes to you with fever and joint pain. On examining there is pallor and a tic-tac heart rhythm with a soft tender liver and spleen.
    a. What is the complete diagnosis? (Rheumatic fever, infective endocarditis, CCF)
    b. What is the drug of choice and give the dose and duration
    c. Mention 3 other findings which you will look for
    d. What are the essential criteria? (Also refer TOF and congenital heart disease and compare).
13. A 7-year-old female child develops puffiness of the eyes and smoky discoloration of urine. Skin reveals healed pyoderma scars. BP—150/80 mm Hg.
    a. What is your diagnosis? (Post streptococcal glomerulonephritis)
    b. What is the dietary advice you will give?
    c. What are the complications you can expect?

d. What would you consider if she complains of dysentery and malena?
e. What do you infer if she develops seizures? (Also refer nephrotic syndrome and compare)

14. A 6-year-old child presents with muffled voice and trismus. On examination, shows an unilateral bulge in the soft palate and peritonsillar region and uvular deviation to the opposite side.
   a. What is the diagnosis? (Quinsy)
   b. What is the treatment?
   c. What drugs will you prefer?
15. A 4-year-old child presents with biphasic stridor, brassy cough, low grade fever and suprasternal, sternal recessions. cyanosis present.
   a. What is the diagnosis? (Croup)
   b. What is the causative organism?
   c. What is the X-ray finding?
   d. What is the treatment?
16. A 12-year-old child presents with irritability, incessant cry, photophobia, on examination shows neck rigidity, multiple hemorrhagic spots in the body. Investigation shows bleeding and clotting time prolonged.
   a. What is the complete diagnosis? (meningococcal septicemia with DIC)
   b. Other causes for neck rigidity.
17. A 3-year-old child presenting with history of fever, abdominal pain and hematuria. On examination shows mass palpable in the lumbar region.
   a. Diagnosis (Wilms tumor)
   b. Other associated lesions
   c. Treatment
18. A 5-year-old child presenting with bleeding spots in the skin and fatigue. On examination hyperpigmented skin, microcephaly and testicular atrophy with hypoplastic thumb.
   a. Diagnosis (Fanconi's anemia).
   b. What is the treatment?
19. A fully immunized child with grade IV PEM was referred with paralysis of all 4 limbs following an attack of diarrhea. There was no similar complaint in the vicinity. On giving one drug the condition was relieved.
   a. What is the probable cause? (Hyperkalemic paralysis)
   b. What cheap investigation will clinch the diagnosis?
   c. What will be the drug given?
20. A 5-year-old child presents in OP with joint pain radiating to groin. There is also history of recurrent diarrhea and respiratory tract infection.
   a. Which vitamin deficiency can be the cause of this clinical picture? (Vitamin A deficiency)
   b. What is the daily requirement in this child?
   c. Why preterm infants are at high-risk of developing this vitamin deficiency?
   d. Which is the earliest sign and symptom?
21. An Infant's parent presents with complaints that the child is not moving his limbs and with history of bleeding from mouth and subconjunctival hemorrhage. Child cries when ever he is handed by someone. Investigations: bleeding time (BT), prothrombin time (PT), activated partial thromboplastin time (APTT), platelet count normal.
   a. What is the probable cause? (Scurvy)
   b. What is the treatment?
22. A child with grade III PEM is suffering from an attack of acute diarrhea. On giving ORS, condition worsened and the child started passing large amount of stools and was extremely thirsty and dehydrated, on stool examination, it contained large amount of glucose. On discontinuing ORS, stool volume decreased.
   a. What is the line of management? (glucose malabsorption)
23. The mother of a child with recurrent episode of watery diarrhea for several days complained that the child had repeated episodes of convulsion, noisy breathing, with breathlessness and abnormal positioning of hands.
   a. What may be the probable metabolic cause? (Hypocalcemia)
24. A 3-year-old child presents with history of recurrent jaundice. On examination hepatosplenomegaly present. There is similar history in the family. Investigation: Hb-8 g%, PS-microspherocytes. Osmotic fragility increased.
   a. What is the immediate DD with similar blood picture? And what investigation is required to rule it out? (autoimmune hemolytic anemia)
   b. What would be the possible cause of sudden fall in Hb? (crisis)
   c. What vitamin has to be given to the child and for what reason? (folate)

DRUGS

1. **Paracetamol:** 10–15 mg/kg/dose 4 times
   Complications: Hepatic necrosis.
2. **Frusemide:** 0.5–1 mg/kg wt IV, 2-4 mg/kg/day po, 1–2 mg/kg/day IV
   Indications: CCF, left ventricular failure (LVF), nephrotic syndrome (massive edema), renal failure
   Complications: Ototoxicity, hypokalemia, hyperglycemia, hypocalcemia.
3. **Aminophylline:** 5 mg/kg/dose slow IV in 5% dextrose saline every 8th hourly (infusion 0.9 mg/kg/hr).
   It is a phosphodiesterase inhibitor causes increased cyclic AMP and relaxes smooth muscle.
   Used in acute severe asthma.
   Side effects: Restlessness, cardiac arrhythmias, nausea and vomiting, seizure.
   Drug interaction with carbamazepine and cimetidine.
4. **Salbutamol:** 0.15 mg/kg/dose thrice daily orally. 100 mg/puff every 6th hourly.
5. **Terbutaline:** 1–2 puffs of 250 mg 6th hourly inhalation given oral, subcutaneous, nebulizer, IV route, IM (0.1 mg/kg)
   Side effects: Tachyphylaxis, tremor, tachycardia, ankle edema, hypokalemia.
6. **Gentamicin:** 5 mg/kg dose IM 8th hourly
   It is an aminoglycoside.
   Effective against gram (–) organisms (*E. coli, Proteus, Klebsiella*).
   Exclude renal failure before giving.
   Used in UTI, RTI especially in newborn, subacute bacterial endocarditis (SABE), bowel injuries, surgery
   Side effects: Ototoxicity, renal toxicity, renal failure, neuromuscular blockade
7. **Diazepam:** 0.3 mg/kg/dose IV, oral, rectal.
   Uses: Status epilepticus, febrile seizure prophylaxis, relief of spasm in tetanus, as hypotonic and sedative.
   Side effects: Respiratory depression, hypotension, bradycardia and leukopenia.
8. **Phenytoin:** 5–10 mg/kg/day in 1–2 divided doses given slow IV (otherwise hypotension and arrhythmias)
   Used in epilepsy, cardiac arrhythmias.
   Side effects: Hirsutism, gingival hyperplasia, pseudolymphoma, nystagmus, cognitive dysfunction, sedation, ataxia, rickets as it interferes with calcium metabolism
9. **Metoclopramide:** 0.5–2 mg/kg; Used in persistent vomiting
   Side effects: Extrapyramidal side effects.
10. **Ranitidine:** 150 mg bd, 2 mg/kg/day orally/IM/IV every 12 hours.
    a. Given prior to surgery
    b. Given along with NSAIDs and steroids.
11. **Dexamethasone:** 0.15 mg/kg/dose every 6th hourly IV
    Uses: TB meningitis, fetal lung maturity, H. *influenzae* meningitis (should precede antibiotics by 15 minutes)
    Side effects: Hypothalamopituitary axis depression, Obesity, Prone for infections, delayed wound healing, Osteoporosis, precipitates diabetes, Gastritis, Pancreatitis, striae, proximal myopathy
12. **$NaHCO_3$:** Used in severe acidosis both metabolic and respiratory (1–2 mEq/kg/dose) (avail in 7.5% and 8.4% solution)
13. **KCl**
    Uses: Hypokalemia and alkalosis, PEM, diarrhea; (due to hypokalemia) (9–12) mEq/kg/day every 8th hourly orally (15 mL oral solution = 20 mEq)
14. **Dopamine:** 0.3–0.5 mg/kg
    a. Used in CCF (2–5 mg/kg/min) (up to 20 mg/kg/min)
    b. It increases the renal blood flow and causes peripheral vasodilation.
15. **Crystalline penicillin**
    a. For newborns < 2 kg 50,000 units/kg/day every 12th hourly
    b. For newborns > 2 kg 75,000 units/kg/day every 12th hourly
    c. Older children 25,000–50,000 units/kg in 4–6 divided doses
    d. In meningitis 4 lakh units/kg/day in 6 divided doses
    e. In ARI 2 lakh units/kg/day in 4 divided doses
16. **Cefotaxime:** 100–200 mg/kg/day IM/IV Q6–8 hourly
    Indicated: In meningitis.

VACCINES

Immunization Schedule

Age	Vaccine			
At birth	BCG	OPV(0)	Hepatitis B(0)	
6 weeks	DPT1	OPV1	Hepatitis B_1	Hib1
10 weeks	DPT2	OPV2	Hepatitis B_2	Hib2
14 weeks	DPT3	OPV3	Hepatitis B_3	Hib3
9 months	Measles		Vitamin A	
15 months	MMR			
18 months	DPT booster	OPV4	Vitamin A	Hib booster
24 months			Vitamin A	Typhoid
30 months			Vitamin A	
36 months			Vitamin A	
5 years	DT	OPV5		Typhoid
10 years	TT			Typhoid

Types of Vaccines

Description	Agent	Example
Live attenuated organism	Bacterial	BCG, oral typhoid (Ty 21a)
	Viral	OPV, MMR, measles, varicella
Killed or inactivated organism	Bacterial	DTPw, whole cell killed typhoid
	Viral	Inactivated polio vaccine, rabies, hepatitis A vaccine
Modified bacterial toxins		Diphtheria toxoid, TT
Subunit	Bacterial capsular polysaccharide	*S. typhi* (Vi), *Haemophilus influenzae* type B, meningococcal, pneumococcal
	Viral	Hepatitis B (surface antigen)

Diphtheria Vaccine

1. Anti-toxin level required is 0.1 IU/mL
2. Immunization does not eliminate *C. diphtheria* from skin or nasopharynx
3. Toxoid vaccine-adsorbed on $Al(OH)_3$ combined with tetanus and pertussis vaccine
4. Schedule—6, 10, 14 weeks, 18 months, 4.5 years (DT)
5. In case primary immunization is to be carried out in older children or adults, adult type toxoid containing (dT) less quantities of antigen should be used (not available in India).

Pertussis Vaccine

1. Adverse reactions are:
   a. Prolonged screaming episodes
   b. Convulsions due to fever or encephalopathy syndrome
   c. Hypotonic hyporesponsive stage
   (In these situations stop DPT and give DT or TT only)

2. Contraindicated in neurodegenerative conditions
3. But we can give it safely in cerebral palsy (CP) and febrile seizures
4. Paracetamol is usually given after DPT to control fever
5. *Newer vaccines*: Acellular pertussis vaccine (aP). It contains inactivated pertussis toxin and is less reactogenic but is costlier (DaPT).

Tetanus Toxoid

1. Unimmunized mothers do not transfer antibodies to the baby. So pregnant women are immunized to prevent neonatal tetanus. In this vaccine, toxin is inactivated by formaldehyde and adsorbed to $Al(OH)_3$ to increase the antigenicity. It can withstand 37°C for a few weeks without losing potency. Single toxoid preparation of TT is used in older children and adults. Protective level of anti-toxin needed is 0.01 IU/mL of serum. An attack of tetanus does not give any protection in the future. So immunization is a must
2. DPT (Diphtheria toxin-2 lf, tetanus-5 lf, pertusis-4 IU)
3. Not to be frozen
4. Storage at 4° to 5°C
5. Given deep IM on the anterolateral aspect of the thigh.

Polio Vaccines

1. *Two types*: Killed IPV (Salk) and live attenuated OPV (Sabin)
2. *Oral Polio Vaccine (OPV)*: Contains 105–106 median cell culture infectious discs of 3 types of attenuated poliovirus
   a. In its each liquid dose—2 drops given
   b. Vaccine pink in color due to phenolphthalein
   c. Vaccine vial monitor to know the potency of vaccine
   d. OPV—3 doses produces vaccine failure so 5 doses are given
   e. *Complications*: Vaccine associated paralytic polio (VAPP) due to mutation of virus
   f. Contraindications of OPV:
      i. Acute infectious fever
      ii. Diarrhea/dysentery
      iii. Immunocompromised states.

NIDs: National Immunization Days
PPI: Pulse polio immunization.

   g. *Mopping up*: Last stage of eradication consists of house-to-house administration of OPV
   h. Magnesium chloride is the stabilizing agent used in OPV
   i. *Cold chain*: It is a system of storage and transport of vaccines at low temperature from manufacturer to the actual vaccination site. OPV can be stored for 1 month at 4–5°C. Polio usually stored at 20°C
   j. *In freezer compartment*: Polio; measles, BCG
   k. Not allowed to freeze, but in cold part—T series vaccine (DPT, TT, typhoid)
   l. *In the lowest part*: Diluents
   m. *Walk in cold rooms*: Deep freezers and ILR cold boxes—vaccine carriers—day carriers
   n. Reverse cold chain. Two stool samples 24–48 hours apart a thumb size (8 g) amount or a rectal swab labeled refrigerated at 48°C and send for examination.
2. Inactivated poliovirus vaccination
   a. Cell culture grown formalin inactivated purified poliovirus suspension contains 20, 2, 4 units of types 1, 2, 3 poliovirus
   b. Three doses 4 to 8 weeks apart give subcutaneous (SC) or intramuscular (IM)
   c. It can be combined with DPT (Quadruple vaccine). It does not give any local immunity unlike OPV
   d. Can be used in immunocompromised children, those with AIDS, poor facilities of cold chain, family members of immunocompromised persons and unimmunized adults.

Bacillus Calmette Guerin

1. It is a live attenuated vaccine administered intradermally in the left deltoids. Its dose is 0.05 mL in neonates and 0.1 mL in all ages. It protects from progressive primary and disseminated tuberculosis (Tb) including meningitis but not against secondary adult type TB. It is contraindicated in immunocompromised individuals.
2. Changes after BCG; after 2–3 weeks papule appears at the site, which gradually heals leaving a scar, regional lymph nodes enlarge. Sometimes they may soften and form a sinus.
3. *Complications*:
   a. Ulceration at the BCG site
   b. Suppurative lymphadenitis
   c. Osteomyelitis
   d. Disseminated BCG infection (Rx by giving isoniazid)
   e. Normal saline is used as a diluent in reconstituting the vaccine.

Measles Vaccine

1. Edmonston Zagreb strain (live attenuated) and Schwartz strain
2. May be given subcutaneous or intramuscular
3. After reconstitution potency drops quickly. Moreover several cases of staphylococcal toxic shock syndrome with high mortality have occured in India after giving reconstituted vaccines stored for one or more days. Hence, for these two reasons reconstituted vaccine should be used the same day. Left over must be discarded
4. Given after completing 9 months
5. However, during epidemics, it can be given at 6 months, but maternal antibody neutralizes the virus, hence another dose is recommended at 12 months in these cases
6. Contraindications:
   a. Malignancies associated with immunosuppression
   b. Children on corticosteroids.
7. *SE*: Measles like illness, subacute sclerosing panencephalitis (SSPE)
8. *Newer vaccine*: Aerosolized measles vaccine can be given even before 6 months because it avoids neutralization by maternal antibodies.

Rubella Vaccine

1. It is a live attenuated vaccine with 3 virus strains available. It is given between 12 and 15 months
2. *Contraindications*: Pregnancy, immunosuppression
3. *Adverse reactions*: Rash, lymphadenopathy
4. *Congenital rubella infection*: Deafness, cataract, PDA, microcephaly, MR.

Mumps Vaccine

1. Live attenuated vaccine from Jeryl-Lynn strain
2. Measles-mumps-rubella (MMR) usually given at 15–18 months.

HBV

1. *Two types*: From pooled human plasma and recombinant variety
2. Given 0,1,6 months 0.5 mL/IM.

Hib Vaccine

H. influenzae type B (Polysaccharide vaccine conjugated with proteins)

1. < 6 months—3 doses + 1 booster at 12–18 months
2. (6 months–1 year)—2 doses + 1 booster at 12–18 months
3. (> 1 year) 1 dose given at 2 months of age and the next dose after a 2-month interval IM, booster dose given at 12–18 months.

Chicken Pox Vaccine

1. Vaccine prepared from Oka strain given between 1 and 2 years 2 doses 1 month apart
2. < 2 year 1 dose
3. > 2 year 2 dose.

Pneumococcal Vaccine

1. 0.5 mL IM or subcutaneous
2. Vaccine consists of 25 mg each of purified capsular polysaccharide antigen of 23 pneumococcal serotypes
3. *Indications*: Child > 2 years having asplenia, sickle cell anemia. Nephrotic syndrome, CRF, immunosuppression.

X-RAY AND INSTRUMENTS

X-rays

1. Cardiomegaly (Cardiothoracic ratio > 50%)
2. Tetralogy of Fallot (boot shaped heart, pulmonary oligemia, main pulmonary trunk is thin)
3. Rickets healing rickets (Peripheral zone of calcification seen)
4. Collapse
5. Hydropneumothorax
6. Foreign body
7. Pneumatocele
8. Consolidation
9. Pleural effusion
10. Hilar lymph nodes
11. Situs inversus.

Instruments

1. **Infant feeding tube**
   Different from Ryles tube as there are no lead balls at the tip.
   Indications
   a. Aspirate gastric contents in poison intake
   b. Aspirate gastric contents in hematemesis to prevent encephalopathy
   c. Decompress intestinal obstruction
   d. Decompress stomach in bag and mask ventilation
   e. Aspiration to prevent aspiration to respiratory tract in altered mental state
   f. To feed a child not taking orally
   g. Giving O_2 through nose
   h. Exchange transfusion
   i. To put in charcoal
   j. Suprapubic catheterization
   k. Intrarectal diazepam.
   Procedure
   Measure length from nose to ear, then to subxiphoid notch, this is the length. Lubricate the tube and ask older children to swallow the tube. To confirm that the tube is put in place; push air into the tube and auscultate for bubbling sounds. Should not be kept in position for more than 48 hours. While taking out the tube the opening must be pinched to prevent aspiration.
2. **Scalp vein set**
   Uses
   a. To give medications
   b. To withdraw blood
   Complications: Infection and hemorrhage
3. **LP needle**
   a. *Site*: Between L3 and L4 or between L4 and L5
   b. *Indications*:

Diagnostic	Therapeutic
Meningitis	To give drugs
First episode of convulsions	Spinal anesthesia
Hydrocephalus	
Demyelinating diseases	
Cisternal puncture	

c. To differentiate between traumatic tap and subarachnoid hemorrhage (SAH) via cerebrospinal fluid (CSF) study; collect CSF in 2 test tubes, the presence of more blood in one indicates trauma whereas it will be uniformly stained in SAH.

d. *Complications*:
   i. Infection
   ii. Coning
   iii. Headache
   iv. Backache.

e. *Contraindications*:
   i. Severe cardiopulmonary compromise
   ii. Relative thrombocytopenia
   iii. Infection at the puncture site
   iv. Masked spinal deformity
   v. Raised intracranial tension (ICT). In such cases LP can be done after giving mannitol (Cushings reflex-seen in raised ICT-bradycardia, irregular respiration, hypertension).

Xanthochromia on CSF

a. SAH (supernatant)
b. GBS
c. Jaundice
d. Spinal tumor syndrome.

(To differentiate spinal block from others we do a Queckenstedt's test; i.e. on pressing the jugular veins, there is an increase in the CSF pressure. So CSF comes out of the LP site. But it is not so in spinal block as the pathway is blocked (as in metastasis).

4. **Bone marrow aspiration needle (Salas needle)**
   (Identify by its guard which helps in preventing overpenetration)
   a. *Indications*:
      i. Bone marrow suppression:
         - Leukemias
         - Megaloblastic anemias
         - Storage diseases.
      ii. Bone marrow infiltration:
         - Lymphomas
         - Other malignancies
   b. *Contraindications*:
      i. Infection at the site
      ii. Bleeding disorders.

   It can also be used to give intraosseous infusion of fluids, in case fluids cannot be given by IV cannula. The site used is tibial tuberosity in children less than 2 years and iliac crest in older children.

5. **Jamshidi-Swain bone marrow trephine biopsy needle**
   Used in aplastic anemia when bone marrow aspiration yields a dry tap.

6. **3 way tap**
   Uses:
   a. Pleural aspiration
   b. Exchange transfusion
   c. Blood transfusion/IV fluids.

   Pleural fluid drained in the 7th or 8th axillary space in the mid axillary line at the site of maximum dullness, usually drained through the lower part of the ribs to avoid damage to neurovascular bundle. In empyema there is development of high grade fever, intercostal tenderness and clubbing. In such cases continuous ICT drainage is required. Usually caused by *Staphylococcus aureus.*

7. **Liver biopsy needle**
   a. Vim-Silverman needle (split end)
   b. Menghini needle (4 parts inside a small pin)
   c. Trucut biopsy needle.

   Indications
   a. Undiagnosed liver disease
   b. Wilson's disease
   c. Storage diseases
   d. Cirrhosis
   e. Alpha 1 antitrypsin deficiency.
   f. Lymphomas, leukemias.

   Prerequisites
   a. PT not prolonged beyond 4 sec
   b. Platelets > 1 lakh
   c. Cooperative patient.

   Contraindications
   a. Biliary obstruction
   b. Thrombocytopenia
   c. Masked ascites and edema
   d. Prolonged PT
   e. Infection at the site.

   Complications
   a. Abdominal/shoulder pain
   b. Infections
   c. Bleeding
   d. Biliary peritonitis
      i. Make PT normal by giving vitamin K before liver biopsy
      ii. *Site*: 10th intercostal space (ICS) in midaxillary line (MAL) in the supine position.
8. **Tuberculin syringe**
   1 cc syringe, 10 divisions, blue piston.
   Uses: To give PPO intradermally on the volar aspect; standard dose 5TU
   A weal of 5 mm should be raised. Read after 48 to 72 hours.
   False (–)ve results are seen in:
   a. Following measles
   b. On steroid therapy
   c. Severe malnutrition
   d. Inactive PPD
   e. Incubation period of TB
   f. Overwhelming TB infection
   g. Wrong technique.

   Inference:
   a. *< 5 mm*: (–)ve
   b. *> 10 mm*: Strongly (+)ve
   c. *> 15 mm*: Very strongly (+)ve
   d. 5 mm or more (+)ve in close contacts, HIV (+)ve cases and those with X-ray findings consistent with old healed tuberculosis.

   False (+)ve:
   a. Atypical mycobacteria
   b. BCG inoculation (usually up to 1–2 years).

   BCG test:
   BCG is used instead of PPD, an induration of 5 to 6 mm after 3 days of BCG vaccine indicates a (+)ve test.
   Other uses of this syringe
   a. To deliver insulin
   b. To give other medications subcutaneous, e.g. adrenaline 0.15 mg/kg.
9. **AMBU bag (Ambulatory mobile breathing unit)**
   Uses: To give bag and mask ventilation or through endotracheal tube or through tracheostomy tube.
   Contraindication: Diaphragmatic hernia
   Used when:
   a. There is apnea
   b. Spontaneous respiration but HR < 100/min.
10. **Three way cannula—uses**
   a. To aspirate fluid from pleural, peritoneal or pericardial sac (fluid is withdrawn through one inlet by connecting a syringe with the cannula and by adjusting the screw, fluid in the syringe may be pushed into the kidney tray via the outlet).
   b. Through one inlet IV fluids can be given and the other inlet may be used for medication or monitoring central venous pressure.

11. **Tongue depressor—uses**
    a. Examination of throat and oral cavity
    b. Spatula test in tetanus
    c. Detection of posterior nasal bleeding
    d. Oral surgery
    e. Removal of foreign body from tonsil, throat or posterior part of tongue
    f. Elicitation of gag reflex
    g. Indirect laryngoscopy
    h. Helps to open the mouth for oral toilet or suction in a comatose patient.
12. **Metered dose inhaler**
    Advantages:
    a. Rapid onset of action
    b. Very small dose of the drug is required to have desired effect
    c. Very little medicine is allowed to reach other parts of the body (i.e. chances of side effects tend to be minimum)
    Disadvantages:
    a. The major limitation of mode of administration is that training and skills are required to coordinate actuation of drug from metered dose inhaler (MDI)
    b. Pharyngeal infection (e.g. candidiasis with inhaled corticosteroids) if the device is not properly cleaned at a regular interval.
13. Endotracheal tube—indications
    a. Respiratory failure as a result of chronic obstructive pulmonary disease (COPD), massive pneumonia or respiratory muscle paralysis in an attempt to give positive pressure ventilation
    b. To carry out artificial respiration in a patient of cardiorespiratory arrest
    c. Respiratory difficulty in an unconscious patient—clear the airway and prevent aspiration
    d. Administration of anesthesia.

DEVELOPMENTAL MILESTONES

Gross Motor

Head control	3–4 months
Turning over	
Prone to supine	
Supine to prone	
Crawling	8 months
Sitting with support	5 months
Sitting without support	8 months
Standing with support	10 months
Standing without support	12 months
Walking with support	12 months
Walking without support	13 months
Cruising	10 months
Pivoting	11 months
Walk sideways and backwards	15 months
Running	18 months
Climbs stairs 2 feet/step	2 years
Walks on tip toes	30 months
Climbs up stairs 1 foot/step	3 years
Climbs down stairs 2 feet/step	3 years
Climbs down stairs 1 foot/step	4 years
Skipping	5 years

Fine Motor

Eye fixation	1 month
Follow up to 180 degrees	2 months
Making limb movements	3 months
Reaches out for objects (overshoots)	4 months
Reaches out with both hands	5 months
Takes feet to mouth	5 months
Transfers objects	7 months
Palmar grasp	7 months
Hits 2 cubes together	9 months
Pincer grasp assisted	7–8 months
Pincer grasp unassisted	9–10 months
Releases objects on request	1 year
Makes a tower of 2 cubes	1 year
Can feed without much spilling	15 months
Turns pages 2–3 at a time	13 months
Turns page by page	2 years
Handedness	2 years
Scribbling	1 year
Vertical line	18 months
Horizontal line	2 years
Circle	3 years
Rectangle/+	4 years
Triangle	5 years
Hexagon	6 years
Makes postural adjustments for dressing	1 year
Wears shoes 2 years	2 years
Dress and undress	3 years
Tower of 3 cubes	1 year
Tower of 3 cubes	18 months
Tower of 6 cubes	2 years

Social

Regards face	1 month
Social smile	2 months
Smile of recognition	3 months
Recognizes mother	3 months
Smiling at mirror	5 months
Stranger anxiety	7 months
Waves bye-bye	10 months
Simple ball game	1 year
Imitates others	1 year
Knows gender	3 years

Language

Turns head to sound	1 month
Cooing	3 months
Laughs loud	4 months
Monosyllables	6 months
Bisyllables	9 months

Responds to name	7 months
Two words with meaning	12 months
Ten words with meaning	18 months

Bowel and Bladder

Made to sit in toilet	10 months
Walks to toilet	18 months
Toilet trainable completely	2 years
Bowel control	3 years
Bladder control dry by day	2 years
Bladder control dry by night	3 years

NEWBORN PERIOD

Primitive neonatal reflexes are unique in the newborn period, a consequence of the continued development of the CNS after birth. Any asymmetry, increase, or decrease in tone elicited by passive movement may indicate a significant CNS abnormality and requires further evaluation. Similarly a delay in the expected disappearance of the reflexes may warrant an evaluation of the CNS. The most important reflexes to assess during the newborn period are as follows:

1. *The Moro reflex* is elicited by allowing the infant's head gently to move back suddenly (from a few inches off the crib mattress). This results in abduction and upward movement of the arms followed by adduction and flexion. The Moro reflex disappears by 4–6 months
2. *The rooting reflex* is elicited by touching the corner of the infant's mouth, resulting in the lowering of the lower lip on the same side with tongue movement toward the stimulus. The face may turn to the stimulus. The rooting reflex disappears at 4–6 months
3. *The sucking reflex* occurs with almost any object placed in the newborn's mouth. The infant responds with vigorous sucking. The sucking reflex is replaced later by voluntary sucking only
4. *The grasp reflex* occurs when placing an object, such as a finger, onto the infant's palm (palmar grasp) or sole (plantar grasp). The infant responds by flexing fingers or curling the toes. The palmar grasp usually disappears by 3–4 months and the plantar grasp by 6–8 months
5. *The asymmetric tonic neck reflex* is elicited by placing the infant supine and turning the head to the side. This placement results in ipsilateral extension of the arm and the leg into a "fencing" position. The contralateral side flexes as well. This reflex disappears by 2–3 months of age.

Age	Gross motor	Fine motor—adaptive	Personal-social	Language
2 weeks	Moves head side to side		Regards face	Alerts to bell
1 month	Holds chin up, turns head while prone		Watches person	Follows moving object
2 months	Lifts shoulder while prone	Tracks past midline	Social Smile	Cooing searches for sound with eyes 180
3 months	ATNR disappears Lifts head and chest with arms extended Bears weight on forearm Moro and grasp lost	Reaches towards and misses object Movements on seeing object	Recognizes mother	
4 months	Lifts up on hands Rolls front to back If pulled to sit from supine, no head lag	Reaches for object Raking grasp	Looks at hand Begins to work toward toy	Laughs and squeals

Contd...

Contd...

6 months	Sits alone	Transfers object hand to hand Holds bottle	Feeds self	Babbles
9 months	Pulls to stand Gets into sitting position	Starting to pincer grasp Bangs 2 blocks together	Waves bye-bye Plays pat-a-cake	Says *dada* and *mama*, but nonspecific 2-syllable sounds
12 months	Walks Stoops and stands	Puts block in cup	Drinks from a cup Imitates others	Says *mama* and *dada*, specific Says 1–2 other words
15 months	Walks backward	Scribbles Stacks 2 blocks	Uses spoon and fork Helps in housework	Says 3–6 words Follows commands
18 months	Runs Kicks a ball	Stacks four blocks "Feeds" doll	Removes garment	Says at least 6 words
2 years	Walks up and down stairs Throws overhand	Stacks 6 blocks Copies line	Washes and dries hands Brushes teeth Puts on clothes	Puts 2 words together Points to pictures Knows body parts
3 years	Walks steps alternating feet Broad jump	Stacks 8 blocks Wiggles thumb	Uses spoon well, spilling little Puts on T-shirt	Names pictures Speech understandable to stranger 75% Says 3-word sentences
4 years	Balances well on each foot Hops on one foot	Copies rectangle or plus sign Draws person with 3 parts	Brushes teeth without help Dresses without help	Names colors Understands adjectives
5 years	Skips Heal-to-toe walks	Copies triangle or multiplication sign		Counts Understands opposites
6 years	Balances on each foot 6 sec	Copies hexagon Draws person with 6 parts		Defines words

Appendix

HEMATOLOGY AND COAGULATION

Differential blood count	WB	
Neutrophils		40–70%
Bands		0–5%
Lymphocytes		20–50%
Monocytes		4–8%
Eosinophils		0–6%
Basophils		0–2%
Eosinophil count	WB	150–300/mm^3
Erythrocyte count	WB	
Adult males		4.30–5.60 × 10^6/mm^3
Adult females		4.00–5.20 × 10^6/mm^3
Erythrocyte life span	WB	
Normal survival		120 days
Erythrocyte sedimentation rate	WB	
Females		0–20 mm/h
Males		0–15 mm/h
Hematocrit	WB	
Adult males		38.8–46.4
Adult females		35.4–44.4
Hemoglobin		
Plasma	P	0.6–5.0 mg/dL
Whole blood	WB	
Adult males		13.3–16.2 g/dL
Adult females		12.0–15.8 g/dL
Hemoglobin electrophoresis		WB
Hemoglobin A		95–98%
Hemoglobin A2		1.5–3.1%
Hemoglobin F		0–2.0%
Hemoglobin other than A, A2/F		Absent
Leukocytes		
Count (WBC)	WB	3.54–9.06 × 10^3/mm^3
MCH	WB	26.7–31.9 pg/cell
MCHC	WB	32.3–35.9 g/dL
MCV	WB	79–93.3 fL
MPV	WB	9.00–12.95 fL
Osmotic fragility of RBCs	WB	
Direct		0.35–0.45%
Index		0.30–0.65%
Partial thromboplastin time, activated	P	26.3–39.4 s
Platelet count	WB	165–415 × 10^3/mm^3
Platelet, mean volume	WB	6.4–11 fL
Prothrombin time	P	12.7–15.4 s
Reticulocyte count	WB	
Adult males		0.8–2.3% red cells
Adult females		0.8–2.0% red cells
Thrombin time	P	15.3–18.5 s
Total eosinophils	WB	150–300/mm^3
Transferrin receptor	S, P	9.6–29.6 nmol/L
Viscosity		
Plasma	P	1.7–2.1
Serum	S	1.4–1.8

CLINICAL CHEMISTRY AND IMMUNOLOGY

Alanine aminotransferase (AST, SGPT)	S	7–41 U/L
Albumin	S	
Female		4.1–5.3 g/dL
Male		4.0–5.0 g/L
Alpha fetoprotein (adult)	S	0–8.5 ng/mL
Alpha-1 antitrypsin	S	100–200 mg/dL
Ammonia, as NH_3	P	19–60 g/dL
Amylase (method dependent)	S	20–96 U/L
Anion gap	S	7–16 mmol/L
Arterial blood gases		
[HCO_3^-]		22–30 mEq/L
PCO_2		32–45 mm Hg
pH		7.35–7.45
PO_2		72–104 mm Hg
Aspartate aminotransferase (AST, SGOT)	S	12–38 U/L
B type natriuretic peptide (BNP)	P	< 167 pg/mL
Bilirubin	S	
Total		0.3–1.3 mg/dL
Direct		0.1–0.4 mg/dL
Indirect		0.2–0.9 mg/dL
CA 125	S	0–35 U/mL
CA 19-9	S	0–37 U/mL
CA 15-3	S	0–34 U/mL

Test	Specimen	Reference range
CA 27-29		0–40 U/mL
Calcitonin	S	
Male		3–26 pg/mL
Female		2–17 pg/mL
Calcium	S	8.7–10.2 mg/dL
Calcium, ionized	WB	4.5–5.3 mg/dL
Carbon dioxide content (TCO_2)	P (sea level)	22–30 mEq/L
Carboxyhemoglobin (carbon monoxide content)	WB	
Nonsmokers		0–4%
Smokers		4–9%
Onset of symptoms		15–20%
Loss of consciousness and death		> 50%
Carcinoembryonic antigen (CEA)		
Nonsmokers		0.0–3.0 ng/mL
Smokers	S	0.0–5.0 ng/mL
Ceruloplasmin	S	25–63 mg/dL
Chloride	S	102–109 mEq/L
Complement		
C3	S	83–177 mg/dL
C4	S	16–47 mg/dL
Cortisol		
Fasting, 8 AM–12 noon	S	5–25 g/dL
12 noon–8 PM		5–15 g/dL
8 PM–8 AM		0–10 g/dL
Cortisol, free	U	20–70 g/24 hours
Creactive protein	S	0.2–3.0 mg/L
Creatine kinase (total)	S	
Females		39–238 U/L
Males		51–294 U/L
Creatine kinase-MB	S	
Mass		0.0–5.5 ng/mL
Fraction of total activity (by electrophoresis)		0–0.04, 0–4.0%
Creatinine	S	
Female		0.5–0.9 ng/mL
Male		0.6–1.2 ng/mL
Erythropoietin	S	4–27 U/L
Ferritin	S	
Female		10–150 ng/mL
Male		29–248 ng/mL
Fructosamine	S	< 285 mol/L
Gamma glutamyl transferase	S	9–58 U/L
Gastrin	S	< 100 pg/mL
Glucagon	P	20–100 pg/mL
Glucose (fasting)	P	
Normal		75–110 mg/dL
Impaired glucose tolerance		111–125 mg/dL
Diabetes mellitus		> 125 mg/dL

Test	Specimen	Reference range
Glucose, 2 hours postprandial	P	70–120 mg/dL
Hemoglobin A_{1c}	WB	4.0–6.0%
Human chorionic-gonadotropin (hCG)	S	
Nonpregnant female		< 5 mIU/mL
1–2 weeks postconception		9–130 mIU/mL
2–3 weeks postconception		75–2600 mIU/mL
3–4 weeks postconception		850–20,800 mIU/mL
4–5 weeks postconception		4000–100,200 mIU/mL
5–10 weeks postconception		11,500–289,000 mIU/mL
10–14 weeks postconception		18,300–137,000 mIU/mL
Second trimester		1400–53,000 mIU/mL
Third trimester		940–60,000 mIU/mL
Insulin	S, P	2–20 U/mL
Iron	S	41–141 g/dL
Iron-binding capacity	S	251–406 g/dL
Iron-binding capacity saturation	S	16–35%
Ketone (acetone)	S, U	Negative
Lactate	P, arterial	4.5–14.4 mg/dL
	P, venous	4.5–19.8 mg/dL
Lactate dehydrogenase	S	115–221 U/L
Lipase (method dependent)	S	3–43 U/L
Lipoprotein (a)	S	0–30 mg/dL
Magnesium	S	1.5–2.3 mg/dL
Methemoglobin	WB	0–1%
Osmolality	P	275–295 mOsmol/kg serum water
	U	500–800 mOsmol/kg water
Oxygen content	WB	
Arterial (sea level)		17–21 vol%
Venous (sea level)		10–16 vol%
Oxygen percent saturation (sea level)	WB	
Arterial		94–100%
Venous, arm		60–85%
Parathyroid hormone (intact)	S	8–51 pg/mL
Phosphatase, alkaline	S	33–96 U/L
Potassium	S	3.5–5.0 mEq/L
Prealbumin	S	17–34 mg/dL
Prolactin	S	0–20 ng/mL
Prostate-specific antigen (PSA)	S	
Male		
< 40 years		0.0–2.0 ng/mL
> 40 years		0.0–4.0 ng/mL

PSA, free; in males 45–75 years, with PSA values between 4 and 20 g/mL	S	> 25% associated with benign prostatic hyperplasia
Protein fractions	S	
Albumin		3.5–5.5 g/dL (50–60%)
Globulin		2.0–3.5 g/dL (40–50%)
Alpha-1		0.2–0.4 g/dL (4.2–7.2%)
Alpha-2		0.5–0.9 g/dL (6.8–12%)
Beta		0.6–1.1 g/dL (9.3–15%)
Gamma		0.7–1.7 g/dL (13–23%)
Protein, total	S	6.7–8.6 g/dL
Pyruvate	P, arterial	0.35–1.14 mg/dL
	P, venous	0.35–1.14 mg/dL
Rheumatoid factor	S, JF	< 30 IU/mL
Sodium	S	136–146 mEq/L
Thyroglobulin	S	0.5–53 ng/mL
Thyroid-binding globulin	S	1.3–3.0 mg/dL
Thyroid-stimulating hormone	S	0.34–4.25 IU/mL
Thyroxine, free (fT4)	S	0.8–1.7 ng/dL
Thyroxine, total (T4)	S	5.4–11.7 g/dL
(Free) thyroxine index	S	6.7–10.9
Transferrin	S	200–400 mg/dL
Triglycerides	S	30–200 mg/dL
Triiodothyronine, free (fT3)	S	2.4–4.2 pg/mL
Triiodothyronine, total (T3)	S	77–135 ng/dL
Troponin I	S	
Normal population, 99% tile		0–0.08 ng/mL
Cut-off for MI		> 0.4 ng/mL
Troponin T	S	
Normal population, 99% tile		0–0.01 ng/mL
Cut-off for MI		0–0.1 ng/mL
Urea nitrogen	S	7–20 mg/dL
Uric acid	S	
Females		2.5–5.6 mg/dL
Males		3.1–7.0 mg/dL
Urobilinogen	U	0.05–25 mg/24 hours
Vanillylmandelic acid (VMA)	U, 24 hours	< 6 mg/day

CLASSIFICATION OF LDL, TOTAL, AND HDL CHOLESTEROL

LDL cholesterol, mg/dL	
< 70	Therapeutic option for very high-risk patients
< 100	Optimal
100–129	Near optimal/above optimal
130–159	Borderline high
160–189	High
190	Very high
Total cholesterol, mg/dL	
< 200	Desirable
200–239	Borderline high
240	High
High density lipoprotein cholesterol, mg/dL	
< 40	Low
60	High

CEREBROSPINAL FLUID (CSF)

Osmolarity	292–297 mOsmol/L
Electrolytes	
Sodium	137–145 mEq/L
Potassium	2.7–3.9 mEq/L
Calcium	2.1–3.0 mEq/L
Magnesium	2.0–2.5 mEq/L
Chloride	116–122 mEq/L
CO_2 content	20–24 mEq/L
PCO_2	45–49 mm Hg
pH	7.31–7.34
Glucose	40–70 mg/dL
Lactate	10–20 mg/dL
Total protein	
Lumbar	15–50 mg/dL
Cisternal	15–25 mg/dL
Ventricular	6–15 mg/dL
Albumin	6.6–44.2 mg/dL
Ammonia	25–80 g/dL
Creatinine	0.5–1.9 mg/dL
Myelin basic protein	< 4 g/L
CSF pressure	50–180 mm H_2O
CSF volume (adult)	~150 mL
Red blood cells	0
Leukocytes	
Total	0–5 mononuclear cells per mm^3
Differential	
Lymphocytes	60–70%
Monocytes	30–50%
Neutrophils	None

URINE ANALYSIS

Acidity, titratable	20–40 mEq/day
Ammonia	30–50 mEq/day
Amylase	4–400 U/L
Amylase/creatinine clearance ratio [(Clam/CLcr) × 100]	1–5
Calcium (200 mg/day dietary calcium)	< 300 mg/day

Creatine, as creatinine	
Female	< 100 mg/day
Male	< 50 mg/day
Creatinine	1.0–1.6 g/day
Eosinophils	< 100 eosinophils/mL
Glucose	
(glucose oxidase method)	50–300 mg/day
5-Hydroxy indole acetic acid	2–9 mg/day
Microalbumin	
Normal	0–30 mg/day
Microalbuminuria	30–300 mg/day
Clinical albuminuria	> 300 mg/day
Microalbumin/creatinine ratio	
Normal	0–30 g/mg creatinine
Microalbuminuria	30–300 g/mg creatinine
Clinical albuminuria	> 300 g/mg creatinine
Oxalate	
Male	7–44 mg/day
Female	4–31 mg/day
pH	5.0–9.0
Phosphate	400–1300 mg/day
Potassium	25–100 mEq/day
Protein	< 150 mg/day
Sediment	
Red blood cells	0–2/high power field
White blood cells	0–2/high power field
Bacteria	None
Crystals	None
Bladder cells	None
Squamous cells	None
Tubular cells	None
Broad casts	None
Epithelial cell casts	None
Granular casts	None
Hyaline casts	0–5/low power field
Red blood cell casts	None
Waxy casts	None
White cell casts	None
Sodium	100–260 mEq/day
Specific gravity	1.001–1.035
Urea nitrogen	6–17 g/day
Uric acid (normal diet)	250–800 mg/day

Abbreviations: WB: Whole blood; P: Plasma; S: Serum; U: Urine; JF: Joint fluid

Diagrams

MEDICINE

Common Murmurs

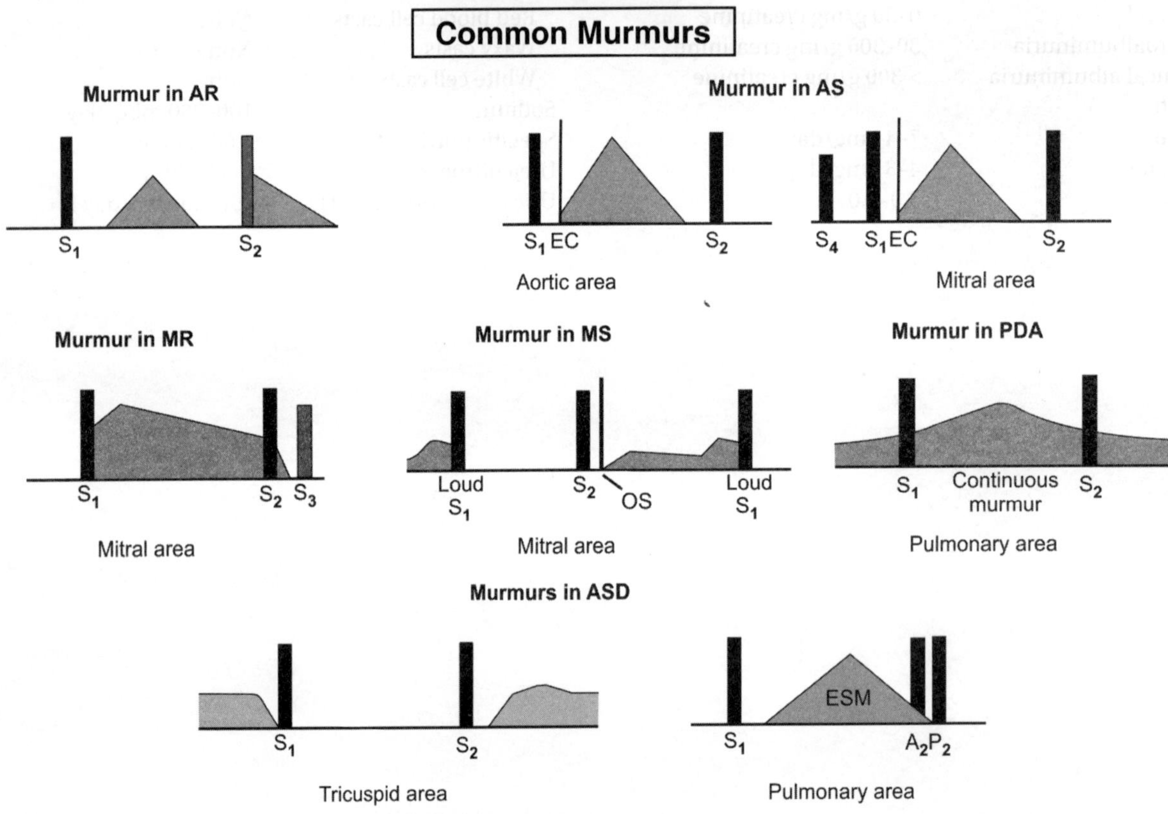

Conduction System of Heart

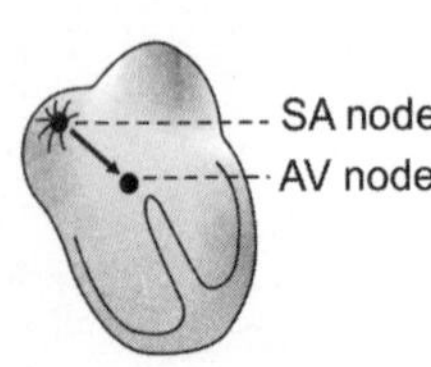

Atrial activation

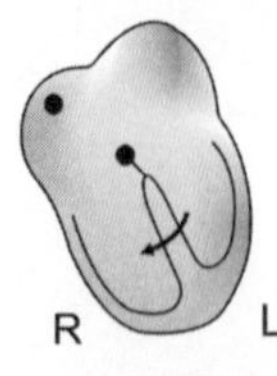

Septal activation from left to right

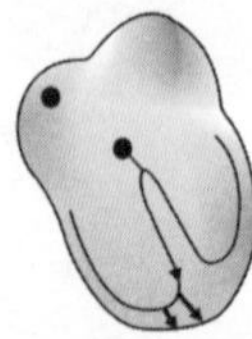

Activation of anteroseptal region of the ventricular myocardium

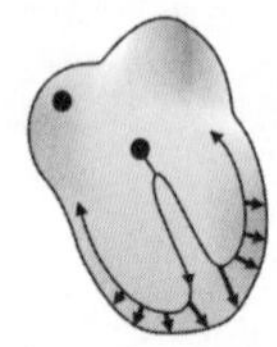

Activation of major portion of ventricular myocardium from endocardial surfaces

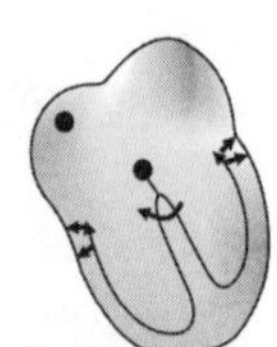

Late activation of posterobasal portion of the left ventricle and the pulmonary conus

Normal ECG

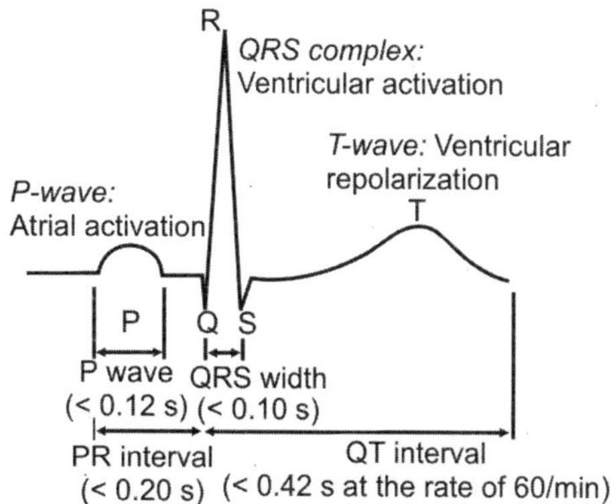

Aortic Dissection

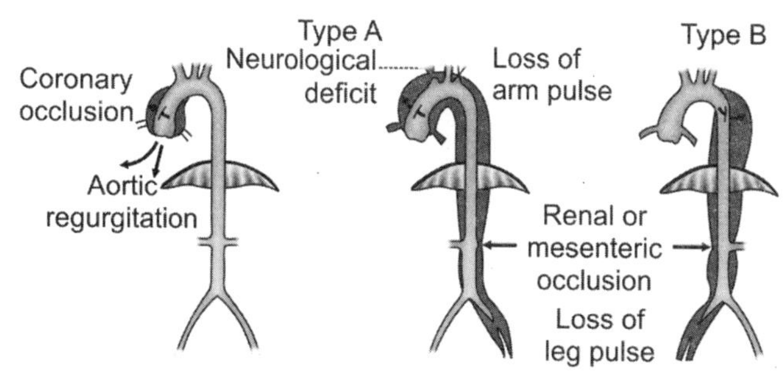

Aortic Aneurysm

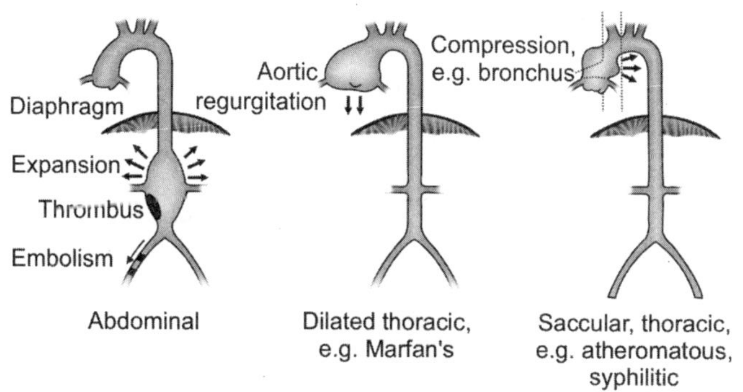

Jugular Venous Pressure

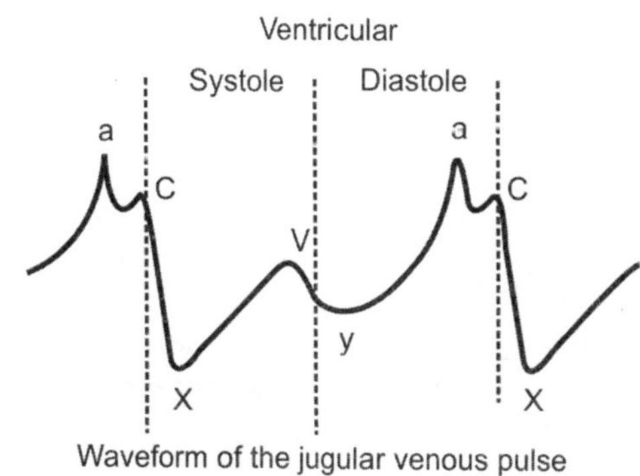

Waveform of the jugular venous pulse

Mitral Stenosis and Mitral Regurgitation

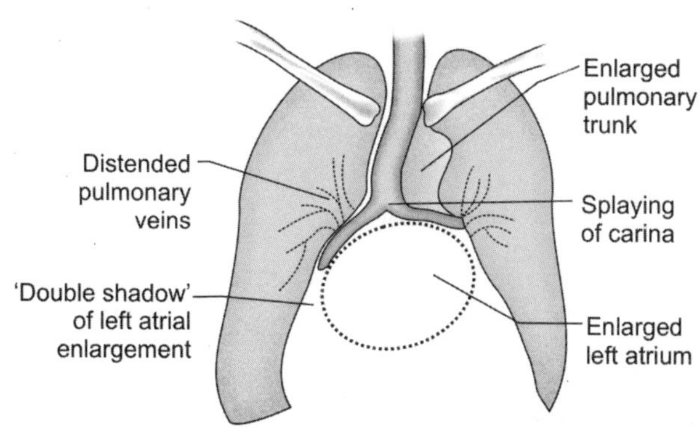

Mitral stenosis and regurgitation indicating enlargement of the left atrium and prominence of the pulmonary artery

Fallot's Tetralogy

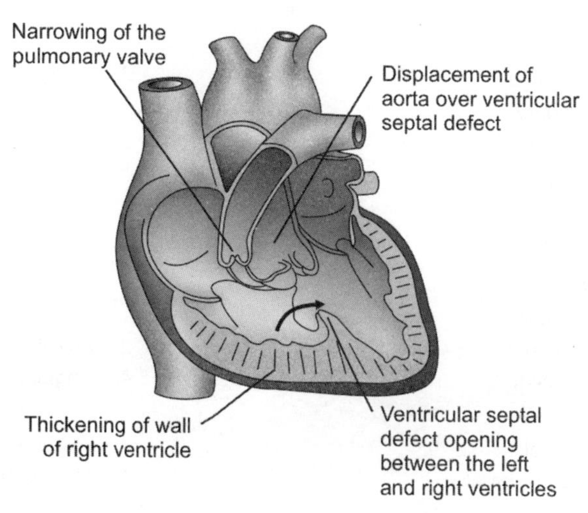

Aortic Regurgitation

Dilated ascending aorta

Normal-sized aortic arch

Large left ventricle

Aortic regurgitation, left ventricular enlargement and dilatation of the ascending aorta

Changes in Enzyme Concentration after Myocardial Infarction

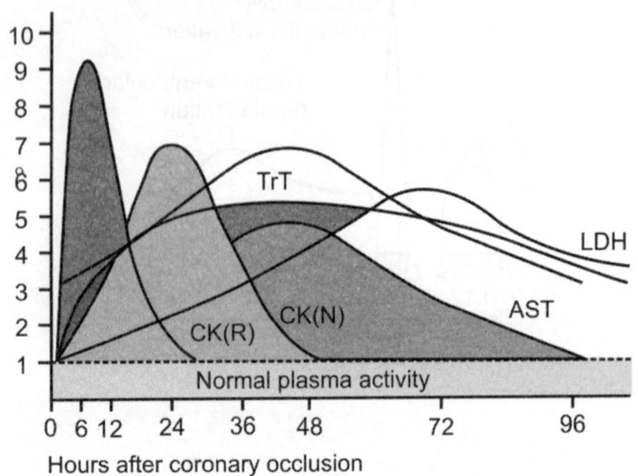

Bronchopulmonary Segments

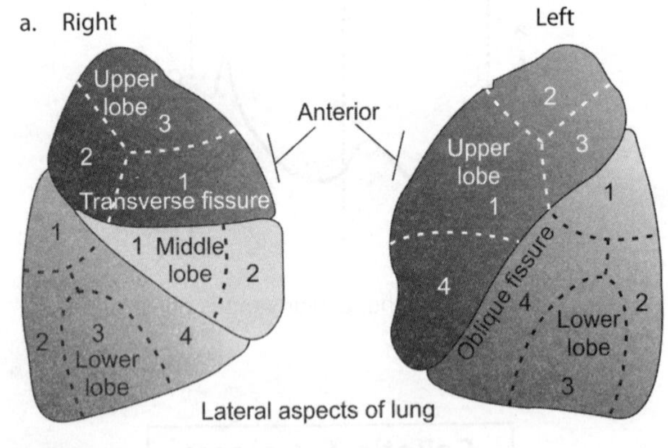

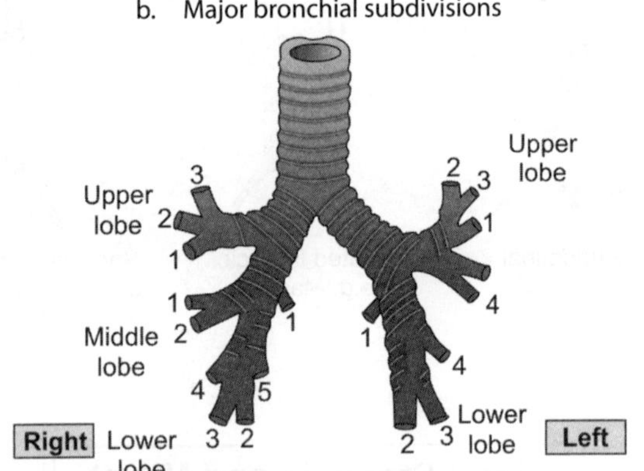

Bronchopulmonary Segments

Right

Upper lobe

1. Anterior
2. Posterior
3. Apical.

Middle lobe

1. Lateral
2. Medial.

Lower lobe

1. Apical
2. Posterior basal
3. Lateral basal
4. Anterior basal
5. Medial basal.

Left

Upper lobe

1. Anterior
2. Apical
3. Posterior
4. Lingular.

Lower lobe

1. Apical
2. Posterior basal
3. Lateral basal
4. Anterior basal.

Types of Spontaneous Pneumothorax

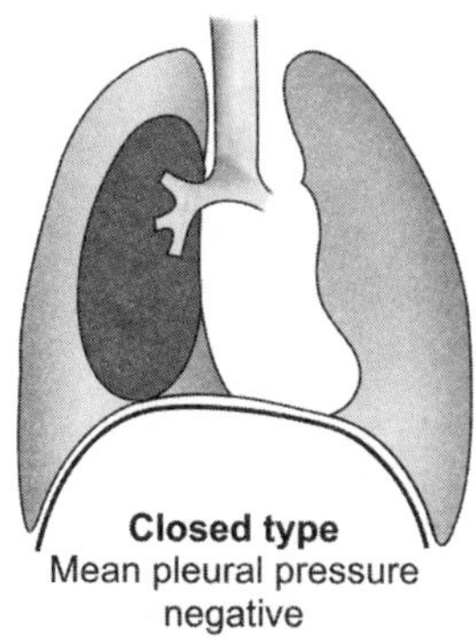

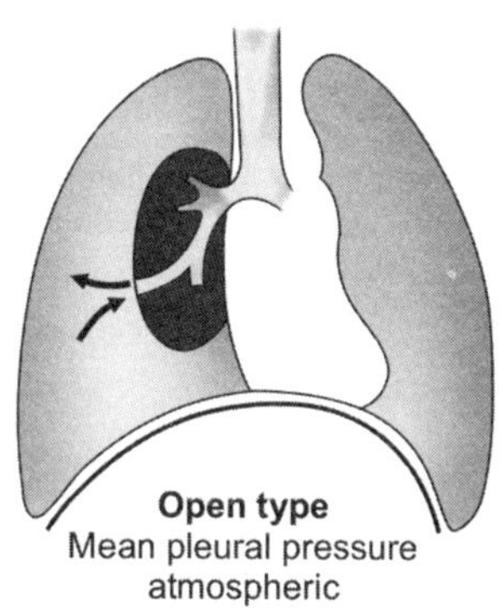

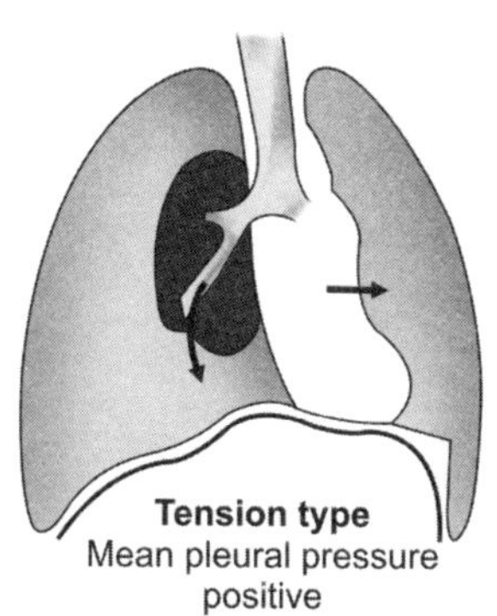

Asbestosis: The Range of Effects on Respiratory Tract

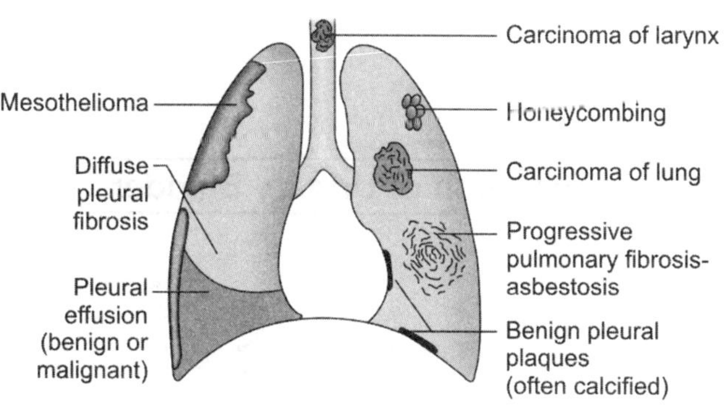

Pulmonary Edema

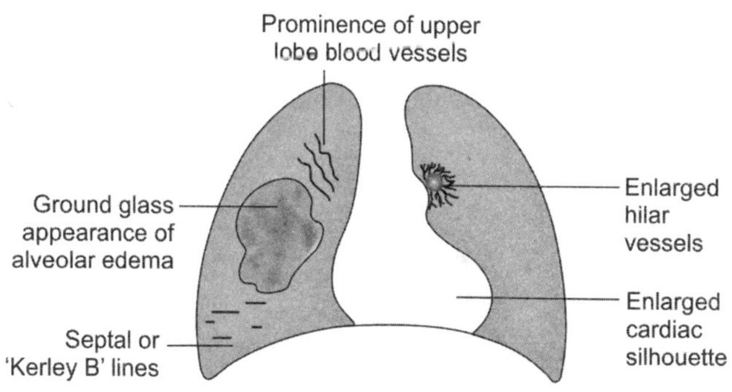

Spirometry

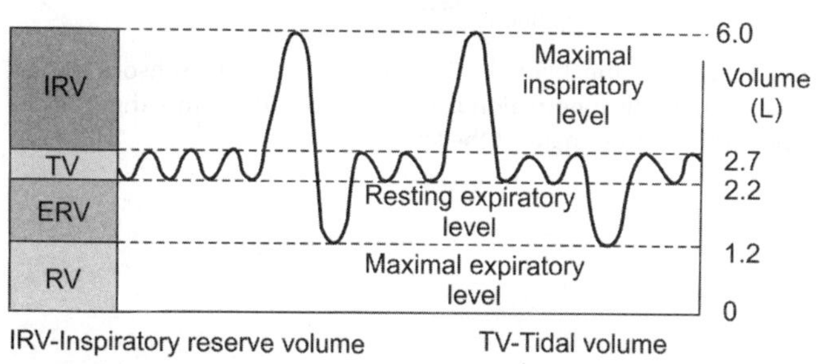

Virological and Immunological Progression of HIV Infection

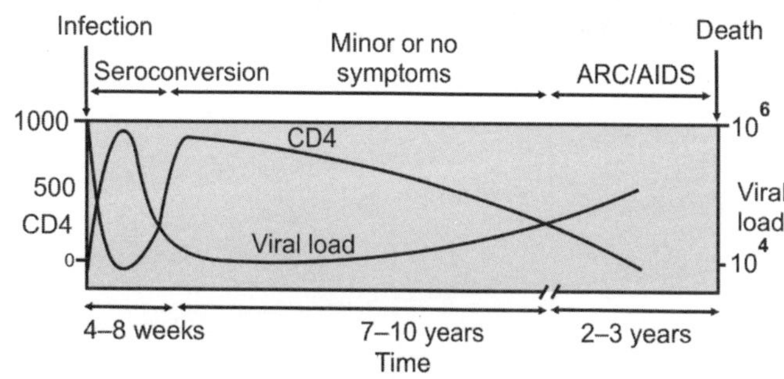

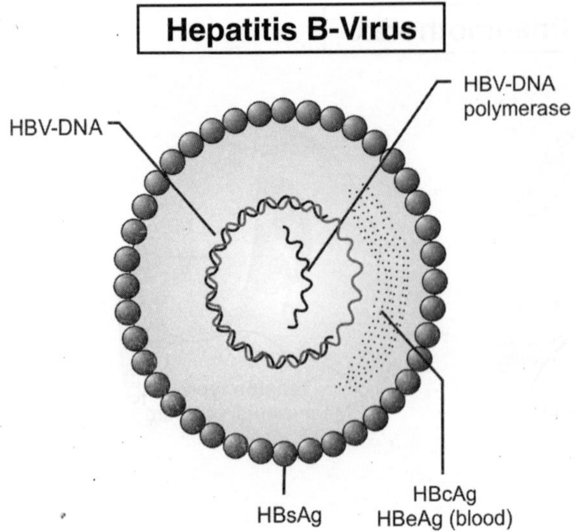

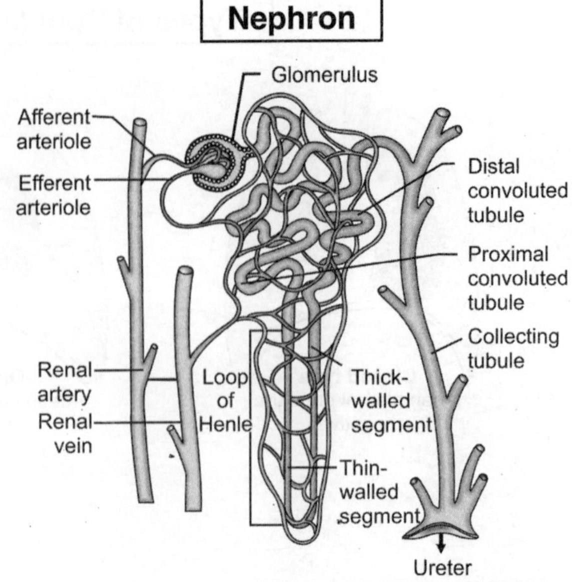

HIV

GP 120

Reverse transcriptase

RNA

Lipid bilayer

Innervation of Urinary Bladder

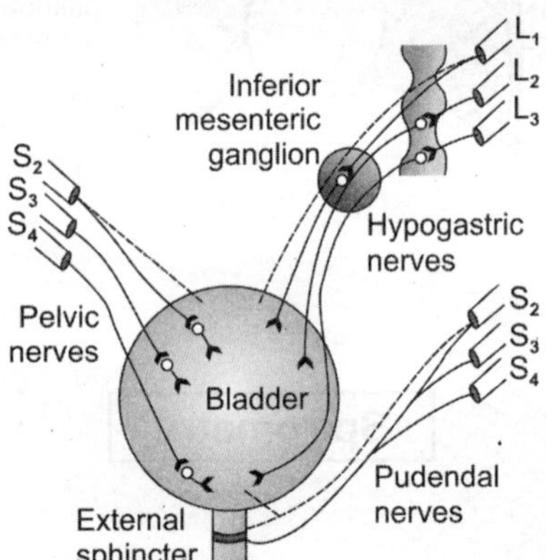

Innervation of the bladder. Dashed lines indicate sensory nerves. Parasympathetic innervation is shown at the left, sympathetic at the upper right, and somatic at the lower right

Corticospinal Tract

Precentral gyrus (area 4, etc.)
Corticospinal tract
Internal capsule
Pyramids
Decussation of the pyramids
Ventral cortico-spinal tract (20% of fibers)
Lateral cortico-spinal tract (80% of fibers)
Anterior horn cell
Interneuron
Spinal nerve
Distal muscle
Proximal muscle

Visual Pathway

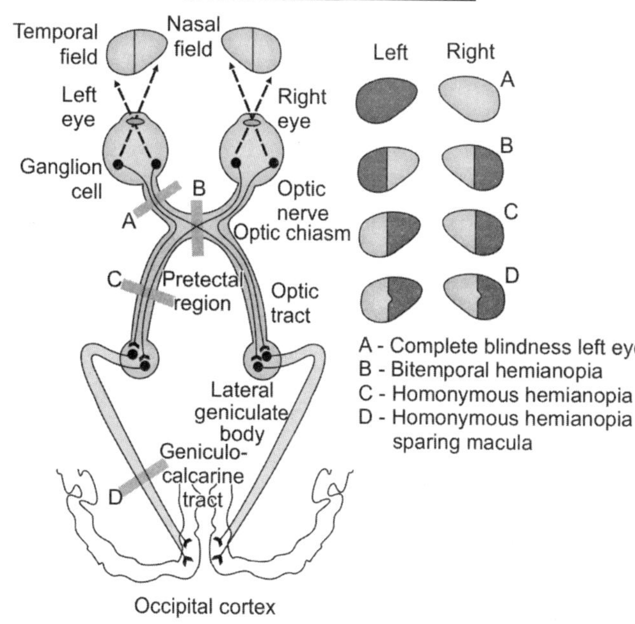

Stretch Reflex

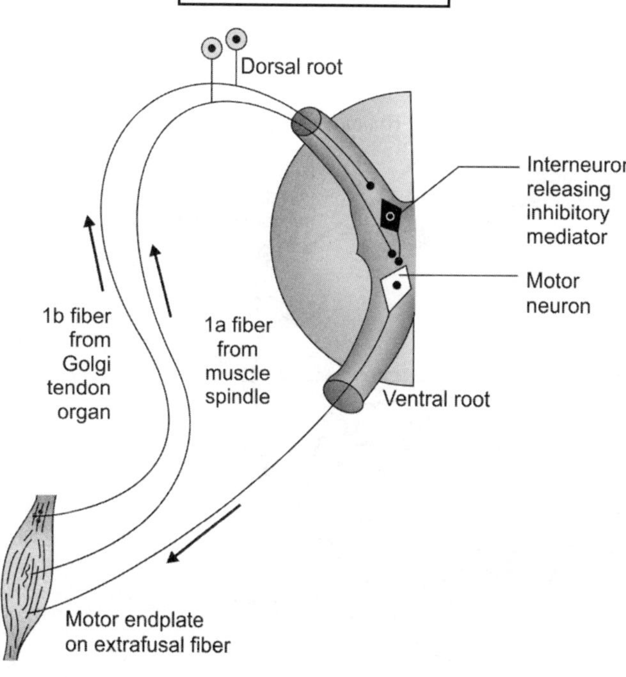

Clotting Pathway

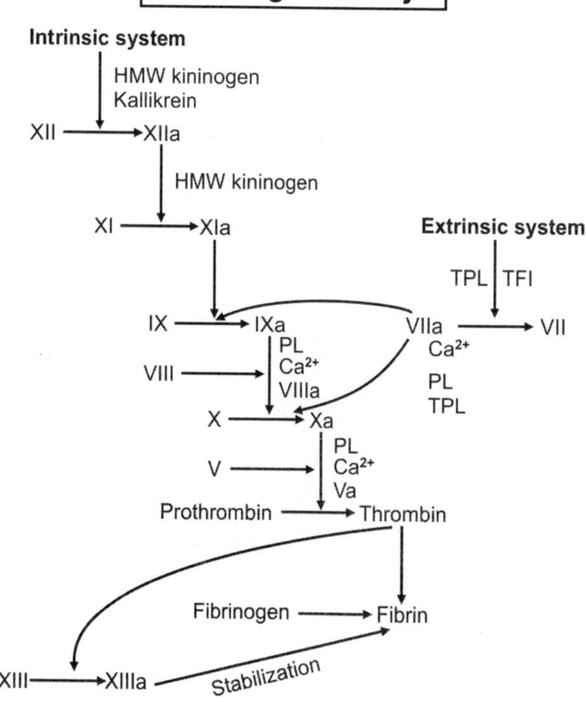

Scheme of the Fetal Circulation

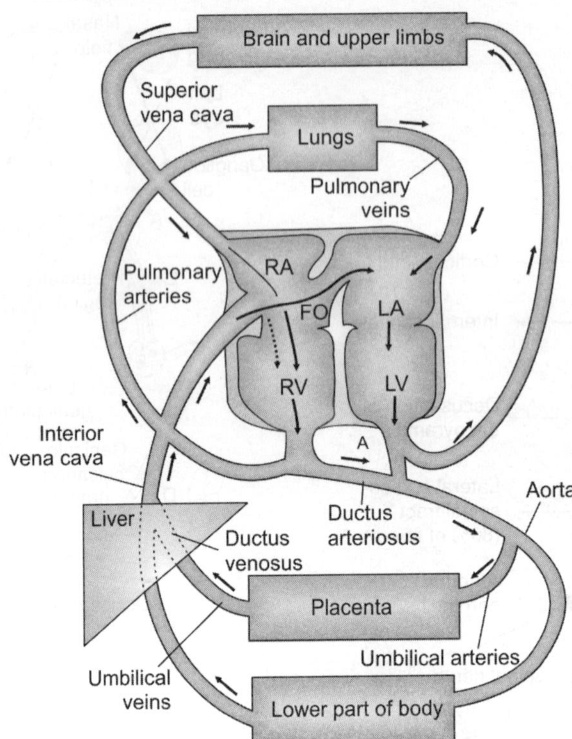

The degree of deoxygenation is shown by the intensity of shading.

1. RA = Right atrium
2. LA = Left atrium
3. RV = Right ventricle
4. LV = Left ventricle
5. FO = Foramen ovale
6. P = Pulmonary trunk
7. A = Aorta

PARASITOLOGY

Malarial Parasite's Life Cycle

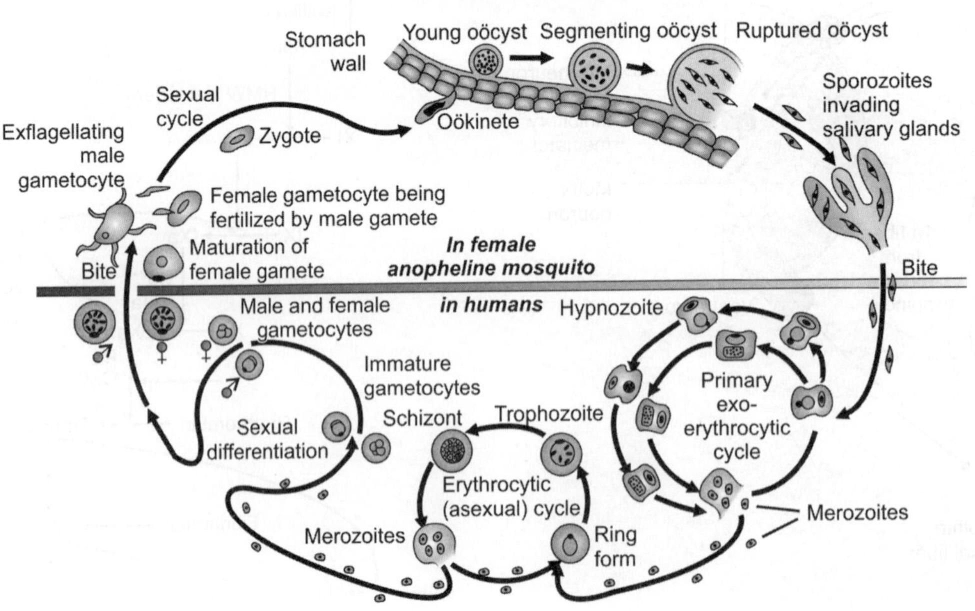

Microfilaria

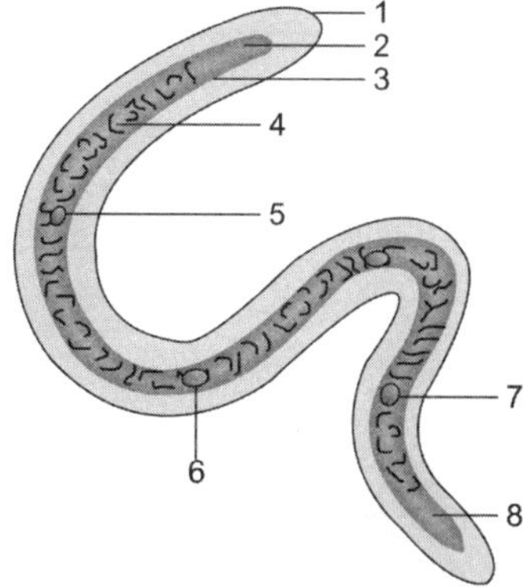

Morphology of *Microfilaria bancrofti*

1. Sheath
2. Stylet
3. Cephalic space
4. Nuclei
5. Nerve ring
6. Anterior V-spot
7. Posterior V-spot
8. Tail

Schistosome Eggs

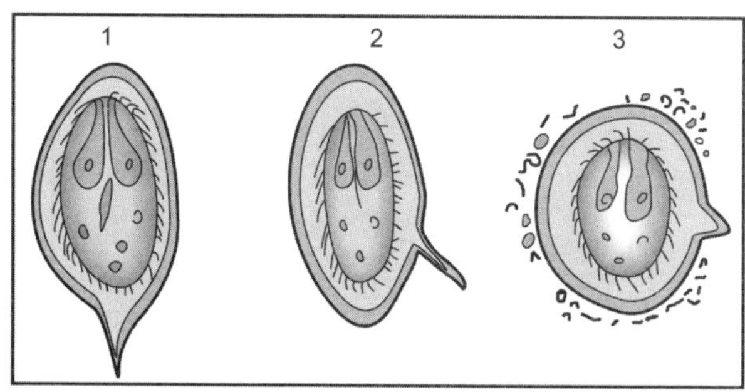

1. *S. haematobium*—oval with terminal spine
2. *S. mansoni*—oval, with lateral spine
3. *S. japonicum*—roundish with lateral knob

Small granules of tissue debris adherent to shell

Giardia lamblia

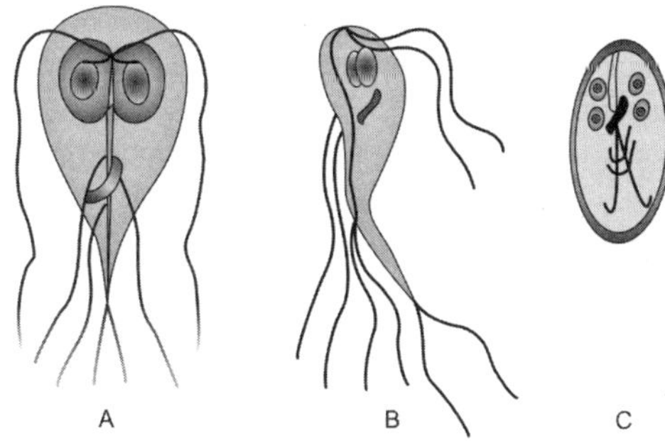

A. Trophozoite–ventral
B. Trophozoite–lateral view
C. Cyst

Oocysts of *Isospora belli*

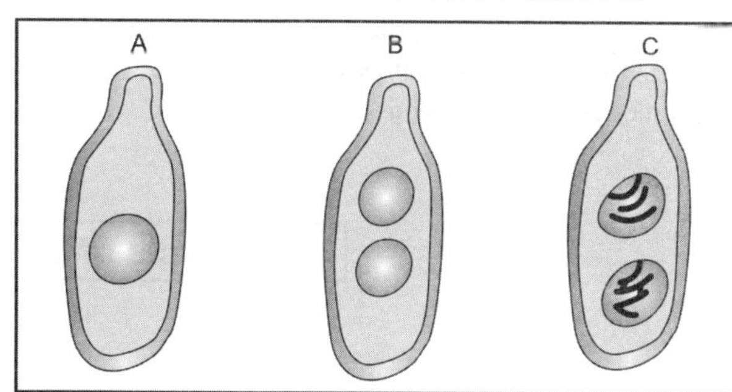

A. Immature oocyst
B. Oocyst showing two sporoblasts
C. Mature oocyst with two sporocysts containing sporozoites

Hydatid Cyst

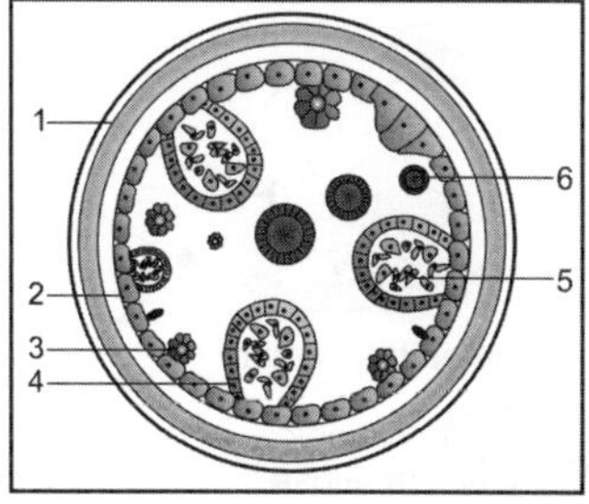

1. Outer laminated layer
2. Germinal layer
3. Gemmule
4. Brood capsule
5. Protoscolex
6. Sterile daughter cyst

Toxoplasma gondii

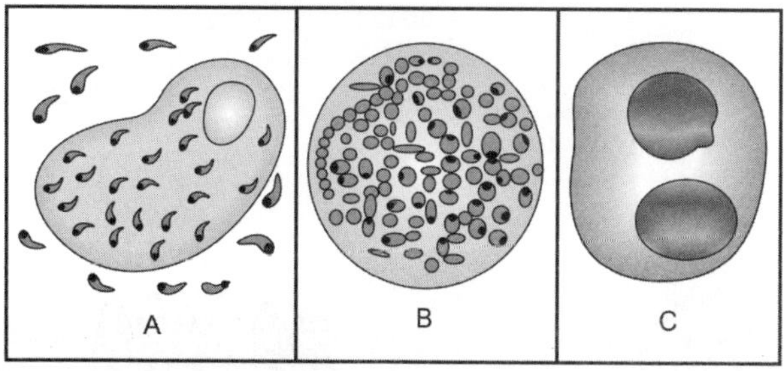

A. Smear from peritoneal fluid of infected mouse, showing crescentic tachyzoites—extracellular trophozoites and intracellular form within macrophage
B. Thick-walled tissue cyst containing rounded forms bradyzoites
C. Oocyst containing two sporocysts with sporozoites inside

Ascaris Eggs

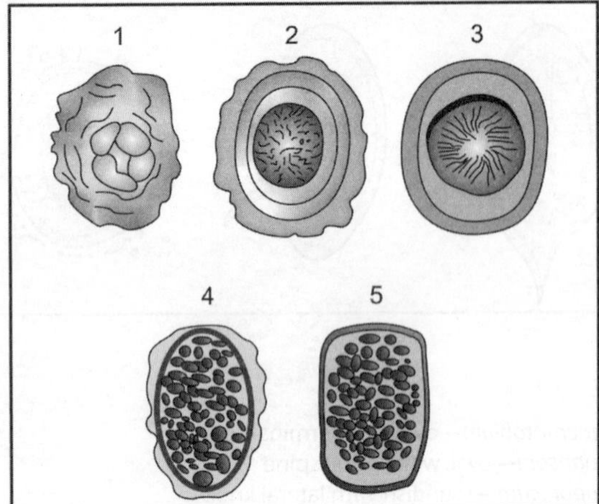

Types of *Ascaris* eggs found in stools:

1. Fertilized egg—surface focus, showing outer mamillary coat
2. Fertilized egg—median focus, showing unsegmented ovum surrounded by three layers of coats
3. Decorticated fertilized egg. The mamillary coat is absent
4. Unfertilized egg—elongated, with atrophic ovum
5. Decorticated unfertilized egg

Tapeworm Larvae

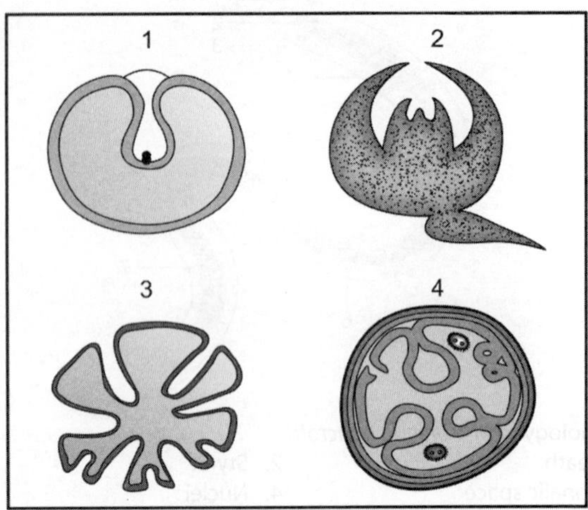

Larvae of cyclophyllidean tapeworms:

1. Cysticercus, a typical bladder with the invaginated protoscolex, e.g. *T. solium*
2. Cysticercoid, a fleshy larva with the head withdrawn and surrounded by a double fold of integument, e.g. *H. nana*
3. Coenurus larva with multiple invaginated protoscolices, e.g. *M. multiceps*
4. *Echinococcus*—hydatid cyst with internal budding

Life Cycle of *Entamoeba histolytica*

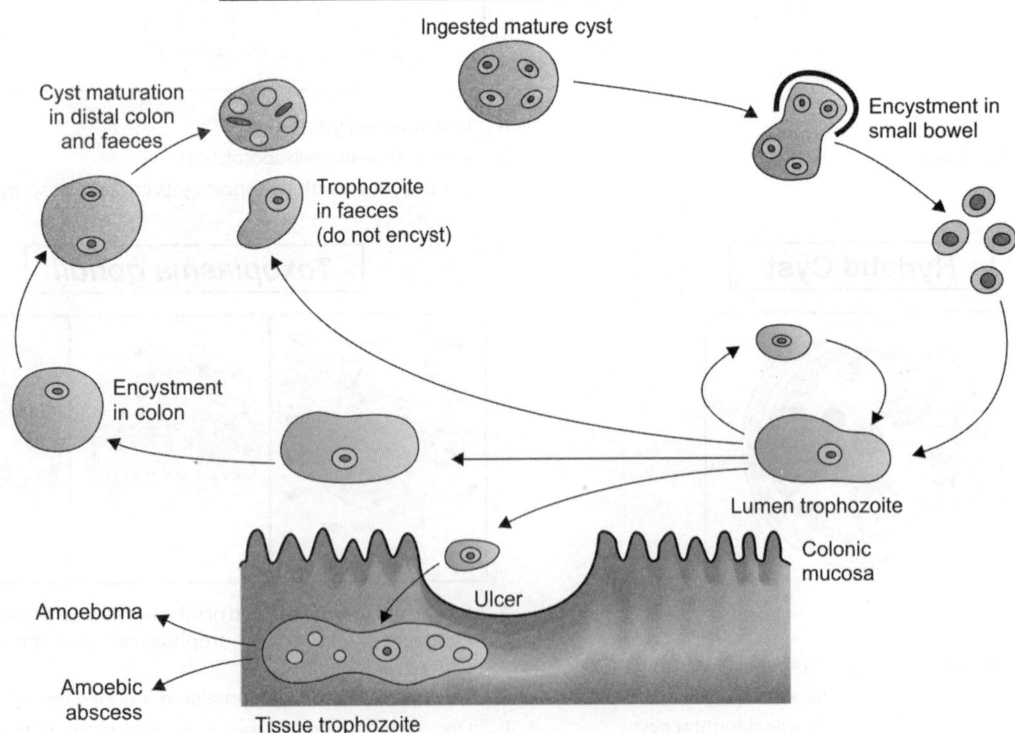

Trichomonas

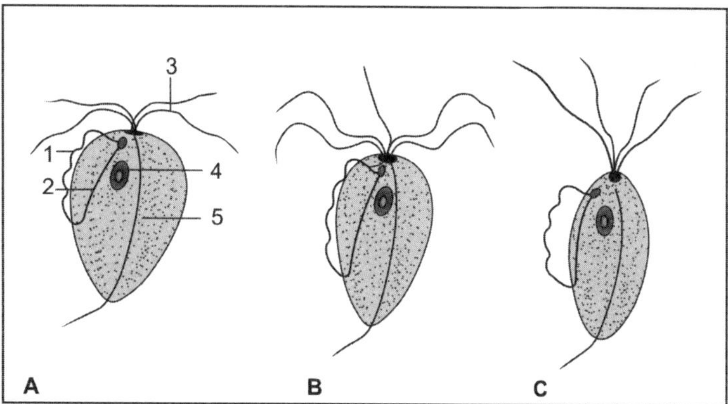

Trichomonas species: A. *T. vaginalis*; B. *T. hominis*; C. *T. tenax*.
1. Undulating membrane
2. Costa
3. Flagella
4. Nucleus
5. Axostyle

Plasmodium vivax

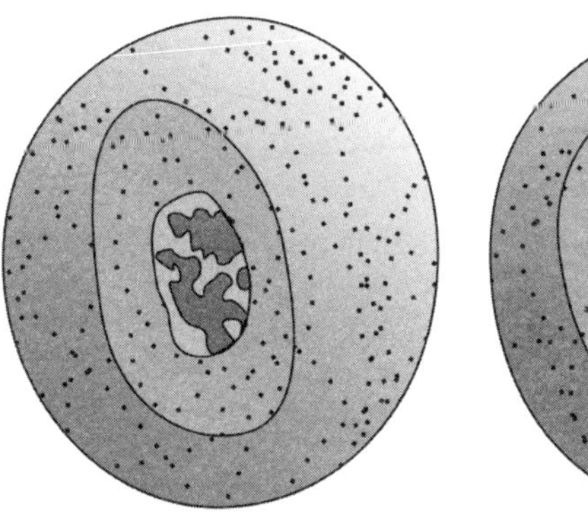

Male gametocyte

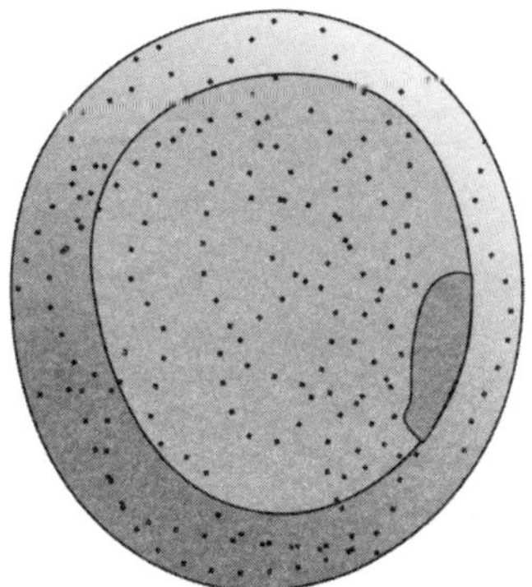

Female gametocyte

Plasmodium ovale

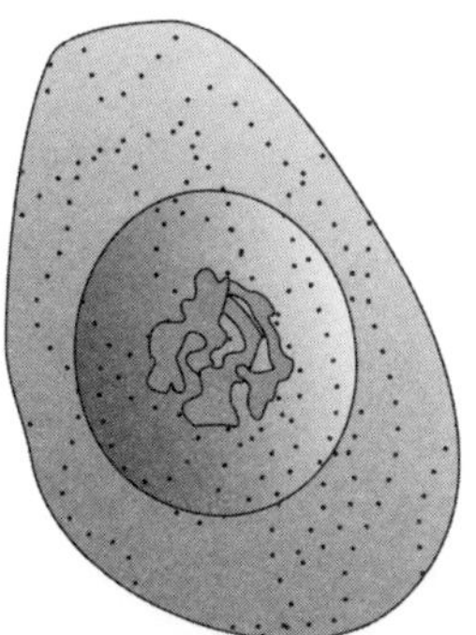

Male gametocyte

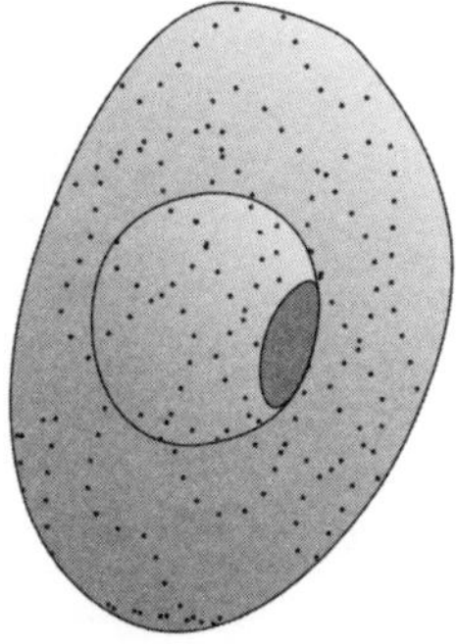

Female gametocyte

Plasmodium malariae

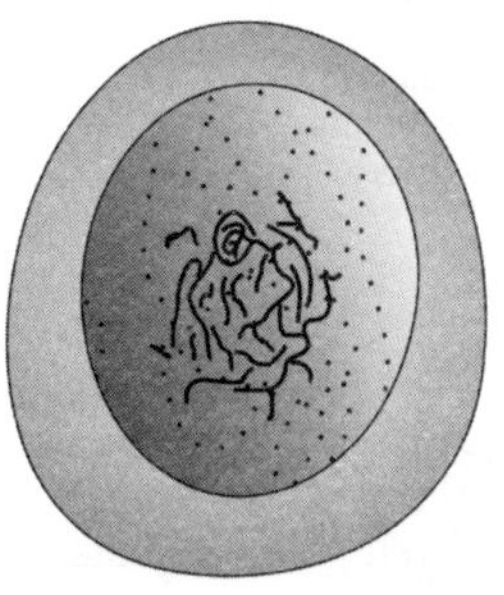

Male gametocyte

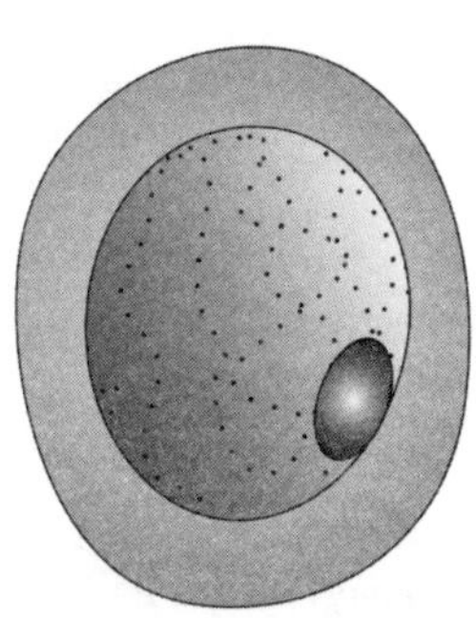

Female gametocyte

SURGERY

Situations for Residual Abscesses

Common situations for residual abscesses:

1. Subphrenic
2. Paracolic
3. Right iliac fossa
4. Pelvic

Types of Anorectal Abscess

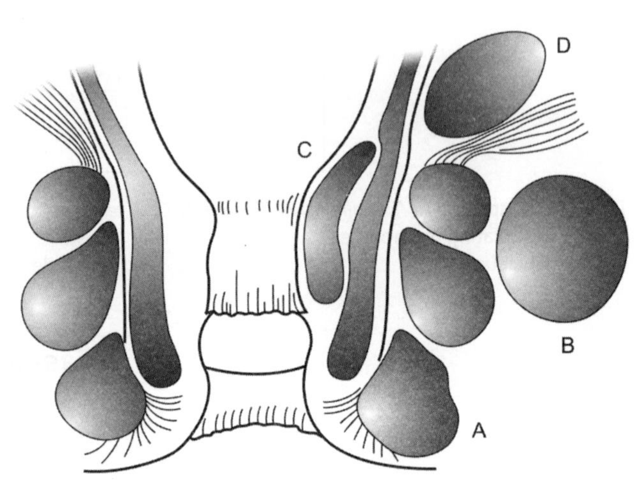

The four types of anorectal abscess:

A. Perianal
B. Ischiorectal
C. Submucous
D. Pelvirectal (after WFW Southwood, Bath, England)

Arterial Supply of Nasal Septum

Anterior ethmoidal artery

Posterior ethmoidal artery

Kiesselbach's plexus

Sphenopalatine artery

Greater palatine artery

Facial artery

Various Positions of Appendix

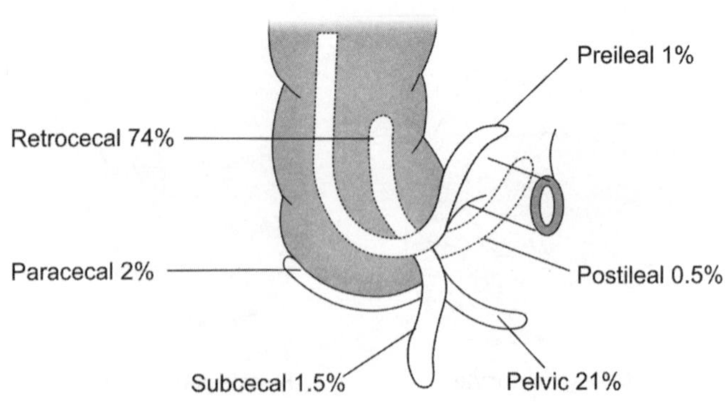

Arterial Supply of Stomach

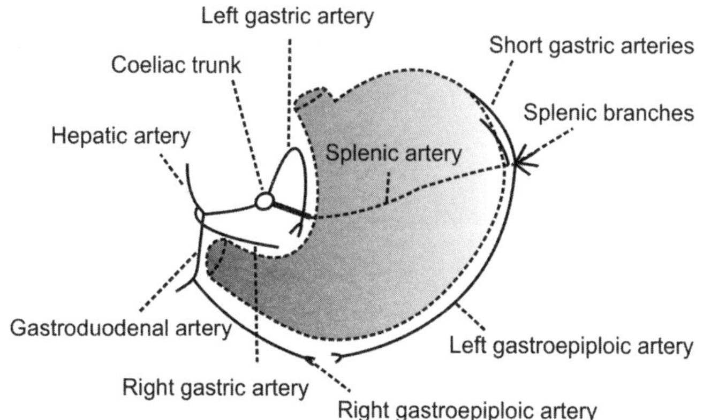

Circle of Willis

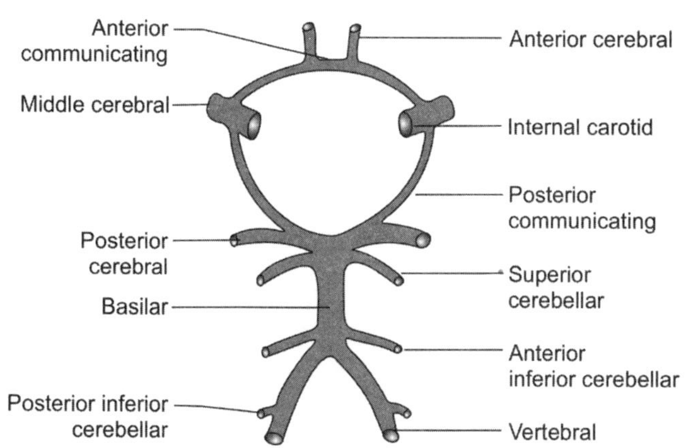

Congenital Biliary Atresia—Type I, II and III

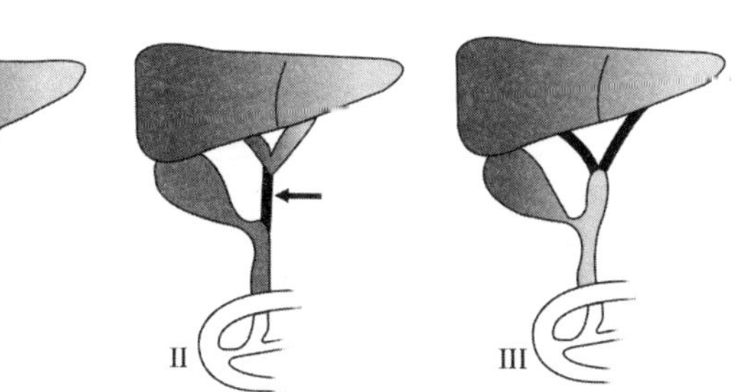

Carcinoma Breast

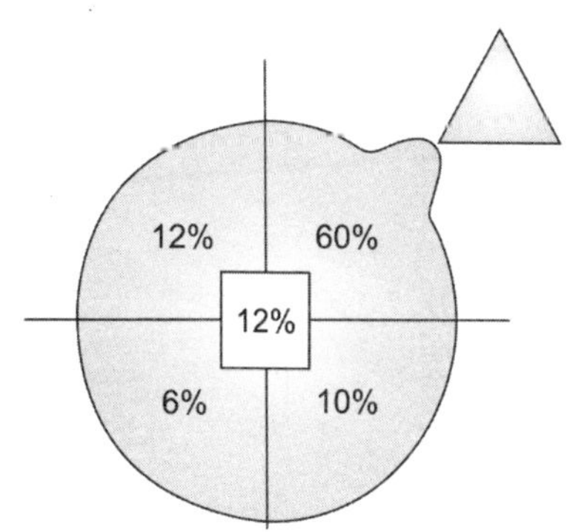

The relationship of carcinoma of the breast to the quadrants of breast

Anatomical Representation of Cleft LIP

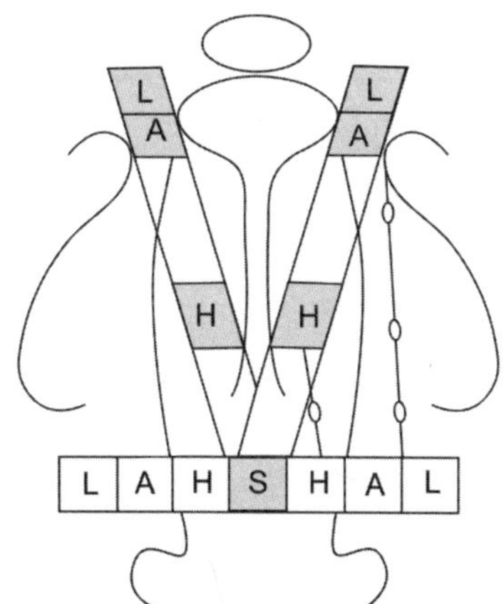

LAHSAL. An anatomical representation of cleft lip (L), alveolus (A), hard (H) and soft palate (S)

Sites of Ectopic Testis

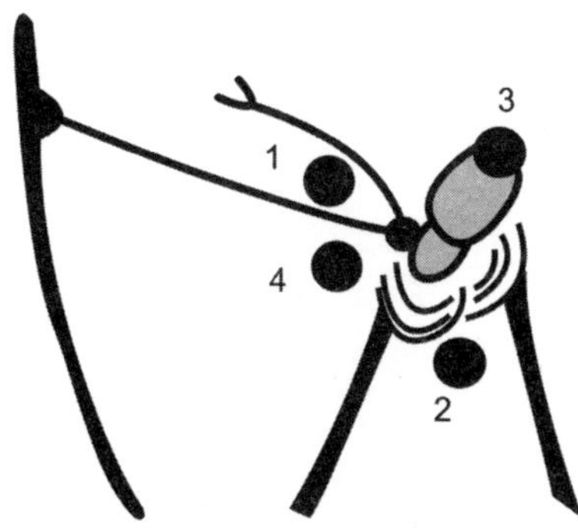

1. Superficial inguinal pouch
2. Perineum
3. Root of penis
4. Femoral triangle (thigh)

Blood Supply of Thyroid Gland

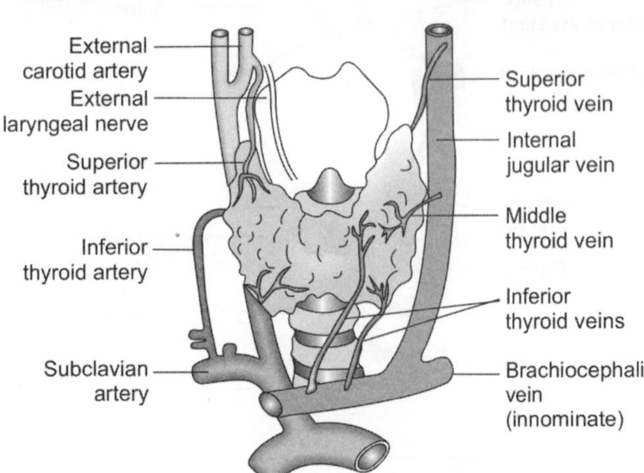

Layers of Scrotum

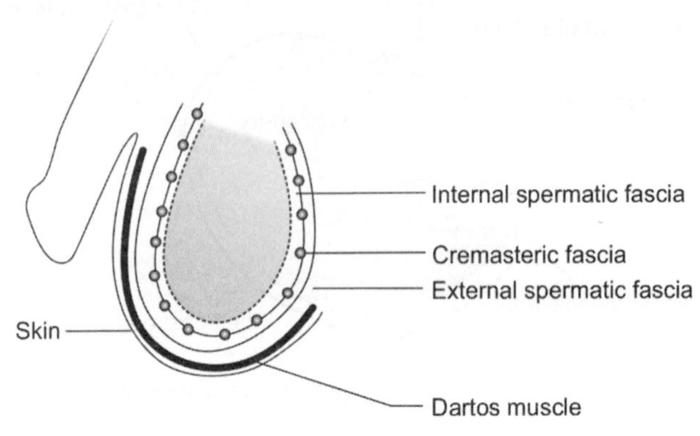

Brachial Plexus

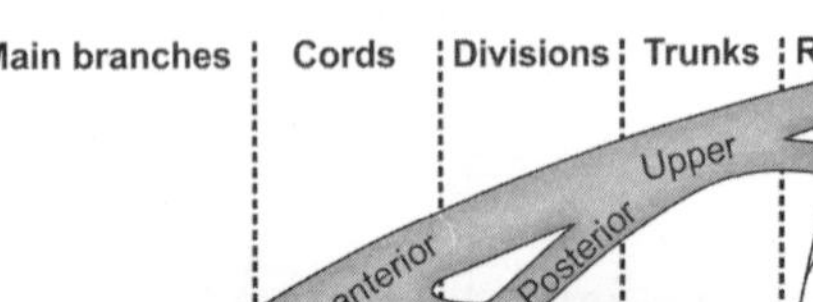

Layers of Scalp

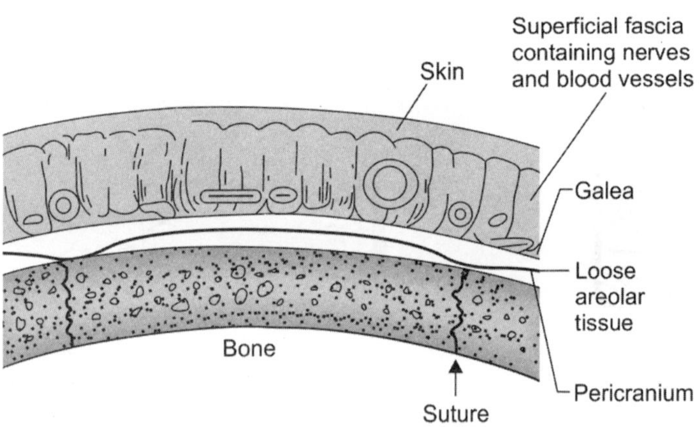

Layers of the scalp: skin, dense connective tissue, galea aponeurotica, loose connective tissue and pericranium

Goodsall's Rule

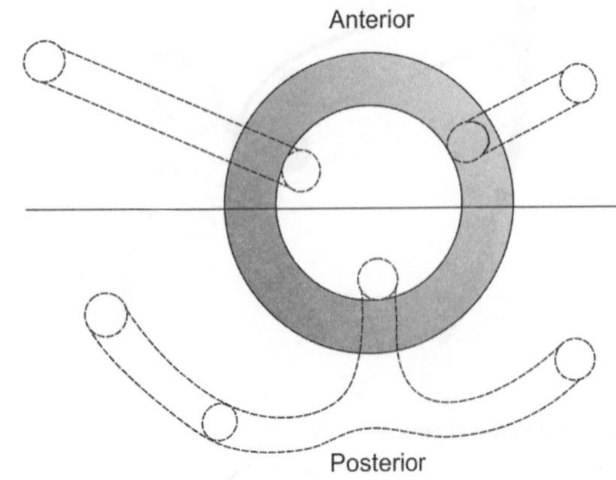

Types of Hypospadias

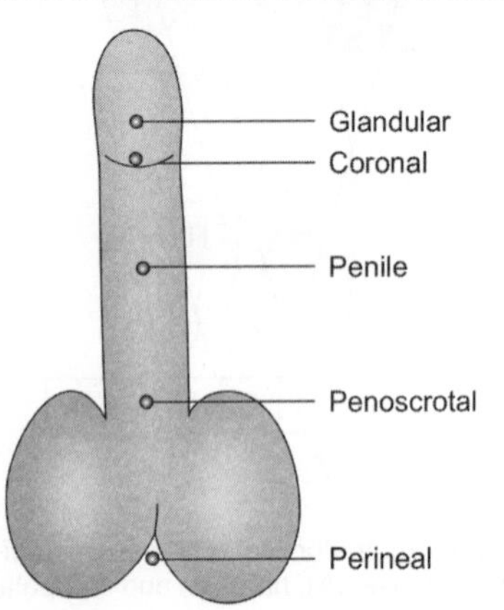

Whipple's Resection and Reconstruction

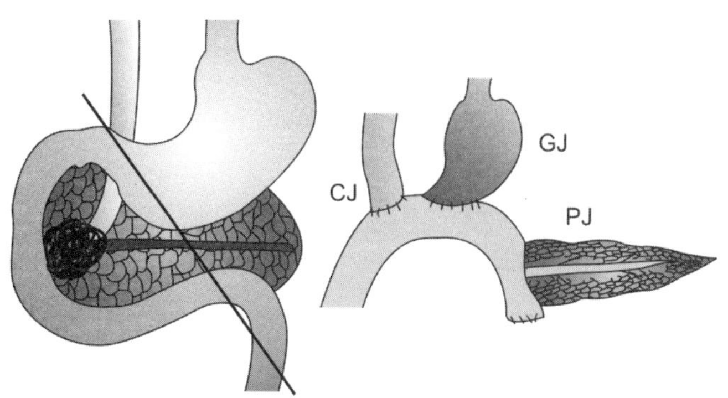

Waldeyer's Ring

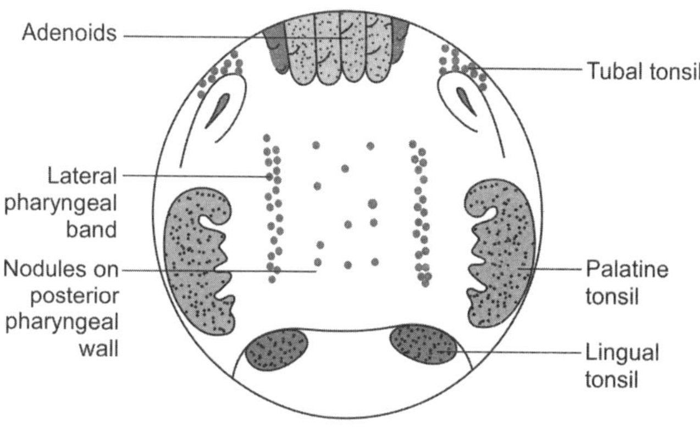

Hydrocele—Types

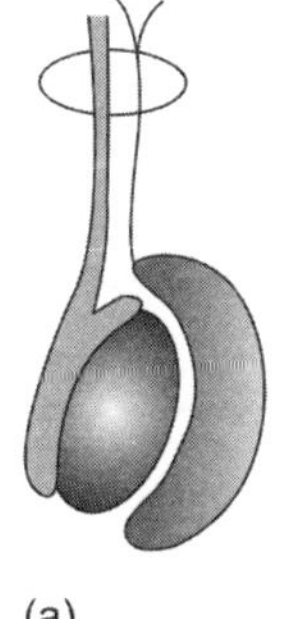
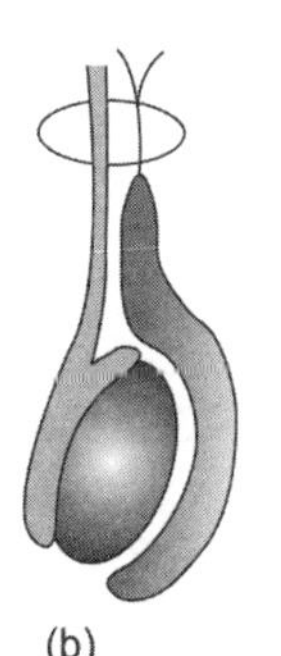
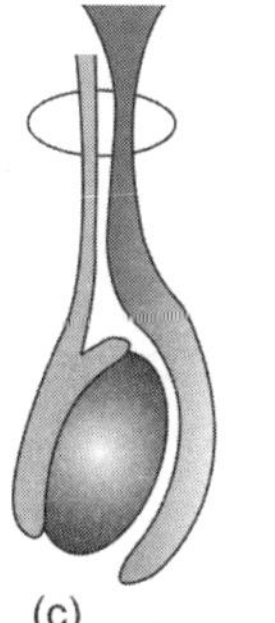
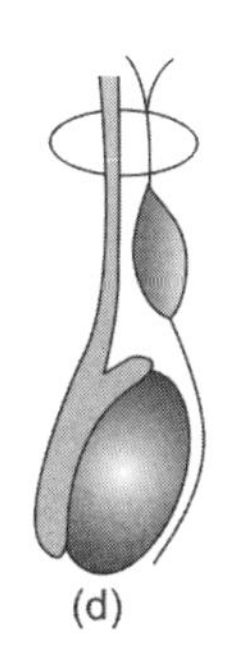

(a) (b) (c) (d)

(a) Vaginal hydrocele (very common)
(b) 'Infantile' hydrocele
(c) Congenital hydrocele
(d) Hydrocele of the cord

Lymph Nodes of Head and Neck

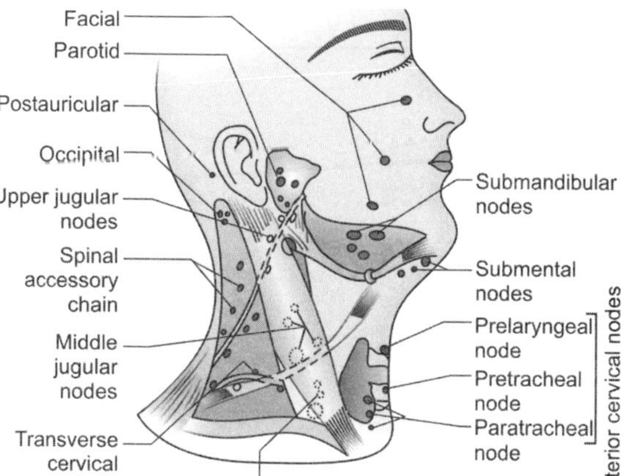

Levels of Lymph Nodes of Head and Neck

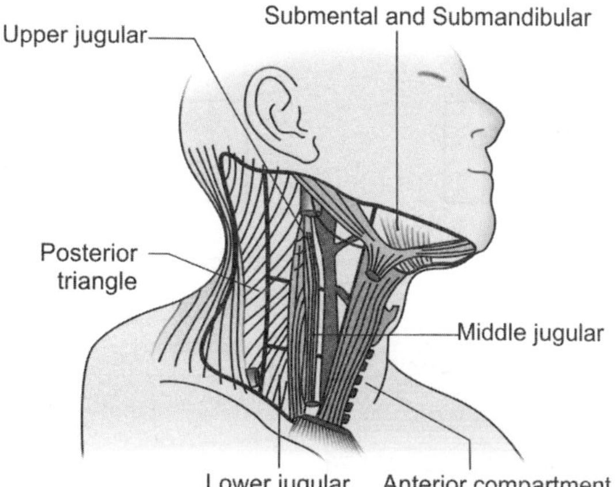

The level system for describing location of lymph nodes in the neck. Level I, submental and submandibular group; level II, upper jugular group; level III, middle jugular; level IV, lower jugular group; level V, posterior triangle group; level VI, anterior compartment group.

Sites of Portosystemic Anastomosis

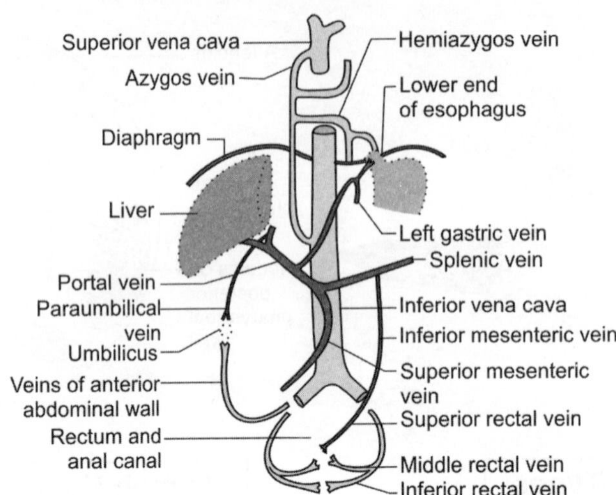

Ulcer—Type of Edges

A B C D E

Diagrammatic representation of different types of edge of ulcers:

(A) Undermined edge
(B) Punched out edge
(C) Stopping edge
(D) Raised and a pearly-white beaded edge of rodent ulcer
(E) Rolled out (everted) edge of an epithelioma

Sites of Subarachnoid Hemorrhages

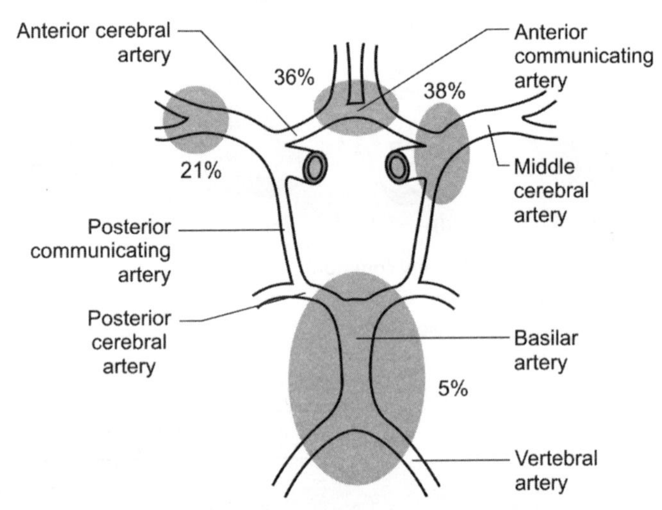

Various Parts of an ulcer-diagrammatic

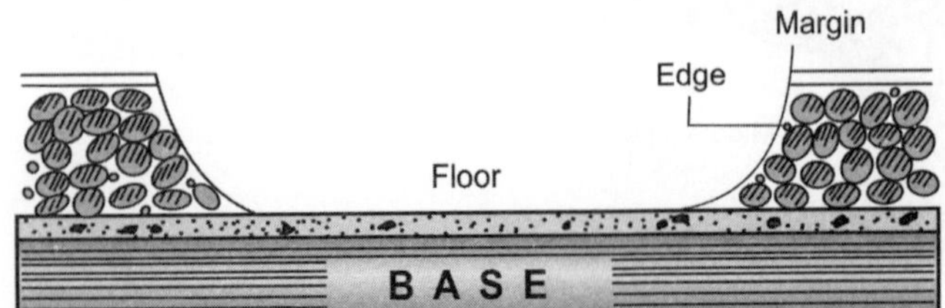

Transjugular Intrahepatic Portosystemic Stent Shunt (TIPSS)

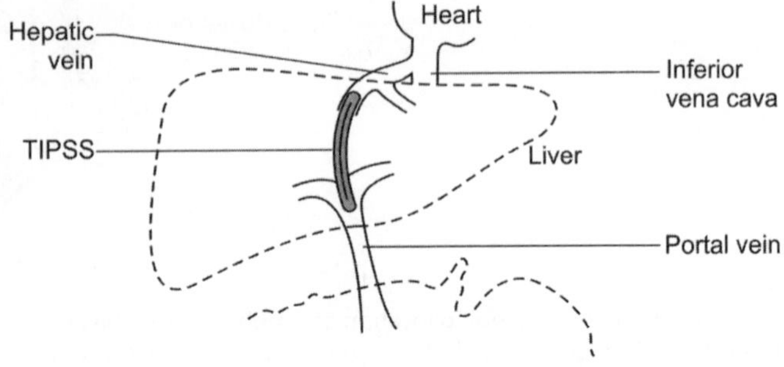

Types of Lesion in Renal Tuberculosis

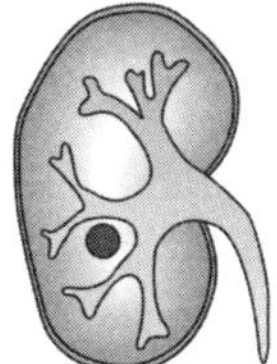

(A) Tuberculous papillary ulcer

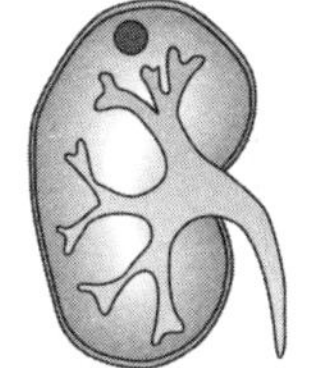

(B) Cavernous form. It tends to burst like a bombshell

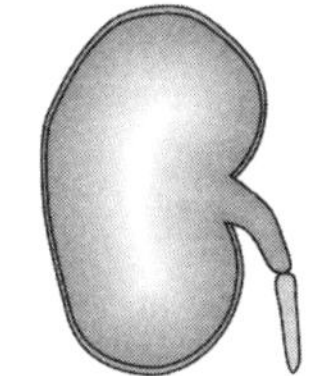

(C) Hydronephrosis (rare)

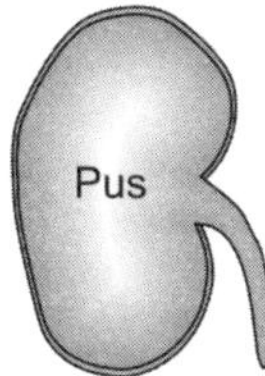

(D) Pyonephrosis secondary infection *E. coli*, etc. very prone to supervene

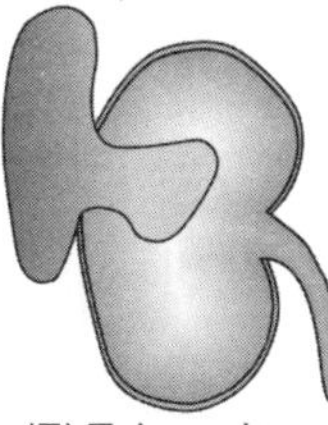

(E) Tuberculous perinephric abscess

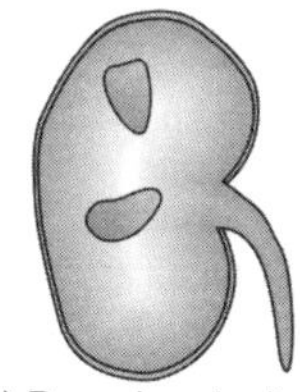

(F) Pseudocalculi on X-ray examination, calcified tuberculous areas in the kidney simulate calculi

(G) Caseous kidney divided by fibrous septa

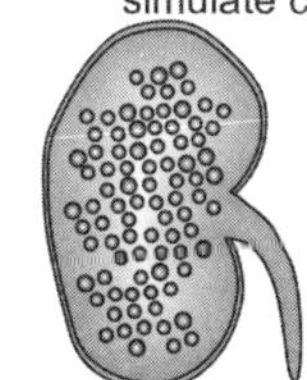

(H) Miliary a part of a general tuberculous process

Intraperitoneal Subphrenic Abscess

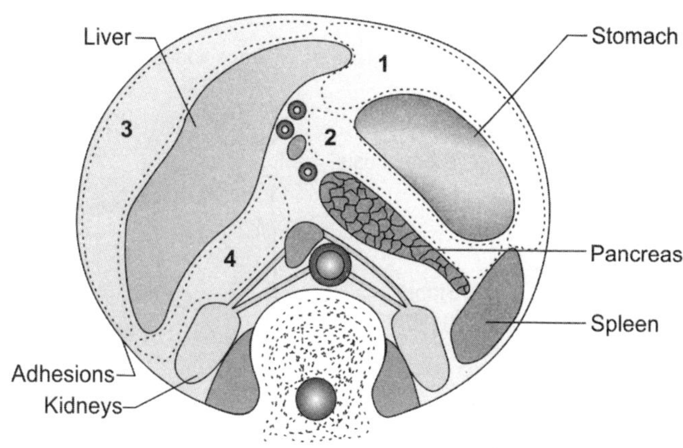

(1) Left superior space
(2) Left inferior space (lesser sac)
(3) Right superior space which becomes shut off by adhesions
(4) Right inferior space

Types of Closed Renal Trauma

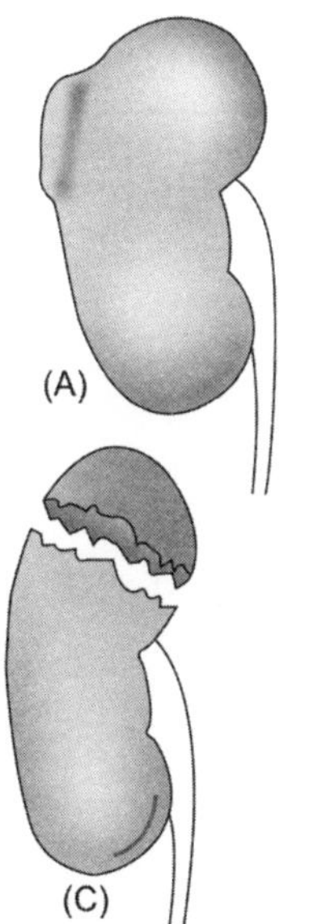

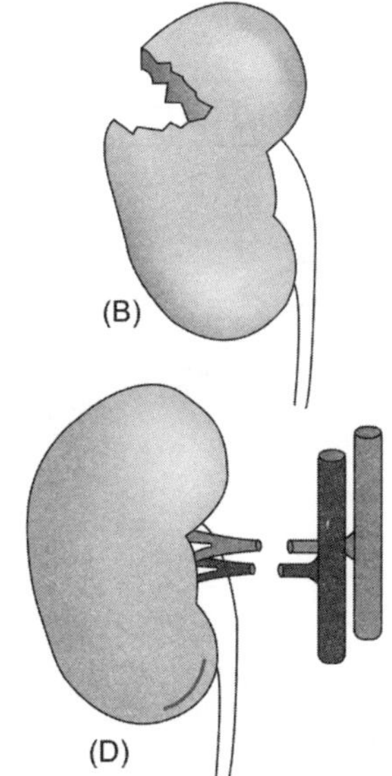

(A) Subscapular hematoma
(B) Laceration
(C) Avulsion of one pole
(D) Avulsion of renal pedicle

Intraperitoneal Subphrenic Abscess—Sagittal Section

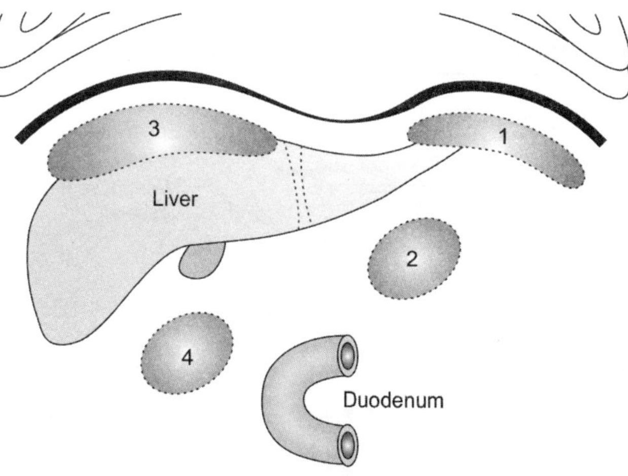

(1) Left superior (anterior) abscess ('left subphrenic')
(2) Left inferior (posterior) abscess ('left subhepatic')
(3) Right superior (anterior) abscess ('right subphrenic')
(4) Right inferior (posterior) abscess ('right subhepatic')

Common Causes of Hematuria

Superficial Veins of Lower Limb

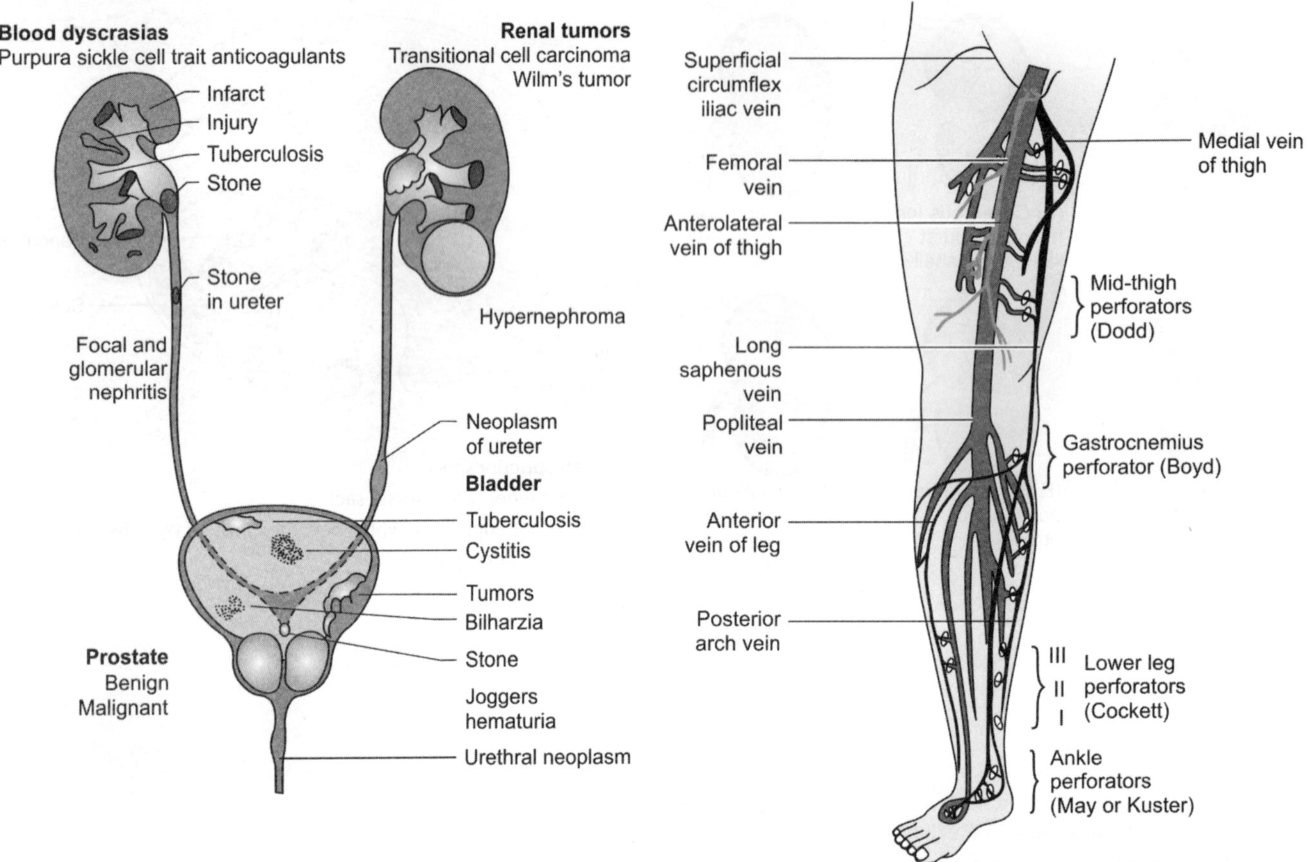

ORTHOPEDICS

Blood Supply of a Typical Long Bone

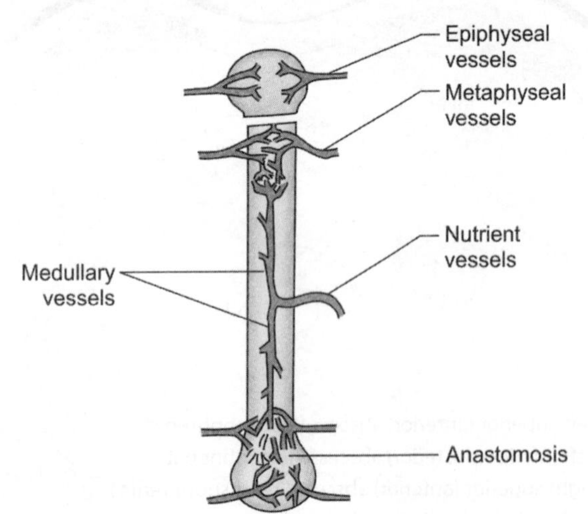

Blood Supply of Head of Femur

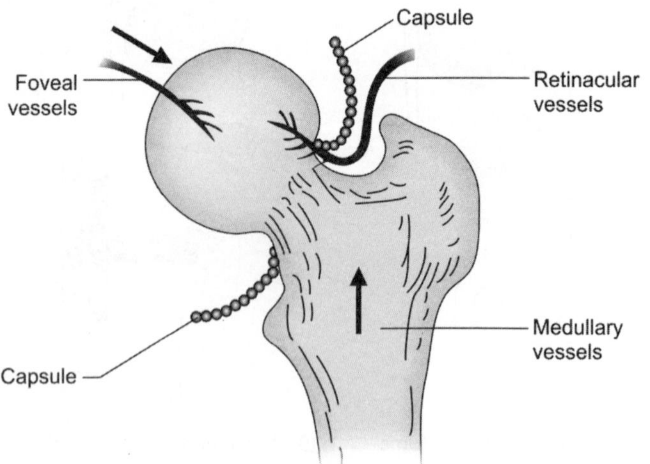

Common Sites of Tuberculosis Hip

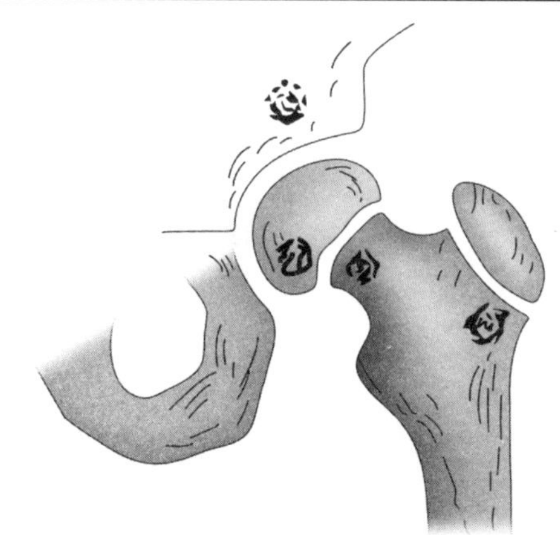

Wandering Acetabulum

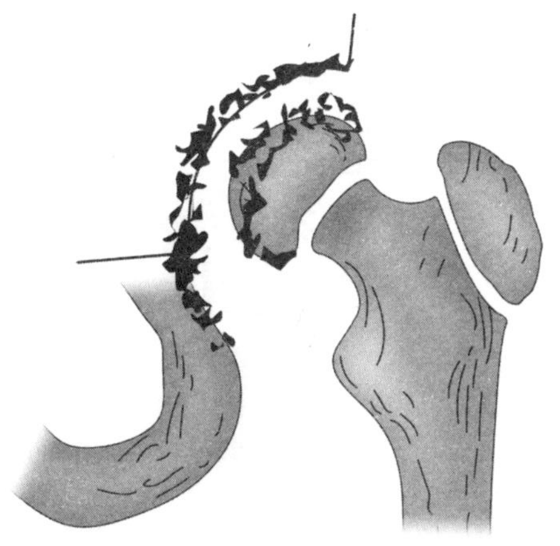

McMurray's Osteotomy

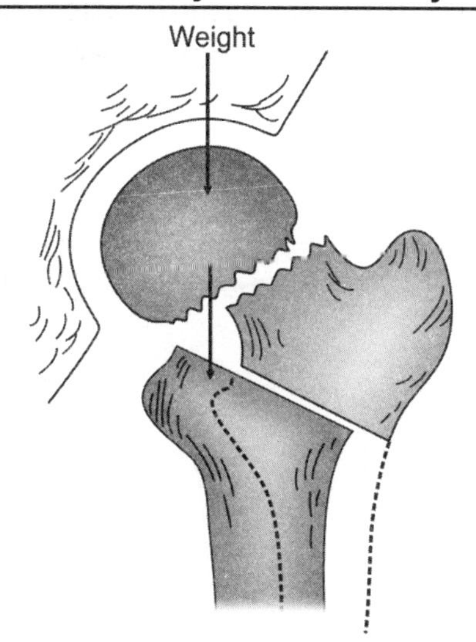

Spread of Pus from Metaphysis

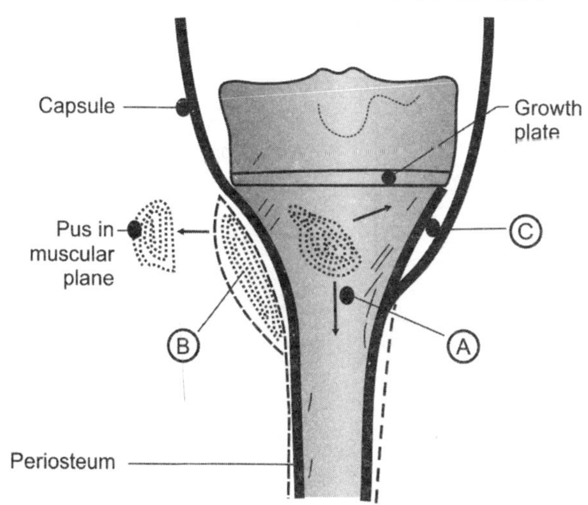

(A) Along medullary cavity; (B) Out of the cortex; (C) To the joint

Carpal Tunnel

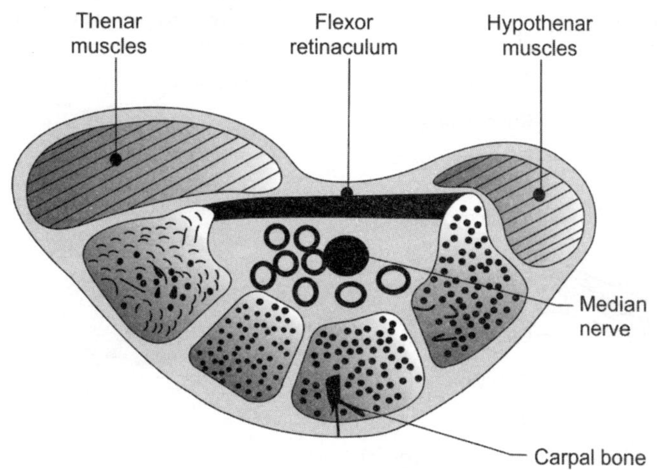

Vascular Arrangement of Metaphysis of Long Bone

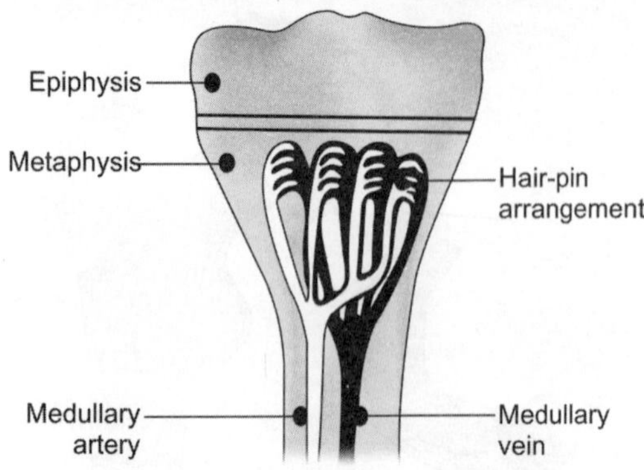

Anatomy of Shoulder

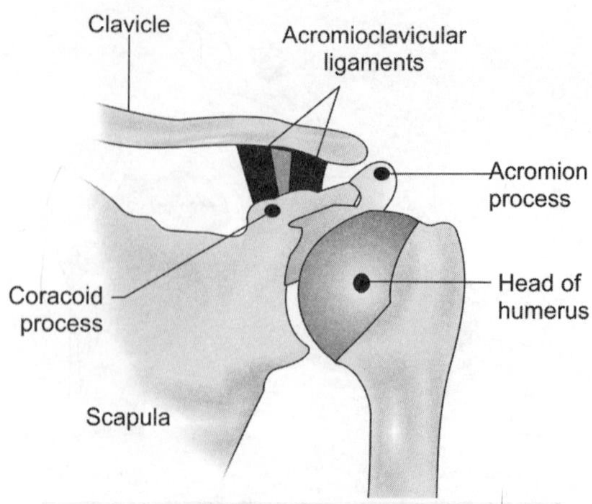

Types of Anterior Dislocation of Shoulder

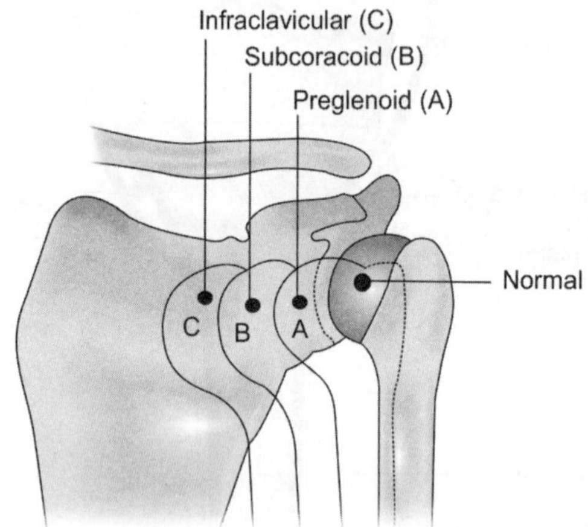

Anatomical Classification of Fractures of Neck of Femur

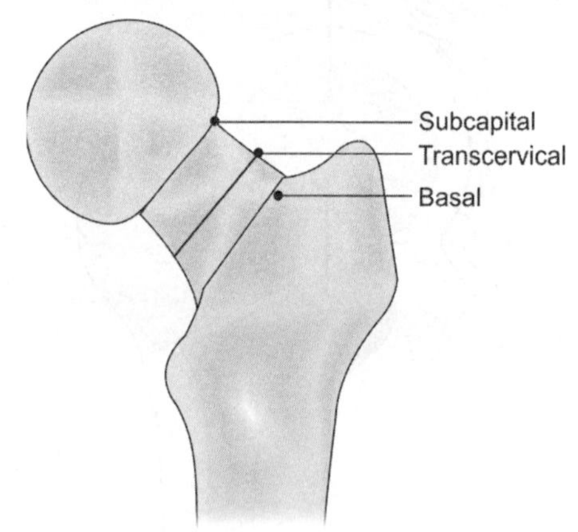

OBSTETRICS

Pelvic Diaphragm

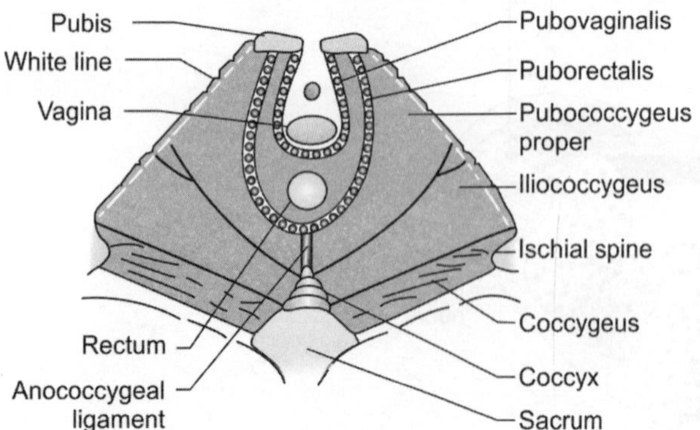

Superior view of the pelvic diaphragm (the levator ani and coccygeus)

Ligamentary Supports of Uterus

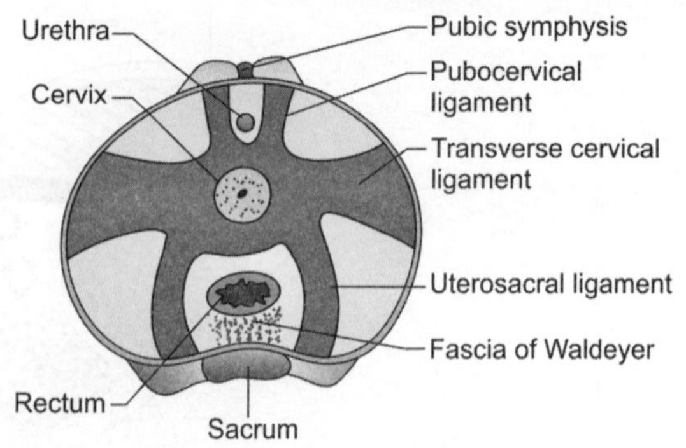

Graafian Follicle

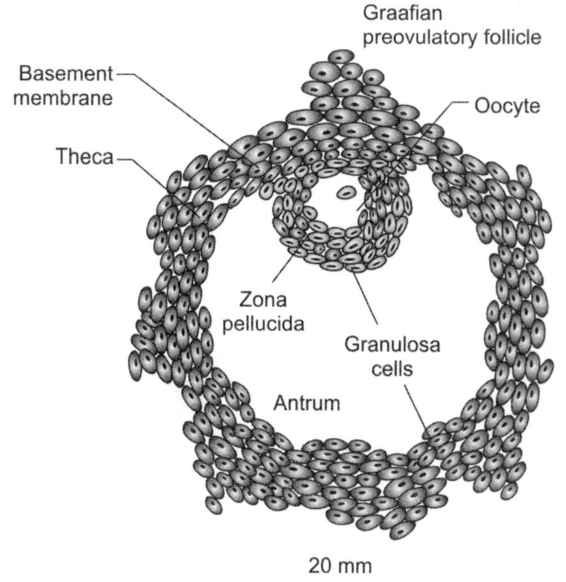

Graafian follicle showing granulosa cells, the ovum, and theca interna cells. Graafian follicle measures 20 mm at ovulation

Staging of Carcinoma Cervix

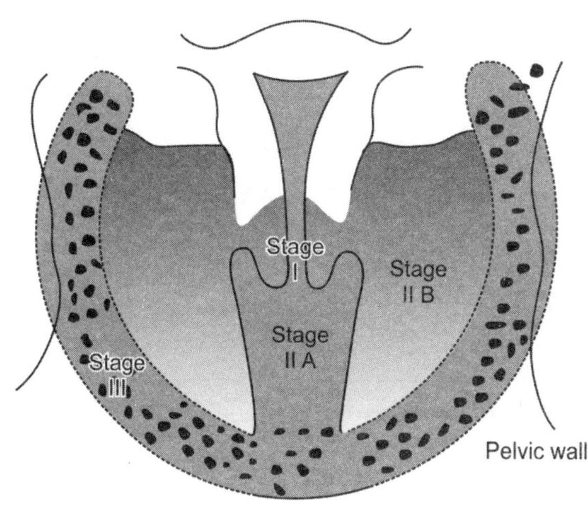

Branches of Right Internal Iliac Artery in Female

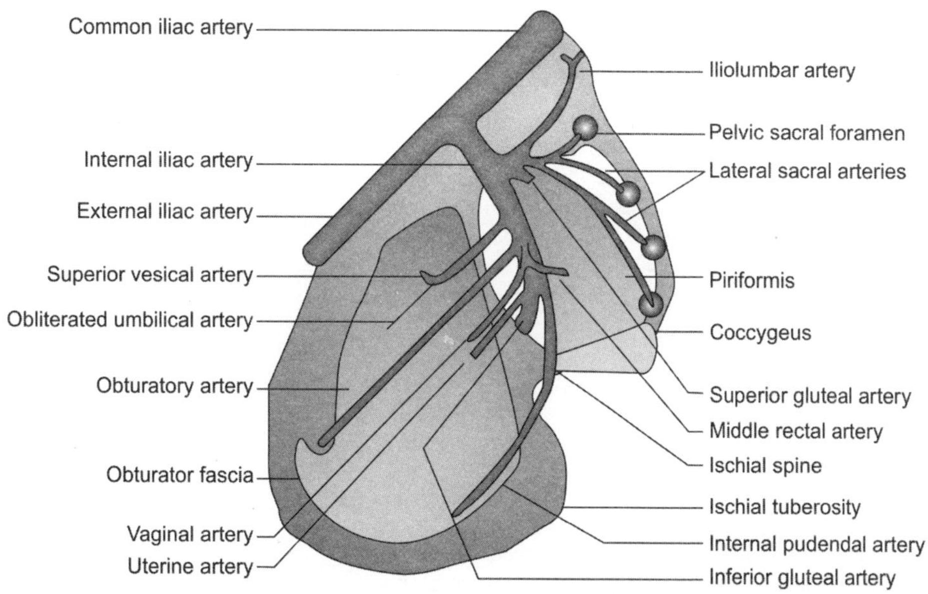

Types of Uterine Prolapse

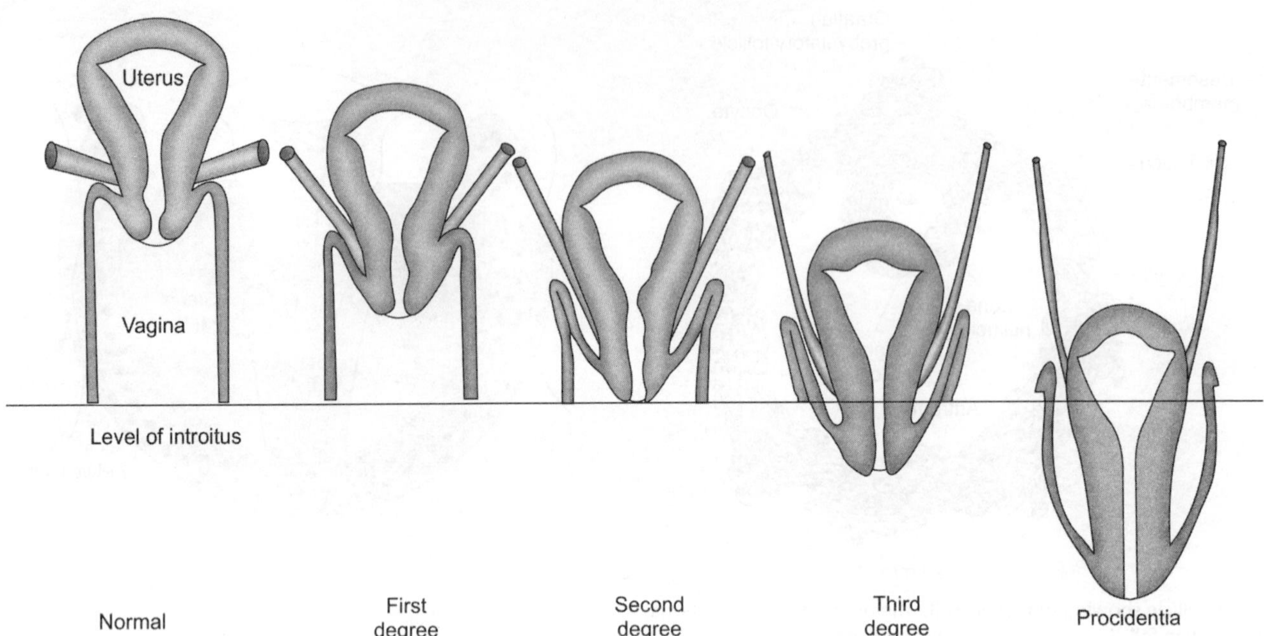

PARTOGRAPH

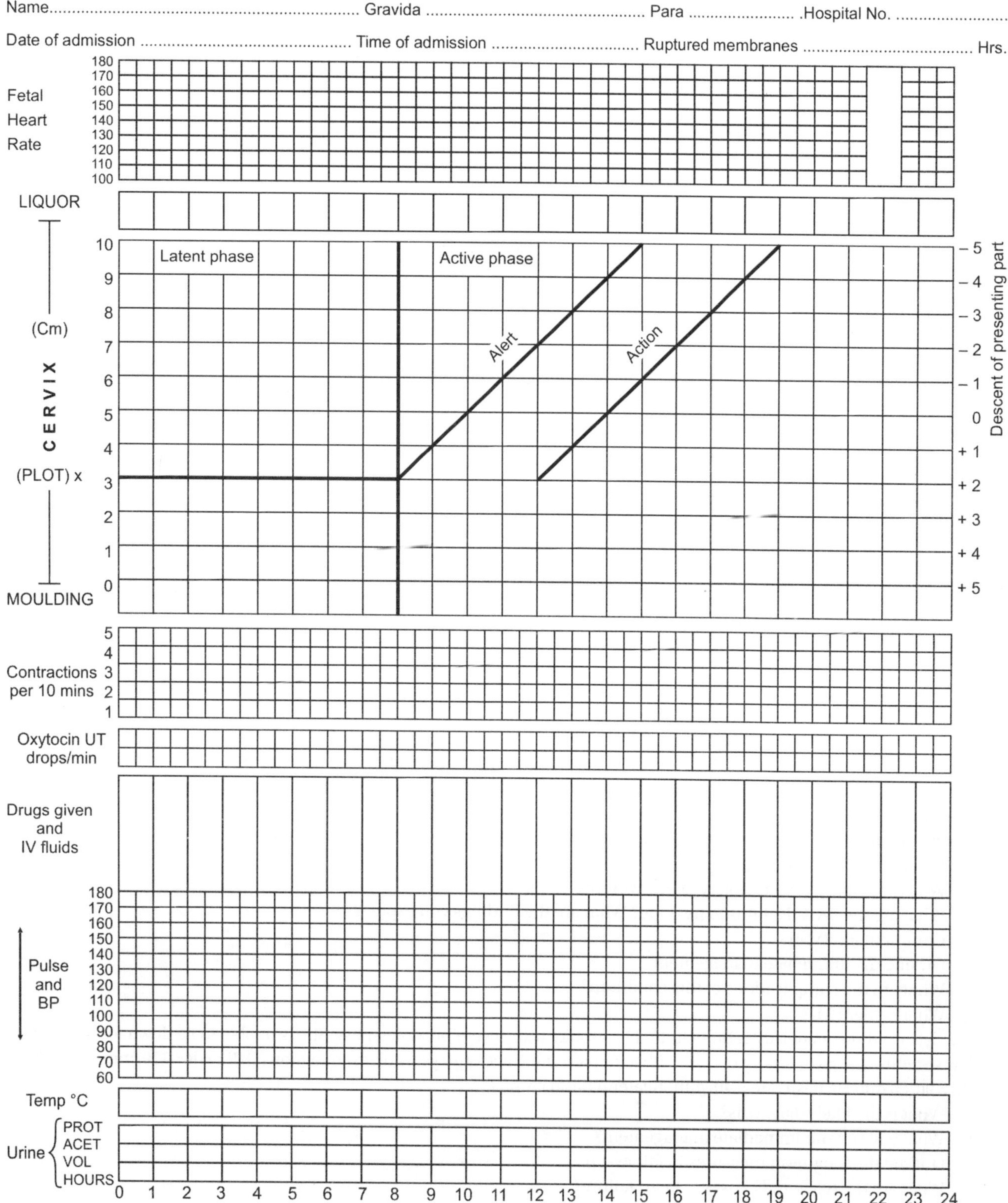
Name........ Gravida .... Para .... .Hospital No. ....
Date of admission .... Time of admission .... Ruptured membranes .... Hrs.
Fetal Heart Rate
180 170 160 150 140 130 120 110 100
LIQUOR
CERVIX
(Cm)
(PLOT) x
MOULDING
10 9 8 7 6 5 4 3 2 1 0
Latent phase
Active phase
Alert
Action
– 5 – 4 – 3 – 2 – 1 0 + 1 + 2 + 3 + 4 + 5
Descent of presenting part
Contractions per 10 mins
5 4 3 2 1
Oxytocin UT drops/min
Drugs given and IV fluids
Pulse and BP
180 170 160 150 140 130 120 110 100 90 80 70 60
Temp °C
Urine
PROT
ACET
VOL
HOURS
0 1 2 3 4 5 6 7 8 9 10 11 12 13 14 15 16 17 18 19 20 21 22 23 24

Question Bank

MEDICINE

Theory Topics:

Paper I	: Clinical Medicine, CVS, GIT, Nephrology, CNS, Endocrine, Hematology, Applied Questions of Basic Sciences	60 Marks
Paper II	: Chest, Dermatology, Psychiatry, Radiodiagnosis, Basic Sciences as Applied Medicine, Genetics, Immunology, Rheumatology, Tropical Infections, Nutrition, Poisoning, Toxicology.	60 Marks

Practical Examinations:

Clinical I	: Long Case (Including Case Sheet)	50 Marks
Clinical II	: Short Case I	20 Marks
Clinical III	: Short Case II	20 Marks
Clinical IV	: OSCE/Spotter	10 Marks

Oral Examinations: X-rays and Instruments, Drugs, Investigation Charts. 20 Marks

Clinical Questions

1. A 50-year-old male, a known diabetic and hypertensive, presents with sudden onset of epigastric pain, nausea and vomiting. He gives history of retrosternal discomfort with pain in the throat and left shoulder on exertion and sexual intercourse.
   On examination (O/E): HR = 50/min, irregular; BP = 110/70 mm Hg.
   a. What is the probable diagnosis?
   b. Which coronary vessel is likely to be involved?
   c. What are the investigations to be done? What are the findings you expect?
   d. Comment on RVMI.
   e. Outline the immediate management.
   f. What are the complications of this condition?
   g. What is silent MI?
2. A 28-year-old pregnant lady is brought to the casualty with severe breathlessness. She is unable to lie down for more than a few seconds. She gives history of fever with joint pain at the age of 10 years on examination (O/E): HR = 120/min, low volume; BP = 90/60 mm Hg Resp rate = 40/min, Bilateral basal creps +
   a. What is the likely diagnosis?
   b. What will be your immediate management?
   c. Outline the long-term measures in follow-up.
   d. What are the types and causes of heart failure?
   e. What is Framingham criteria?

f. What are the causes of high output failure?
g. Comment on digoxin toxicity.

3. A 25-year-old male with DOE, exertional palpitation and frequent chest infections now presents with fever since 3 weeks, loss of appetite and loss of weight; arthralgia. O/E: Pallor: +, Clubbing: +, a PSM at the apex; Splenomegaly:
   a. What is the probable diagnosis?
   b. What other clinical findings will you look for?
   c. Mention the etiological agents responsible for the condition.
   d. What all investigations will you ask for?
   e. How will you manage this case?
   f. What are the indications for surgery in such a case?
4. A 55-year-old chronic smoker presents with history of low grade fever, malaise, fatigue and cough with hemoptysis of 3 weeks duration and loss of weight. O/E: Pallor: +, Post-tussive rales in right supraclavicular, infraclavicular and axillary area.
   a. What is the most likely diagnosis?
   b. What other possibilities will you keep in mind?
   c. What are the clinical features of this disease? (Signs and symptoms)
   d. What are the complications you can expect?
   e. What are the main investigations you will like to ask for? What are the likely findings?
   f. What are the main pathological varieties of the disease?
   g. Outline the main modalities of Rx.
5. A 45-year-old male smoker with history of high grade fever, malaise, headache and dry cough is presenting with increase in dyspnea, vomiting and streaky blood stained sputum.
   a. What is the likely diagnosis?
   b. Mention the predisposing factors for the condition.
   c. What are the other possibilities to be kept in mind?
   d. What investigations are to be asked for?
   e. How will you treat the patient?
   f. Comment on the clinical features and Rx of severe pneumonia.
6. A 38-year-old female presents with sudden onset of weakness of the left half of the body including the face. She gives history of exertional dyspnea, fatigue and palpitation for the past 10 years.
   O/E : pulse = 120/min, irregular with varying volume; BP = 110/70 mm Hg.
   a. What is your clinical diagnosis?
   b. What is the likely predisposing factor in the case? Mention the risk factors and precipitants of stroke.
   c. What is the investigation of choice? What are the likely findings?
   d. How will you manage this case?
   e. What are the complications associated with the disease?
   f. What are the important differential diagnosis of acute stroke?
   g. What are the causes of young stroke?
7. A 60-year-old male presents with recurrent seizures, progressive headache and loss of weight of 1 year duration. He also gives history of slowly progressing weakness of both lower limbs. He also complains of impaired memory and urinary incontinence.
   a. What is the most likely diagnosis?
   b. Mention causes of recurrent seizures.
   c. Mention the clinical features and Rx of raised ICT (intracranial tension).
   d. What are the investigations to be done in this case?
   e. Outline the various modalities of Rx.
   f. What are the different pathological types of the disease?
8. A 10-year-old boy with fever and ear discharge now presents with headache, vomiting and drowsiness. The child is now responding only to pain and has developed seizures. O/E: Pupil dilated on one side, Plantar is b/l extensor.
   a. What is your clinical diagnosis?
   b. How will you explain the various clinical signs and symptoms in the boy?
   c. Mention the various etiological agents responsible.
   d. What are the various investigations to be done?

e. How will you manage this case?
f. Mention the various complications of meningococcal septicemia.

9. A 23-year-old tribal female from Wayanad presented in the casualty with complaints of involuntary movements that started in the morning. O/E: A dirt filled wound prick was there on the sole of the left foot. While recording the BP, the patient threw violent spasmodic movement of whole of the body. Oral temperature could not be recorded since patient was unable to open the mouth properly, axillary temperature was 36.2°C.
   a. What is the most probable diagnosis?
   b. What are the types of the disease?
   c. Name the required investigations, if any.
   d. What treatment will you give?
   e. What advice will you give to the patient on discharge?
   f. Describe the characteristic facial appearance.
10. A 20-year-old female presented with high grade fever and diffuse macular red rash. Her last menstruation which occurred 2 days ago was associated with purulent discharge. Vomiting, myalgia and hypotension were present. There were no other localizing signs.
   a. What diagnosis will you first consider?
   b. What is the characteristic tongue appearance? Name the other diseases that can cause the same.
   c. What are the differential diagnosis?
   d. What skin finding do you expect during convalescence?
   e. What advice will you give to prevent recurrence?
   f. How will you treat the patient?
11. A 13-year-old girl presented with fever since 1 week duration associated with bifrontal headache, malaise, constipation and bodyache. O/E: spleen tip was palpable.
   a. What is the likely diagnosis?
   b. Describe the course of the disease, if untreated.
   c. What are the investigations to be done for diagnosis?
   d. How will you treat the patient?
   e. What are the preventive measures?
   f. What are the neuropsychiatry symptoms that can occur?
   g. What are the expected complications?
12. A 20-year-old manual laborer came with complaints of low grade fever, weight loss, sweating, loss of appetite since 1 month; cough with blood stained sputum; multiple swellings in the neck; headache, altered behavior, weakness of lower limbs (or other focal deficits), cranial nerve palsies; knee pain more at night. O/E: severe wasting of muscles around the knee.
   a. Comment on the diagnosis of TB.
   b. Write briefly on the treatment- drugs and durations.
   c. How will you interpret Mantoux test?
   d. Specific side effects of drug therapy.
   e. Comment on the prevention of TB.
   f. How will you categorize TB?
   g. CSF picture of TB meningitis.
   h. Clinical features of cavitary lesions.
   i. Microscopic appearance of granuloma.
   j. X-ray appearance of pulmonary TB.
   k. Ziehl-Neelsen technique.
   l. Atypical *Mycobacterium*.
13. A 30-year-old farmer presents with high grade fever, myalgia and headache, conjunctival suffusion, diminished urine output. O/E: icterus+; liver palpable.
   a. What is your diagnosis?
   b. How will you confirm your diagnosis?
   c. What are the types of the disease?
   d. How will you treat the patient?
   e. What prophylaxis will you advice?
14. A 20-year-old lady from Karnataka was brought to the casualty in an unconscious state. There was no proper history available except that her neighbor had similar illness and died last year. O/E: she was febrile; spleen tip was palpable. There were no localizing signs, no signs of meningeal irritation.
   a. What diagnosis will you consider first?
   b. How will you confirm your diagnosis?
   c. How will you treat the lady?
   d. What are the types of the disease?

e. What complications can occur?
f. Draw the characteristic hematological picture.

15. A 40-year-old man presented with c/o weakness of both upper limbs. O/E: there were painless burns over the right hand. Fasciculations were present in the small muscles of the hand. B/L claw hand +; there was a large hypopigmented patch over the trunk which showed diminished sensation.
    a. What may be the cause?
    b. What clinical finding will you specifically look for?
    c. How will you confirm your diagnosis?
    d. What are the types of the disease?
    e. Describe the characteristic facial appearance.
    f. How will you take care of the limbs?
16. A 16-year-old female presented with low grade fever of 2 weeks duration and joint pain involving most of the peripheral joints. There was tenderness and swelling of the knee joints. The patient's hair was rough with loss of texture and patchy hair loss.
    a. What is the probable diagnosis?
    b. What specific history will you like to elicit?
    c. What investigation will you like to undertake?
    d. Name 2 drugs that can cause this disease.
    e. Briefly outline the treatment of the disease.
    f. Name 4 systemic complications.
    g. Draw the characteristic peripheral smear finding.
17. A 45-year-old lady presents with pain of the small joints of the hand of 6 months duration. There is a history of joint stiffness when the patient wakes up from sleep. Recently patient developed knee joint swelling O/E: popliteal cyst+
    a. What is the most probable diagnosis?
    b. What all will you consider in the differential diagnosis?
    c. How will you clinically distinguish the above?
    d. What investigations will you do?
    e. What all deformities do you expect in the hand?
    f. Outline the treatment.
18. A 40-year-old man presented with hoarseness of voice which occurred insidiously. He also gave a history of frequently bumping into objects situated on either side. He also notices progressive tightening of his shoes. His lower jaw was slightly protuberant.
    a. What is the diagnosis?
    b. What findings do you expect in the face?
    c. What metabolic abnormality do you expect?
    d. What visual abnormality is likely to be present?
    e. What abnormalities may be seen in the teeth of the patient?
    f. Mention the investigations to be done?
    g. Outline the treatment.
19. A 50-year-old lady under treatment for severe asthma for a long time presented with back pain which was severe. Her face was puffy and she had protuberant abdomen. BP was 160/90 mm Hg.
    a. What is the likely diagnosis?
    b. What may be the cause of back pain?
    c. What metabolic abnormality do you expect?
    d. What are the types of the disease?
    e. What investigations will you like to perform ?
    f. How will you manage the patient?
20. A 30-year-old man was brought to the casualty in a drowsy state. O/E: both pupils were small. Respiration was depressed. His breath and gastric lavage were odorless.
    a. What is the likely diagnosis?
    b. What other possibilities will you consider?
    c. How will you confirm the diagnosis?
    d. How will you manage the patient?
21. A 25-year-old man was brought to the casualty with vomiting, sweating and froth coming from the mouth. O/E: there was wheezing. Pupils are pin point, muscle fasciculation +
    a. What is the diagnosis?
    b. How can you confirm the diagnosis?
    c. How will you manage the case?
    d. What is the major cause of death?
    e. How will you monitor the case?
22. An 18-year-old boy was brought to the casualty with history of snake bite. Examination revealed 2 fang marks.
    a. What all things will you observe during clinical examination?
    b. How can you identify the species of snake?
    c. What bedside investigations will you perform?

d. What other investigations can be done?
e. How will you monitor?
f. Comment on management.
g. What are the causes of death?

23. A 24-year-old diabetic male on insulin presented with history of loose watery stools since 3 days and progressive drowsiness since 2 days. He had omitted his insulin doses due to diarrhea. O/E patient drowsy, tachypneic, dehydrated. BP 80/60 mm Hg. PR 104 feeble.
    a. What are the problems you consider in this patient?
    b. What investigations will you do?
    c. How will you treat the patient?
    d. What are the probable causes of death in this patient?

Short Notes

I. Genetics

1. Oncogenes
2. Tumor suppressor genes
3. Leukocyte adhesion deficiency
4. Innate and adaptive immunity
5. Hypersensitivity reactions
6. Primary immunodeficiency
7. Define-mutation
   a. Polymorphism
   b. Epigenetics and imprinting
8. Karyotyping
9. Southern blotting
10. PCR
11. Positional cloning
12. Gene therapy

II. Infectious Diseases

1. Define PUO
2. Causes of PUO
3. Traveller's diarrhea
4. Chemoprophylaxis
5. Causes of high grade fevers
6. Clinical features, diagnosis of yellow fever
7. Clinical features, of dengue HF
8. Complications of measles
9. Herpes labialis (or cold sore)
10. Complications of HSV infections
11. Complications of chicken pox
12. Management of HSV
13. Viral warts
14. Types and etiological agents of rickettsial infections
15. Clinical features of parvoviral infections
16. Clinical features of IMN
17. Erysipelas
18. TSS
19. Clinical features of anthrax
20. Causes of food poisoning
21. cd4 count in HIV
22. Diagnosis of HIV
23. HAART
24. Clinical features of HIV disease
25. ARC (AIDS related complex)
26. TB and AIDS
27. CMV in AIDS
28. Neoplasms in AIDS
29. Skin diseases in HIV
30. Oral diseases in HIV
31. *Pneumocystis carinii pneumonia*
32. GI disease in AIDS
33. AIDS neurological manifestations
34. Widal test
35. Rx of *Shigella* dysentery
36. Clinical features of brucellosis
37. Clinical features of plague
38. Rx of cholera
39. Upgrading and downgrading (reversal) reactions
40. Lepra reaction
41. Lucio's phenomenon
42. Borderline leprosy
43. Diagnosis of leprosy
44. Lepromin test
45. Dharmendra antigen
46. What is leonine facies?
47. Complications of leprosy
48. Erythema nodosum leprosum
49. Rx of leprosy
50. What is fite-faraco staining?
51. Clinical features and complications of Weil's disease
52. Relapsing fever
53. What is ring worm?
54. What is kerion reaction?
55. What are Id eruptions (auto eczematization)?
56. What is favus?
57. Mycetoma
58. Clinical features of histoplasmosis

59. Complications of malaria
60. What is tropical splenomegaly?
61. Rx of malaria
62. Rx of cerebral malaria
63. Malaria prophylaxis
64. What is amoeboma?
65. Complications of amoebiasis
66. Rx of amoebiasis
67. Diagnosis of giardiasis
68. What is entero-test?
69. Leishmanin test
70. Rx of kala-azar
71. What is xenodiagnosis?
72. What is mega disease ?
73. Clinical features of toxoplasmosis
74. What is Katayama syndrome?
75. Bladder schistosomiasis
76. Diagnosis and Rx of schistosomiasis
77. What is endemic hemoptysis?
78. Cysticercosis
79. Rx of teniosis
80. What is ground itch?
81. Clinical features of strongyloidiasis
82. What is larva currens?
83. Tropical pulmonary eosinophilia
84. Complications of lymphatic filariasis
85. Rx of lymphatic filariasis
86. What is calabar swelling?
87. What is river blindness ?
88. Management of onchocerciasis
89. What is larva migrans?
90. Clinical features of guinea worm infection
91. Loeffler's syndrome
92. Rx of scabies
93. Rx of lice infestation
94. What is myiasis?
95. What are gummata ?
96. What are snail track ulcers?
97. What are condyloma lata?
98. Congenital syphilis
99. NGU (non-gonococcal urethritis)

III. CVS

1. AF (atrial fibrillation)
2. Wolff-Parkinson-White syndrome
3. VT
4. Pulsus bigeminus
5. Fusion (or capture) beat
6. Digoxin
7. AV Block
8. Wenckebach's phenomenon
9. Complete heart block
10. BBB (bundle branch block)
11. Risk factors of CAD
12. Clinical features of angina
13. Management of angina
14. Enzymes in MI
15. Unstable angina
16. Thrombolysis/streptokinase
17. Complications of MI
18. What is cannon wave?
19. What is pulsus paradoxus?
20. What is pulsus bisferiens?
21. Kussmaul's sign
22. Myocardial stunning?
23. Common causes of chest pain
24. Causes of acute valve failure
25. Rx of acute pulmonary edema
26. Starling's law
27. Causes of heart failure
28. What is cardiac cachexia?
29. Complications of heart failure
30. Management of heart failure
31. Causes of hypertension
32. Investigations in hypertension
33. Refractory hypertension
34. Malignant hypertension
35. Causes of syncope
36. Sinus brady/tachy cardia
37. Sudden death
38. Aortic dissection-clinical features
39. Aortic dissection-management
40. Acute rheumatic fever-Rx
41. Jones's criteria
42. Management of mitral stenosis
43. X-ray in MS
44. Causes of MR
45. MVP (mitral valve prolapse)
46. Causes of ankylosing spondylitis
47. Causes of AR
48. What is Hill's sign?
49. Austin flint murmur
50. Carey Coombs murmur
51. Graham Steel's murmur
52. Peripheral signs of AR
53. Clinical features of tricuspid valve disease
54. Infective endocarditis-clinical features
55. Etiology
56. Investigations
57. Prophylaxis
58. Libman-Sacks endocarditis?
59. HOCM
60. Myxoma
61. Causes of pericarditis
62. TB pericarditis
63. Clinical features of chronic constrictive pericarditis
64. Classify aortic dissection

IV. Respiratory System

1. V/Q Scan
2. Lung defences
3. Tracheal tug?
4. Causes of respiratory failure
5. Management of failure
6. Causes of hemoptysis
7. Causes of acute severe dyspnea
8. COPD–investigations
9. COPD–complications
10. Rx of a/c exacerbation of COPD
11. Rx of bronchial asthma
12. Rx of acute severe asthma
13. Clinical features of bronchial asthma
14. Status asthmaticus
15. Causes of bronchiectasis
16. Clinical features and complications of bronchiectasis
17. Management-bronchiectasis
18. What is bronchiectasis sicca?
19. Rx of community acquired pneumonia
20. Complications of pneumonia
21. Lung abscess
22. Hospital acquired pneumonia
23. Sequelae of primary tuberculosis
24. Miliary TB
25. Cryptic TB
26. What is program pulmonary TB?
27. What is postprimary pulmonary TB
28. BCG vaccination pulmonary TB
29. Tuberculin tests
30. Side effects of ATT
31. ATT
32. Chemoprophylaxis of TB
33. Aspergillosis
34. Clinical features of bronchial carcinoma
35. Radiological features
36. Bronchial adenoma
37. Bronchial carcinoid
38. Bronchoalveolar cell carcinoma
39. Clinical features of sarcoidosis
40. ILD-investigations
41. Organic lung diseases
42. What is byssinosis?
43. What is honey comb lung?
44. Coal worker's pneumoconiosis
45. Asbestosis
46. Caplan's syndrome
47. Rheumatoid lung
48. What is hidebound chest?
49. Clinical features of pulmonary thromboembolism
50. Management of thromboembolism
51. Causes of pleural effusion
52. Investigations-pleural effusion
53. Spontaneous pneumothorax
54. Tension pneumothorax

V. Renal System

1. Define ARF
2. Management of ARF
3. Causes of chronic renal failure
4. Define CRF
5. Clinical features of CRF
6. Bone changes in CRF
7. Renal artery stenosis
8. Alport's syndrome
9. Ig A nephropathy
10. Causes of ATN
11. Causes of AIN
12. Polycystic kidney disease (PKD)
13. RTA (renal tubular acidosis)
14. Kidney in SLE
15. Diabetic nephropathy
16. Asymptomatic bacteriuria
17. What is urethral syndrome?
18. Complications of nephritic syndrome

VI. Diabetes and Nutrition

1. Clinical features of DM
2. Dietary modifications in DM
3. Side effects of insulin therapy
4. HbA_{1c}
5. Clinical features of hypoglycemia
6. Management of hypoglycemia
7. Diagnosis of DM
8. What is Somogyi effect?
9. What is dawn phenomenon?
10. What is potential diabetes?
11. What is latent diabetes?
12. Plate model of diabetes
13. Clinical features of DKA
14. Management-DKA
15. Acute complications of diabetes
16. Chronic complications of diabetes
17. Metabolic X syndrome
18. Grading of diabetic retinopathy
19. Diabetic amyotrophy
20. What is neuropathic cachexia?
21. Clinical features of diabetic neuropathy
22. Rx of diabetic neuropathy
23. What is glycemic index?
24. Wernicke-Korsakoff syndrome
25. BMI (body mass index)
26. Etiology of obesity
27. Complications of obesity
28. Drug therapy in Rx of obesity
29. What is apronectomy?

VII. Endocrinology

1. MEN 1 and 2
2. Clinical features of hypothyroidism
3. Classification of hypothyroidism
4. Clinical features of hyperthyroidism
5. Management of hyperthyroidism
6. Clinical features of Graves' disease
7. What is pretibial myxedema?
8. deQuervain's thyroiditis
9. Thyrocardiac
10. Hyperthyroid crisis
11. Management of hypothyroidism
12. Pendred syndrome
13. Myxedema coma
14. Riedel's thyroiditis
15. Gynecomastia
16. Hirsutism
17. Hypercalcemia
18. Management of malignant hypercalcemia
19. Tetany
20. Latent tetany
21. Hyperparathyroidism
22. Radiological changes
23. Side effects of steroid therapy
24. Classify Cushing's disease?
25. What is Cushing's syndrome
26. Clinical features of Cushing's syndrome
27. Investigations in Cushing syndrome
28. Waterhouse-Friderichsen syndrome
29. Causes of adrenal insufficiency
30. Causes of hyperaldosteronism
31. Pheochromocytoma
32. What is Conn's syndrome?
33. Replacement therapy in hypoadrenalism
34. Hyperprolactinemia
35. Spontaneous hypocalcemia
36. Causes of hypocalcemia
37. Clinical features of hypopituitarism
38. What is pituitary apoplexy?
39. Visual defects in pituitary disease
40. Synacthen test
41. Diabetes insipidus

VIII. Gastrointestinal tract

1. Causes of dyspepsia
2. Causes of GI bleeding
3. Causes—villous atrophy
4. Causes- protein losing enteropathy
5. Causes—small intestinal bacterial overgrowth
6. Malabsorption
7. Autoimmune gastritis
8. Ménétrier's disease
9. Vincent's angina
10. Plummer-Vinson syndrome
11. GI lymphoma
12. Celiac disease
13. Tropical sprue
14. Whipple's disease
15. Complications of intestinal irradiation
16. Complications-pancreatitis
17. Complications-inflammatory bowel disease
18. Pathological features IBD
19. Clinical features of IBD (Inflammatory bowel disease)
20. Drug therapy in IBD
21. Peutz-Jeghers syndrome
22. What is Gardner's syndrome?
23. Turcot's syndrome
24. Pseudomembranous colitis
25. Risk factors for colorectal Ca
26. Ogilvie's syndrome

IX. Hepatobiliary Disease

1. Liver biopsy
2. Gilbert's syndrome
3. Causes of portal hypertension
4. Causes of portal ascites
5. Precipitants of hepatic encephalopathy
6. Causes of steatosis
7. Causes of cirrhosis
8. Causes of biliary cirrhosis
9. Clinical features and complications of portal hypertension
10. Management of variceal bleeding
11. Investigations of ascites
12. Spontaneous bacterial peritonitis
13. Clinical features of hepatic encephalopathy
14. Management of encephalopathy
15. What is fulminant hepatic failure?
16. Causes of fulminant hepatic failure
17. Complications of fulminant hepatic failure?
18. What are councilman bodies?
19. What are Mallory bodies?
20. What is bridging necrosis?
21. What is piecemeal necrosis?
22. What is interface hepatitis?
23. Clinical features of cirrhosis
24. Complications of viral hepatitis
25. Management of viral hepatitis
26. Complications of autoimmune hepatitis
27. Alcoholic liver disease
28. Hemochromatosis
29. Wilson's disease
30. Budd-Chiari syndrome
31. Hepatic cysts
32. Post-cholecystectomy syndrome

X. Hematology

1. Howell-Jolly bodies
2. Basophilic stippling
3. Target cells
4. Causes of polycythemia
5. Causes of lymphadenopathy
6. Causes of splenomegaly
7. Causes of thrombocytopenia
8. Adverse effects of transfusion
9. Causes of Fe deficiency anemia
10. Oral iron therapy
11. Indications of parenteral Fe
12. Diagnosis of megaloblastic anemia
13. Causes of megaloblastic anemia
14. Pernicious anemia
15. Subacute combined degeneration (SACD)
16. Anemia of chronic disease
17. Features of intravascular hemolysis
18. Schilling test
19. G6PD deficiency
20. Heinz bodies
21. Crises in hemolytic anemia
22. What is march hemoglobinuria?
23. Supportive therapy in leukemia
24. Philadelphia chromosome
25. Clinical features of chronic myeloid leukemia (CML)
26. Blood picture in chronic myelogenous leukemia (CML)
27. Management of c/c leukemia
28. Hairy cell leukemia
29. Myelodysplastic syndrome
30. Reed Sternberg cell
31. Staging of Hodgkin's lymphoma/Ann Arbor Staging
32. Management of Hodgkin's lymphoma/Ann Arbor Staging
33. Hypersplenism
34. Bence Jones proteins
35. Waldenstrom's macroglobulinemia
36. Clinical features of multiple myeloma
37. Diagnosis of multiple myeloma
38. Causes of DIC
39. Myelofibrosis
40. Polycythemia rubra vera
41. Anticoagulant therapy

XI. Connective Tissue Disorders

1. Acute phase response
2. Rheumatoid factor
3. Anti-nuclear antibody (ANA)
4. Antiphospholipid antibody syndrome
5. Diagnosis of rheumatoid arthritis
6. Hand in rheumatoid arthritis
7. Rheumatoid nodules
8. Extra-articular features
9. Felty's syndrome
10. DMARD therapy
11. Clinical features of ankylosing spondylitis
12. Radiological features of AS (ankylosing spondylitis)
13. Reactive arthritis
14. Psoriatic arthropathy
15. Podagra
16. Gouty tophus
17. Clinical features of gout
18. Management of gout
19. Osteoporosis
20. Biochemical features of osteoporosis, osteomalacia and hyperparathyroidism
21. Diagnosis of osteomalacia
22. Diagnosis of SLE
23. Jaccoud's arthropathy
24. Discoid lupus erythematosis
25. CREST syndrome
26. Polymyositis
27. Giant cell arteritis
28. Polyarteritis nodosa
29. Takayasu's arteritis
30. Wegener's granulomatosis
31. Charcot's joint

XII. Skin

1. Petechia, purpura, ecchymosis,
2. Hematoma, telengectasia
3. Pruritus
4. Scabies
5. Urticaria vs angioedema
6. Pemphigus {Nikolski's sign}
7. Alopecia
8. Eczema
9. Psoriasis-histology
10. Nail changes in psoriasis
11. Types of psoriasis
12. Rx of psoriasis
13. Lichen planus
14. Acne
15. Koebner phenomenon
16. Clubbing
17. Erythema nodosum

XIII. Drugs

1. Penicillin
2. Cephalosporin
3. Vancomycin/MRSA
4. Erythromycin

5. Ciprofloxacin
6. Anti-tubercular treatment (ATT)
7. Dapsone
8. Clofazimine
9. Aminoglycoside
10. Metronidazole
11. Acyclovir
12. Albendazole
13. Jarisch-Herxheimer reaction
14. Steroids
15. Insulin
16. Oral hypoglycemic agents (OHA)
17. Statins
18. Calcium gluconate
19. Paracetamol
20. Nonsteroidal anti-inflammatory drugs (NSAIDs)
21. Phenobarbitone
22. Phenytoin
23. Carbamazepine
24. Valproate
25. Aminophylline
26. Adrenaline
27. Frusemide
28. Loop diuretics
29. Nifedipine
30. Digoxin
31. Lignocaine
32. ACE inhibitors
33. Octreotide
34. Lactulose
35. Methotrexate
36. Heparin
37. Aspirin
38. Streptokinase
39. Atropine
40. Dopamine
41. Antiparkinsonian drugs
42. Lithium
43. Haloperidol
44. Potassium chloride (KCl)
45. Diethylcarbamazine (DEC)
46. Quinine
47. Primaquine
48. Atenolol
49. Ivermectin
50. D penicillamine
51. Desferrioxamine

XIV. Nervous System

1. Lumbar puncture (LP)
2. Coning
3. Common causes of headache
4. Cluster headache
5. Rx of migraine
6. Trigeminal neuralgia
7. Central pain syndrome (CPS)
8. Absent seizures
9. What is Jacksonian epilepsy?
10. Todd's palsy
11. Causes of seizures
12. Management of seizures
13. Rx of status epilepticus
14. Narcolepsy
15. Clasp knife phenomenon
16. Cog wheel rigidity
17. Tremor
18. Define chorea, athetosis, ballismus, myoclonus
19. Causes of chorea
20. Causes of asterixis
21. Brown-Sequard syndrome
22. What is causalgia?
23. Causes of coma
24. Glasgow coma scale
25. What is Gegenhalten?
26. Apraxia
27. Aphasia—Wernicke's, Broca's, global, nominal
28. What is pseudodementia?
29. Causes of delirium, dementia
30. Bulbar and pseudobulbar palsy
31. Internuclear ophthalmoplegia
32. One and a half syndrome
33. Horner's syndrome
34. Papilledema
35. Define stroke
36. TIA (transient ischemic attack)
37. Risk factors for stroke
38. Lacunar infarcts
39. Embolic stroke
40. Causes of young stroke
41. Subarachnoid hemorrhage
42. Management of stroke
43. Cerebral venous thrombosis
44. Complications of stroke
45. Clinical features of multiple sclerosis
46. Parkinson's disease
47. Motor neuron disease
48. Causes of peripheral neuropathy
49. Guillain-Barré syndrome (GBS)
50. Froin's syndrome
51. Bell's palsy
52. Duchenne muscular dystrophy
53. Lambert-Eaton syndrome
54. Syringomyelia
55. TB meningitis
56. Rx of pyogenic meningitis
57. HSV encephalitis

58. Subacute sclerosing panencephalitis (SSPE)
59. Herpes zoster
60. Risus sardonicus
61. Neurosyphilis
62. Prion disease
63. Neurofibromatosis
64. Visual pathway and lesions
65. CSF circulation
66. Bladder—innervation and lesions
67. Berry aneurysm—sites

XV. Psychiatry

1. Define delusion, hallucinations
2. Psychotherapy
3. ECT (electroconvulsive therapy)
4. Disulfiram
5. Clinical features of alcohol abuse
6. Irritable bowel syndrome
7. Phobic disorder
8. Somatoform disorder
9. Anorexia nervosa
10. Munchausen syndrome
11. Post-traumatic stress disorder
12. Manic depressive psychosis
13. Catatonic schizophrenia
14. Paranoid schizophrenia

XVI. Poisoning

1. Gut decontamination
2. Charcoal
3. Universal antidote
4. Gut dialysis
5. Organophosphorus poisoning
6. Rx of snake bite
7. Management of paracetamol poisoning
8. N-acetyl cysteine
9. Salicylate poisoning
10. Barbiturate, benzodiazepine poisoning

XVII. Critical Care

1. Systemic inflammatory response syndrome (SIRS)
2. Acute respiratory distress syndrome (ARDS)
3. Define sepsis
4. Management of septic shock
5. Indication of mechanical ventilation

SURGERY

Theory Topics :

Paper I	:	GIT and Orthopedics	40 Marks
Paper II	:	Whole of General Surgery Except GIT, Anesthesia, Dental and Radiotherapy	40 Marks

Practical Examinations :

Clinical I	:	Surgery Long Case (Including Case Sheet)	50 Marks
Clinical II	:	Surgery Short Case	20 Marks
Clinical III	:	Ortho Short Case	20 Marks
Clinical IV	:	OSCE/Spotter	10 Marks

Oral Examinations : X-rays and Instruments, Specimens, Operative Surgery, General Surgery. 20 Marks

Clinical Questions

1. A 40-year-old man presents with loss of weight, irregular fever, and altered bowel symptoms. He also complains of abdominal pain, colicky in nature. The only relevant clinical finding in abdomen is a mass in right lower abdomen during colic and disappearing with relief of pain.
   a. What are the probabilities you will keep in mind?
   b. What are the investigations you will call for, for confirming your diagnosis?
   c. What complications do you expect with this condition?
   d. How do you treat the different conditions you consider?
2. 15-years-following a truncal vagotomy and drainage procedure, a patient presents with fever, right sided abdominal pain not relieved by posture or food. It disappeared the next morning as dramatically as it had appeared.
   a. What is the most probable diagnosis?
   b. What is the reason for relief of symptoms?
   c. What is the reason for the development of this condition?
   d. What are the methods of treating such conditions?
3. Following a minor trauma to the foot with a thorn, a 45-year-old man presents with fever, rigor, swelling and pain of the lower limb with redness and shiny skin.
   a. What is the most probable diagnosis?
   b. What are the predisposing factors for this condition?
   c. What are the most common causative agents?
   d. What is the ideal treatment of the condition?
4. A patient with bleeding primary hemorrhoids and a Hb percent of 4 is admitted under your care. As a measure to stop bleeding, you decide to give sclerotherapy along with replacement of Hb deficit.
   a. What are the necessary instruments you require to do it?
   b. What are the common sclerosants used?
   c. What is Albright's solution?
   d. Where will you inject the sclerosants?
   e. What are the possible complications of the procedure?
5. Following an attempted IV infusion, in the cubital region, patient complains of severe pain in the hand and soon had severe pallor and numbness of the hands.
   a. What is the most likely possibility?
   b. What are the urgent measures you do under these circumstances?
   c. What investigations will be helpful in confirming your diagnosis?
   d. If conservative measures fail, what is the ideal treatment?
6. A psychiatric patient on Rx with lithium salts (not properly monitored) presents with anemia and numbness of hand. On examination, sensory deficit noted in thumb and index finger with wasting of thenar region.
   a. What is your diagnosis?
   b. What is the underlying problem for this condition?
   c. What is the single investigation that clinches the diagnosis?
   d. How will you treat the patient medically?
   e. If the hand problem persists, what is the ideal Rx?

7. Person with intractable peptic ulceration. On examination is found to have a swelling in the neck which moves with deglutition. 1 × 1 cm in size. He also gets profound diarrhea at times and he has persistent hypercalcemia also.
   a. What is the person most likely suffering from?
   b. Can you correlate the neck swelling and the disease process?
   c. What investigations can clinch the diagnosis?
   d. How will you treat the person?
8. Following an attempted catheterization of urethra of a male patient, he presents with severe bleeding, perineal swelling and is unable to pass urine.
   a. What is your diagnosis?
   b. What are the immediate measures you will undertake?
   c. What are the possible complications of this problem?
   d. If these complications develop, how is it diagnosed?
9. A 43-year-old female with cyclical mastalgia presents with a painful breast swelling of 3 days duration. She is afebrile. The swelling is smooth, firm, has restricted mobility. No lymph nodes palpable.
   a. What is the most likely diagnosis?
   b. What are the investigations required to confirm the diagnosis?
   c. What is the treatment you will suggest?
   d. What concerns you when you do this procedure?
   e. What will you advice if your concern is confirmed?
10. A patient with obstructive jaundice is operated upon for removing bile stones.
   a. What are the instruments used to retrieve stones from the bile duct?
   b. How do you make sure peroperatively that there are no more stones in the bile duct?
   c. What are the sequelae of obstructive jaundice due to stones in the bile duct?
   d. What will you do if you find there is a long benign stricture in the distal bile duct following removal of CBD stones?
   e. What is white bile?
11. Three days following total thyroidectomy, a patient develops stridor, glottic edema, tracheal collapse, tension, hematoma, and laryngeal nerve palsies are excluded.
   a. What is the cause for stridor and what do you call this condition?
   b. What are the other findings you look for?
   c. How do you confirm the diagnosis?
   d. How do you treat this emergency condition?
   e. What can be done during surgery to prevent this condition?
12. The anesthetist is preparing to give spinal subarachnoid block.
   a. What are the anesthetic agents used?
   b. Which interspinous space is used?
   c. What are the complications of the procedure?
   d. How do you prevent these complications?
   e. How will you manage the situation of total spinal block?
13. Following hemorrhoidectomy surgery, a 65-year-old male is in extreme agony to pass urine. He is unable to do so:
   a. What are the most likely reasons for this?
   b. What conservative measures will you adopt initially?
   c. If these fail, what will you then do?
   d. What are the complications of this procedure?
   e. What precautions are to be taken to avoid these complications?
14. One week following a hip replacement surgery, a 70-year-old lady develops painful swelling of the entire lower limb associated with low grade fever.
   a. What is the most likely diagnosis?
   b. How will you establish your diagnosis?
   c. What precautions will you take to avoid this condition?
   d. How do you treat this condition?
   e. What are the sequelae of this condition?
15. A 10-year-old presents with history of recurrent mild jaundice and fever. O/E. She has a smooth surfaced rounded swelling 10 × 15 cm size below a uniformly enlarged non-tender liver.
   a. What is the clinical diagnosis?
   b. How do you establish your diagnosis?
   c. How do you classify this condition?
   d. What is the ideal treatment of this condition?
   e. Left alone, what is the most dangerous complication that can develop?
16. A 15-year-old boy underwent emergency appendicectomy for perforated appendicitis with localized peritonitis.
   a. What physical finding confirms localized peritonitis?
   b. What is the most common complication of this surgery?
   c. What will you consider if the boy develops high grade swinging fever, diarrhea and lower abdominal pain?
   d. How do you confirm this condition?
   e. What procedures can be undertaken to treat this condition?

17. 10 days following a blunt injury to abdomen, a person develops a tender smooth surfaced swelling in the epigastrium, not moving with respiration. All borders well defined and do not present expansile pulsations.
    a. What is your diagnosis, why did he develop this swelling?
    b. What 2 tests will you undertake to confirm this diagnosis?
    c. What local complications can occur in this condition?
    d. How do you treat this condition?
18. A young male is brought to the casualty department suspecting blunt injury abdomen. The medical officer requests for DPL (diagnostic peritoneal lavage)
    a. What do you understand by DPL?
    b. What all materials do you need for DPL?
    c. How will you do DPL?
    d. What are the contraindications for DPL?
    e. When do you consider DPL is significant?
19. A middle aged lady presents with history of recurrent lower respiratory infections. She says that she has mild discomfort for swallowing semisolids and liquids.
    a. What is the most likely diagnosis?
    b. Why does she develop respiratory infections?
    c. How will you confirm your diagnosis?
    d. What complications can occur in this condition?
    e. How do you treat this condition?
20. Following head injury subsequent to a fall, you notice ecchymosis over the mastoid region.
    a. What is the reason for this? What do you call this sign?
    b. What are the features in and around the eye in fracture of the anterior cranial fossa?
    c. What is the danger of fracture of the base of the skull?
    d. How do you treat a Pond's depressed fracture in a child? Explain the reasons for your treatment policy.

Short Notes

I. General surgery

1. MRI contraindications
2. Endoluminal ultrasound
3. Drainage of abscess (Hilton's method)
4. Types of biopsy
5. Therapeutic embolization
6. Primary and secondary wound healing
7. Hypertrophic scars vs keloid
8. Blood fractions and substitutes
9. SIRS
10. MODS
11. Gastrostomy feeding
12. Complications of total parenteral feeding
13. Intravenous regional anesthesia (Biers block)
14. Epidural block
15. Cryosurgery
16. A/c vs c/c graft rejection
17. Triage
18. Focussed abdominal sonogram for trauma (FAST)
19. Missile injury
20. Blast lung
21. 1° vs 2° vs 3° hemorrhage
22. Superficial vs deep burns
23. Burns-fluid replacement
24. Wallace—Rule of 9
25. Electric burns
26. Le Forte classification
27. Glasgow coma scale
28. Revised trauma score
29. Lucid interval
30. Coupe and counter coupe injury
31. Subdural hematoma
32. Extradural hematoma
33. Anterior cranial fossa fracture
34. Day surgery unit
35. Diathermy types
36. Ideal theater

II. Tumors, cysts, sinus, ulcers and skin

1. Papilloma
2. Adenoma
3. Lipoma
4. Neuroma
5. Glomus tumor
6. Squamous cell carcinoma
7. Rodent ulcer
8. Soft tissue sarcoma
9. Premalignant lesion of skin
10. Hemangioma
11. Malignant melanoma
12. Clarks grading and Breslows staging
13. Majolins ulcer
14. Wen

15. Hidradenitis suppurativa
16. Tetanus
17. Gas gangrene
18. Cyst classification
19. Persistance of sinus and fistula
20. Types of skin graft
21. Carbuncle
22. Necrotizing fascitis

III. Arterial disorders

1. Intermittent claudication
2. Rest pain
3. Pre-gangrene (Critical limb ischemia)
4. Dry vs wet gangrene
5. Digital subtraction angiography (DSA)
6. Browns vasomotor index
7. Abdominal angina
8. Dissecting aneurysm
9. Thoracic outlet syndrome
10. Diabetic foot (Wagner's classification)
11. Harveys sign
12. Branham's sign
13. Fat embolism
14. Raynaud's phenomenon
15. Thromboangiitis obliterans (TAO)
16. Types of amputation
17. Aortic aneurysm
18. AV fistulae
19. Leriche syndrome
20. Cirsoid aneurysm
21. Pre Ca lesion in SCC
22. Types of aneurysm

IV. Venous disorders

1. Venous drainage of lower limb
2. Complication of varicose veins
3. White cell trapping hypothesis
4. Bisgaard's regimen
5. Acute swollen limb—causes
6. Saphena varix
7. Hook phlebotomy
8. Pulmonary embolism
9. Prevention and treatment of DVT
10. Trendelenburg operation
11. Virchow's triad
12. Plethysmography

V. Lymphatic system

1. Primary lymphedema and Rx
2. Lymphoma
3. Cystic hygroma
4. Chylothorax
5. Milroys disease
6. TB lymphadenitis

VI. Oral cavity and salivary glands

1. Cleft lip and cleft palate
2. Carcinoma (Ca)
3. Premalignant lesions of oral cavity
4. Leukoplakia
5. Erythroplakia
6. Waldeyer's ring
7. Pharyngeal pouch
8. Laryngocele
9. Epulis
10. Odontomas
11. Submucous fibrosis
12. Ranula
13. Sailolithiasis
14. Sailosis
15. Salivary gland tumor classification
16. Pleomorphic adenoma
17. Warthin's tumor
18. Adenoid cystic carcinoma
19. Sjögrens syndrome
20. Mikulicz syndrome
21. Xerostomia

VII. Neck swellings

1. Branchial cyst and fistula
2. Thyroglossal cyst and fistula
3. Cervical rib
4. Adsons test
5. Ludwig's angina
6. Levels of lymph nodes in neck
7. Chemodectoma
8. Types of neck dissection
9. Bezold's abscess
10. Midline swellings of the neck
11. Cold abscess
12. Collar stud abscess

VIII. Thyroid and parathyroids

1. Anatomy and development
2. Lateral aberrant thyroid
3. Myxedema
4. Natural history of goiter
5. Primary and secondary thyrotoxicosis
6. Retrosternal goiter
7. Graves disease
8. Preoperative preparation of a toxic thyroid
9. Complications of thyroidectomy
10. Papillary carcinoma thyroid
11. Medullary Ca thyroid
12. Hashimoto's thyroiditis
13. deQuervain's thyroiditis
14. Hypoparathyroidism

15. MEN 1 and 2
16. Thyroid crisis
17. Thyroid acropachy

IX. Thorax and heart

1. Intercostal drainage
2. Flail chest
3. Stove in chest
4. Tietze's disease
5. Empyema necessitans
6. Tension pneumothorax
7. Pancoasts tumor
8. Cardiac tamponade
9. Sites of herniation in the diaphragm

X. Breast

1. Lymphatic drainage
2. Mammography
3. Triple assessment
4. Retracted nipple
5. Paget's disease vs eczema of nipple
6. Types and causes of nipple discharge
7. Benign breast disease (BBD) classification
8. Breast abscess
9. Mondor's disease
10. Duct ectasia
11. Duct papilloma
12. Aberrations of normal development and involution (ANDI)
13. Fibroadenoma
14. Fibroadenosis
15. Phyllodes tumor
16. Types of mastectomy
17. Quadrantectomy + axillary dissection + radiotherapy (QUART)
18. Sentinel node biopsy
19. Complications of mastectomy
20. Ca breast staging
21. Axillary sampling vs dissection vs clearance
22. Gynecomastia
23. Male Ca breast

XI. Esophagus

1. Tracheoesophageal fistula
2. Dysphagia lusoria
3. Barotrauma (Boerhave's syndrome)
4. Hamman's sign
5. Mallory-Weiss syndrome
6. Gastroesophageal reflux disease (GERD)
7. Barrett's esophagus
8. Sliding hiatus hernia (rolling hernia)
9. Management-Ca esophagus
10. Achalasia cardia
11. Heller's operation
12. Zenker's diverticulum
13. Schatzkis ring
14. Plummer-Vinson syndrome (Patterson-Kelly)

XII. Stomach and duodenum

1. Anatomy, blood supply and lymphatic drainage
2. Types of vagotomy
3. Complications of vagotomy
4. Infantile hypertrophic pyloric stenosis (IHPS)
5. Ramstedt's operation
6. Duodenal atresia
7. *H. pylori*
8. Types of gastritis
9. Duodenal ulcer vs gastric ulcer
10. Periodicity of ulcers
11. Billroth II gastrectomy
12. Complications of gastrectomy
13. Early vs. late dumping syndrome
14. Gastric polyps
15. Carcinoma stomach types and classification
16. ZE syndrome
17. Gastroplasty
18. Trichobezoars
19. Volvulus of stomach

XIII. Liver

1. Segments of liver
2. Sites of portosystemic anastomoses
3. Percutaneous transhepatic cholangiography (PTC)
4. TIPSS
5. Upper GI bleed—causes
6. Budd-Chiari syndrome
7. Primary sclerosing cholangitis
8. Primary biliary cirrhosis
9. Choledochal cyst
10. Pyogenic liver abscess
11. Types of hepatoma
12. Cholangiocarcinoma
13. Klatskin's tumor
14. Liver biopsy procedure

XIV. Spleen

1. Complications of splenectomy
2. Splenic trauma
3. Kehr's sign
4. Splenunculi
5. Splenosis

XV. Gallbladder and bile ducts

1. Calot's triangle
2. Oral cholecystography
3. Endoscopic retrograde cholangiopancreatography (ERCP)
4. Types of biliary atresia
5. Moynihan's hump
6. Pigment stones
7. Cholesterol stones
8. Limey bile
9. Complications of gall stones
10. Mucocele of gallstones
11. Courvoisier's law
12. Mirizzi's syndrome
13. Laparoscopic cholecystectomy
14. Acalculous cholecystitis
15. Gallstone ileus
16. Premalignant lesion of Ca bile duct
17. White Bile

XVI. Pancreas

1. Anatomy
2. Pancreas divisum
3. Octreotide
4. Annular pancreas
5. Pseudocyst of pancreas
6. Complications of acute pancreatitis
7. Ranson's score
8. Clinical features of c/c pancreatitis
9. Wilkie's syndrome (duodenal ileus)
10. Whipples operation
11. Whipples triad

XVII. The peritoneum, omentum, mesentery and retroperitoneal space

1. Spontaneous peritonitis
2. Complications of peritonitis
3. Stages of peritonitis
4. Pelvic abscess
5. Subphrenic space and abscess
6. Pneumococcal peritonitis
7. Types of tuberculous peritonitis
8. Paracentesis abdominis
9. Carcinoma peritonei
10. Pseudomyxoma peritonei
11. Diagnostic peritoneal lavage
12. Seat belt syndrome
13. Mesenteric cyst types
14. Pneumoperitoneum

XVIII. Small, large intestines and intestinal obstruction

1. Hirschsprungs disease
2. Blind loop syndrome
3. Diverticulosis
4. Meckel's diverticulum
5. Ulcerative colitis
6. Crohn's disease
7. Peutz-Jeghers syndrome
8. Familial adenomatous polyposis (FAP)
9. Ca colon types and classification
10. Colectomy types
11. Fecal fistula
12. Types of colostomy
13. Complications of colostomy
14. Sigmoid volvulus
15. Intussusception
16. Closed loop obstruction
17. Cardinal features of intestinal obstruction
18. Paul-Mikulicz procedure
19. Hartmann's operation
20. Enteroclysis
21. Intestinal bands
22. Internal hernia sites
23. Jejunal atresia types
24. Meconium ileus
25. Bishop-Koop procedure
26. Paralytic ileus
27. Causes of intestinal obstruction without constipation
28. Acute mesenteric ischemia
29. Ogilvie's syndrome

XIX. The vermiform appendix

1. Anatomical positions
2. Mucocele of appendix
3. Ochsner-Sherren regimen
4. Sign of appendicitis
5. Appendicular mass
6. Carcinoid tumor
7. Appendicular abscess
8. Laparoscopic appendicectomy

XX. The rectum

1. Tenesmus
2. Spurious diarrhea
3. Grading of prolapse rectum
4. Villous adenoma
5. Dukes staging
6. APR
7. Anorectal malformations
8. Sacrococcygeal teratoma

XXI. The anus and anal canal

1. Pilonidal sinus
2. Fissure in ano
3. Sentinel pile
4. 1° vs 2° vs symptomatic hemorrhoids
5. Goodsal's rule
6. Complications of hemorrhoids
7. Hemorrhoidectomy procedure
8. Anorectal abscess classification
9. Fistula in ano-types
10. Proctalgia fugax

XXII. Hernias, umbilicus and abdominal wall

1. Inguinal canal-anatomy
2. Herniotomy
3. Gastric lymphoma
4. Classification of hernia
5. Richter's hernia
6. Herniorrhaphy
7. Hernioplasty
8. Causes of recurrent hernia
9. Malgaigne's bulges
10. Management of strangulated hernia
11. Sliding hernia
12. Femoral hernia
13. Exomphalos
14. Paraumbilical hernia
15. Mayo's repair
16. Fatty hernia of linea alba (epigastric hernia)
17. Interparietal (interstitial) hernia
18. Phantom hernia
19. Pantaloon hernia
20. Umbilical fistula
21. Raspberry tumor
22. Ventral hernia (incisional hernia)
23. Burst abdomen
24. Divarication of recti
25. Bacterial synergistic gangrene
26. Desmoid tumor (Paget's recurrent fibroid)

XXIII. Urinary symptoms

1. Causes of hematuria
2. Ureteric colic
3. Intravenous pyelogram
4. Micturating cystourethrogram (MCU)
5. Definition of anuria and oliguria
6. Renal cortex-anatomy
7. Percutaneous nephrostomy
8. Painless hematuria
9. Causes of urinary retention

XXIV. The kidneys and ureters

1. Polycystic kidney
2. Horseshoe kidney
3. Crossed dystopia
4. Ureterocele
5. Postcaval ureter
6. Renal trauma classification
7. Boari's operation
8. Hydronephrosis
9. Types of renal calculi
10. ESWL
11. Renal carbuncle
12. Reflux nephropathy (c/c pyelonephritis)
13. Sources of perinephric abscess
14. Lesions in renal TB
15. Wilm's tumor
16. Grawitz tumor

XXV. The urinary bladder

1. Nerve supply
2. Ectopia vesicae
3. Endemic hematuria
4. Rupture bladder
5. Bladder diverticulae
6. Urinary fistula
7. Urethral syndrome
8. Hunner's ulcer (interstitial nephritis)
9. Internal and external urinary diversion
10. Ileal loop conduit
11. Carcinoma bladder
12. Bladder stone—complications
13. Obstructive uropathy

XXVI. The prostate and seminal vesicles

1. Prostatism
2. Prostatism sans prostate
3. Benign prostatic hyperplasia (BPH)
4. Transurethral resection of the prostate (TURP)
5. Carcinoma prostate
6. Prostate specific antigen (PSA)
7. Parts of prostate

XXVII. The urethra and penis

1. Pinhole meatus (meatal stenosis)
2. Posterior urethral valve
3. Hypospadiasis
4. Epispadiasis
5. Rupture of bulbar urethra
6. Rupture of membranous urethra
7. Superficial vs deep extravasation
8. Reiter's syndrome
9. Urethral stricture
10. Periurethral abscess

ORTHOPEDICS

Clinical Questions

1. An elderly female presents in the casualty with history of a fall. She is unable to move her left lower limb. On examination, the limb is found to be externally rotated.
   a. What is the most probable diagnosis giving reasons?
   b. How will you classify this condition?
   c. What is the mode of management?
   d. What are the complications you can anticipate?
2. A headload worker presented in the casualty with history of fall of a heavy load on his left shoulder. He also complains of weakness of his same upper limb. On examination he has difficulty in abduction and external rotation of the same hand.
   a. What is the most probable diagnosis?
   b. Draw and label the brachial plexus showing the site of injury.
   c. What are the groups of muscles that are involved?
   d. What are the causes of claw hand?
3. In a case of fall on outstretched hands
   a. What are the possible injuries you can think of?
   b. If there is pain at the wrist what could be the possible injury, its investigations and management.
   c. If it is a child with pain in the elbow what would you suspect and list its complications?
4. A young footballer following an injury complains of give away, click and locking of his knee joint?
   a. What are the structures liable to be injured?
   b. What are the tests that you will do for reaching a diagnosis?
   c. What is the treatment for meniscal injury?
5. A newborn is bought with b/l club foot
   a. What are the component deformities of club foot?
   b. What is the line of management?
   c. What will you do for late presentations?
   d. Give four corrective operative surgeries?
6. A young patient presented with fever and discharging sinus in the thigh.
   a. What is the most probable diagnosis?
   b. What are the investigation and typical diagnostic findings in radiogram?
   c. What are the complications?
   d. What is the line of management?
7. Following a road traffic injury, a 30-year-old female sustained a fracture shaft of femur.
   a. What are the immediate complications?
   b. What will you think of if she develops breathlessness the next day and how will you manage it?
   c. How will you manage fracture shaft of femur?
   d. What are the late complications?
8. A 21-year-old male complains of pain in the right shoulder following a basketball match. He presented with his right elbow being supported with his other hand. On examination, there was flattening of the right shoulder and fullness of infraclavicular region.
   a. What is the most probable diagnosis?
   b. How will you manage this case?
   c. What are the surgical procedures done?
   d. What are the complications?

Short Notes

I. General orthopedics

1. Pathological fractures
2. Sprain
3. Stages of fracture healing
4. Factors affecting fracture healing
5. Classification of open fractures
6. Thomas splint
7. Internal fixation
8. DCP (dynamic compression plate)
9. Functional bracing
10. Ilizarov's technique
11. Delayed union
12. Non-union
13. Malunion
14. Sudeck's dystrophy

15. Myositis ossificans
16. Salter and Harris classification
17. Green stick fracture
18. Seddons classification
19. Claw hand
20. Ulnar paradox
21. Pointing index
22. Froments sign
23. Cubitus varus (gun stock deformity)
24. Cubitus valgus
25. Dinner fork deformity
26. Mallet finger
27. Osteotomy
28. Arthrodesis
29. Bone graft
30. Plaster of Paris

II. Fractures and dislocations

1. Fracture (#) clavicle
2. Anterior dislocation of shoulder
3. Luxatio erecta
4. Fracture shaft of humerus
5. # Supracondylar
6. VIC
7. Pulled elbow
8. Fracture head of radius
9. Galeazzis fracture dislocation
10. Monteggia fracture dislocation
11. Colles fracture
12. Smiths fracture
13. Bartons fracture
14. Scaphoid fracture
15. Bennets fracture
16. Rolandos fracture
17. Blood supply of head of femur
18. Posterior dislocation of hip
19. Avascular necrosis of hip
20. Fracture Neck of femur
21. McMurray's osteotomy
22. Bryant's triangle
23. Austin moores prosthesis
24. Pseudoarthrosis
25. Intertrochantric fracture
26. Gallows traction
27. Tension band wiring
28. O'Donoghue's triad
29. McMurray test
30. Drawer test
31. Dislocation of patella
32. Phemister grafting
33. Pott's fracture
34. Fracture calcaneum
35. Jones #
36. Fracture spine classification
37. Jeffersons #
38. Hangman's fracture

III. Infections

1. Chronic osteomyelitis
2. Sequestrum
3. Involucrum
4. Garre's osteomyelitis
5. Brodies abscess
6. Tom Smith's arthritis
7. Septic arthritis
8. Caries sicca
9. Types of vertebral TB
10. Pott's paraplegia—causes
11. Wandering acetabulum
12. Spina ventosa

IV. Congenital conditions

1. Congenital talipes equinovarus (CTEV)
2. Barlow's test
3. Ortolanis test
4. Galeazzi's sign
5. Spina bifida

V. Tumors

1. Osteoma
2. Osteoid osteoma
3. Osteoclastoma
4. Osteochondroma
5. Osteosarcoma
6. Premalignant bone lesions
7. Ewing's sarcoma
8. Serum alkaline phosphatase
9. Metastatic bone tumors
10. Enchondromas
11. Fibrous dysplasia
12. Adamantinoma
13. Multiple exostosis
14. Sulcus sign/ledge sign

VI. The vertebral column

1. Pathology of disk prolapse
2. Cobb's angle
3. Scottish dog sign
4. Spondylolisthesis
5. Spondylolysis
6. Sciatica

VII. Connective tissue disorders

1. Deformities in rheumatoid arthritis
2. Ankylosing spondylitis
3. Clinical features of osteoarthritis

VIII. Miscellaneous conditions

1. Tennis elbow
2. deQuervain's tenovaginitis
3. Finkelstein's sign
4. Ganglion
5. Frozen shoulder
6. Painful arc syndrome
7. Heel pain—causes
8. Meralgia paresthetica
9. Osteoporosis
10. Rickets-radiological features
11. Achondroplasia
12. Osteogenesis imperfecta (OI)
13. Osteitis deformans (Paget's disease)
14. Perthe's disease (Coxa plana, pseudocoxalgia)
15. Osgood-Shlatter disease
16. Kienbock's disease
17. Congenital torticollis
18. Coxa vara
19. Slipped capital femoral epiphysis
20. Genu valgum
21. Bow legs (genu varum)
22. Genu recurvatum
23. Baker's cyst
24. Flat foot
25. Loose bodies

IX. The hand

1. Dupuytren's contracture
2. Carpal tunnel syndrome
3. Trigger finger
4. Acute paronychia
5. Apical abscess
6. Felon
7. Middle volar space infections
8. Web space infection
9. Kanavel's sig
10. Acute suppurative tenosynovitis

OBSTETRICS

Theory Topics:

Paper I	: Obstetrics including Social Obstetrics	40 Marks
Paper II	: Gynecology, Family Welfare and Demography	40 Marks

Practical Examinations:

Clinical I	: Obstetrics Case (including Case Sheet)	25 Marks
Clinical II	: Gynecological Case	25 Marks

Oral Examinations: X-rays and CTG, Instruments, Specimens

- Family Planning Methods — 20 Marks
- Case Record — 10 Marks

Clinical Questions

1. A 22-year-old primigravida was detected to have a BP of 150/110 mm Hg during 34 weeks of gestation. She also complains of blurred vision, headache and epigastric pain.
   a. What is your diagnosis?
   b. What are the investigations you would like to do?
   c. Outline the management in this case.
   d. What is HELLP syndrome and mention the drug of choice?
   e. What is the mode of anesthesia in this patient if you opt for a CS?
2. A 23-year-old primigravida with FBS of 104 mg percent and 2 hour postprandial blood sugar 70 mg percent presents at 34 weeks with an over distended abdomen and on examination, the fetal parts are not distinctly felt and the FHS is very feeble.
   a. What is your diagnosis?
   b. How will you manage this patient?
   c. Causes of over distended abdomen during pregnancy?
   d. Give the indications of GTT without GCT.
   e. Fetal complications of diabetes?
3. On examining a 20-year-old primi at 40 weeks of gestation, the fetus is presenting by vertex and the head is found to be nonengaged and is floating high. She does not complain of pain or leaking.
   a. Outline the mode of management in this case.
   b. Enumerate the causes of nonengaged head at term.
   c. How will you assess the pelvis?
   d. How will you deliver a floating head at CS?
   e. Define trial labor.
4. In a 24-year-old primi at 36 weeks of gestation, the fetus was found to be presenting by breech.
   a. List the causes of breech presentation.
   b. What are the methods of breech delivery?
   c. What are the complications of breech delivery?
   d. List the mechanism of labor in breech presentation.
   e. Explain Lovset's maneuver.
5. A 30-year-old second gravida with previous CS (Indication: failed trial) now comes to you for her routine antenatal checkup at 36 week of gestation.
   a. What is the sign you will look for?
   b. How will you manage this patient?
   c. What important procedures will you advice to the patient after delivery?
   d. What are the impending signs of rupture?
   e. List the important steps of CS?
6. A 23-year-old newly married lady (a known: case of rheumatic mitral stenosis) comes to you 2 months after missing her periods. Urine pregnancy test is positive.
   a. How will you functionally grade her heart disease?
   b. When will you admit the patient in a case of
      i. Grade I heart disease
      ii. Grade III heart disease

c. What are the periods during which she is likely to develop heart failure?
d. Discuss the labor room management in this patient.
e. What is the mode of contraception you will advice?

7. A 23-year-old primi was diagnosed to have multiple pregnancy with 2 live fetuses *in utero* comes to you with pain and leaking.
   a. What are the complications you will anticipate during delivery?
   b. Discuss how you will deliver the second of the twin.
   c. What are the postpartum complications you will anticipate?
   d. Explain how you will tackle PPH.
   e. What are the indications for CS in multiple pregnancy?
8. A 30-year-old lady presents at 12 week of amenorrhea with history of vaginal bleeding. O/E BP-160/100 mm Hg, uterus-20 weeks. No fetal parts felt. There is history of excessive vomiting. Pulse rate is 120/minute There is history of palpitation.
   a. What is your diagnosis?
   b. Outline the management and follow-up.
   c. Differential diagnosis if a patient presents at 12 weeks of amenorrhea with vaginal bleeding.
   d. What was the probable cause of tachycardia and palpitation?
   e. List the indications of MTP.
9. A 21-year-old woman with history of one abortion, presents with 12 weeks of amenorrhea, vaginal bleeding and abdominal pain. P/V OS is open, uterus is 8 weeks.
   a. Classify abortion
   b. Causes of recurrent abortion and mention the management of one condition.
   c. What do you mean by missed abortion?
   d. Predisposing factors for ectopic pregnancy.
   e. Write one investigation to diagnose ectopic pregnancy and the findings expected.

Short Notes

I. General obstetrics

1. Functions of zona pellucida
2. Capacitation of sperms
3. Implantation
4. Decidua
5. Chorionic villi
6. Functions of placenta
7. Amniotic fluid
8. Umbilical cord
9. Cardiovascular changes during pregnancy
10. Weight gain during pregnancy

II. Diagnosis of pregnancy

1. Hegars sign
2. Immunological tests for pregnancy detection
3. Sonography in pregnancy
4. Quickening
5. External vs internal ballotment
6. Uterine soufflé vs funic soufflé
7. Methods of estimating gestational age

III. Fetus *in utero*

1. Define lie, presentation, attitude, position, presenting part, denominator and vertex
2. Moulding
3. Caput succedaneum
4. Gynecoid pelvic inlet with diameters

IV. Antenatal care and assessment of fetal well-being

1. Define antenatal care
2. First visit procedures
3. Booking scan (anomaly scan, IInd trimester scan)
4. Biophysical profile
5. Triple test
6. Nonstress test
7. Manning score
8. Amniocentesis
9. Chorionic villi sampling
10. Cordocentesis
11. DFMC and Cardiff count
12. Gravidogram

V. Normal labor and puerperium

1. Define normal labor
2. Cause of onset of labor
3. True vs false labor pain
4. Stages of labor-definition
5. Friedman's partogram
6. Lower uterine segment

7. Methods of placental separation
8. Mechanism of labor
9. Define engagement
10. Define crowning
11. Bishops score
12. Modified Brandt-Andrews technique
13. Define puerperium
14. Lochia
15. Postnatal care

VI. Abortion

1. Define abortion
2. Classify abortion
3. Missed abortion
4. Causes of 1st trimester abortion
5. Causes of IInd trimester abortion
6. MTP Act 1971
7. Threatened abortion
8. Septic abortion
9. Recurrent abortion—causes and investigations
10. Internal Os tightening (cervical encirclage)
11. Methods of inducing abortion in 1st and IInd trimester
12. Menstrual regulation
13. Medical abortion

VII. Multiple pregnancy and polyhydramnios

1. Vanishing twin
2. Twin-to-twin transfusion
3. Complications of multiple pregnancy
4. Management of second of the twin
5. Internal podalic version
6. Chronic polyhydramnios—causes and complications
7. Controlled ARM
8. Amnioreduction

VIII. Antepartum hemorrhage, placenta and cord

1. Classify placenta praevia
2. Placenta previa vs abruptio placenta
3. Grading of abruptio placenta
4. Couvelaire uterus
5. Vasa praevia (Velamentous placenta)
6. Succenturiate lobe
7. Placenta accreta
8. Cord prolapse—management
9. Cord presentation

IX. Pathology of pregnancy

1. Hyperemesis gravidarum
   i. Complications
   ii. Management
2. Pregnancy induced hypertension
   i. Definition
   ii. Complication
   iii. Roll over test
   iv. Impending signs of eclampsia
3. Gestational diabetes mellitus
   i. GCT
   ii. O'Sullivans blood glucose values
   iii. Complications in fetus
   iv. Shoulder dystocia
4. Heart disease complicating pregnancy
   i. Functional grading
   ii. Wet vs dry management
5. Anemia in pregnancy
   i. Estimation of Fe requirement
   ii. Parenteral Fe therapy
   iii. Complications of anemia
6. Urinary tract infections
   i. Asymptomatic bacteriuria
   ii. Complications
7. Fibroids complicating pregnancy
   i. Red degeneration
8. Rh incompatibility
   i. Hydrops fetalis
   ii. Liley curve
   iii. Kleihauer count
   iv. Prevention of Rh isoimmunization
9. *Define*: PROM; PPROM; Preterm labor
10. Drugs used in PROM
11. Causes and Complications of post-term labor
12. Causes of recurrent IUD
13. Term IUD
14. Spalding sign

X. Cesarian section

1. LSCS vs classical CS
2. Steps of LSCS
3. Requisites for VBAC
4. Recurrent indications for CS
5. Evidence of impending rupture
6. Scar dehiscence

XI. Cephalopelvic disproportion

1. Define bad obstetric history
2. Munro-Kerr-Müller method
3. Internal pelvimetry
4. Trial labor
5. Retraction ring (Bandls ring)
6. Constriction ring

XII. Abnormal presentations

1. Deep transverse arrest
2. Face to pubis delivery
3. Mechanism of delivery in face
4. Persistent occipito posterior
5. Mentoposterior
6. Lovset's maneuver
7. Mauriceau-Smellie-Veit procedure
8. Marshall Burns technique
9. Pinard's procedure
10. External cephalic version
11. Neglected shoulder
12. Cephalocentesis

XIII. Complications of 3rd stage of labor

1. Complications of 3rd stage
2. Atonic vs traumatic PPH
3. Management of PPH
4. Causes of retained placenta
5. Placenta accreta
6. Causes of acute inversion
7. O'Sullivan's method
8. Complete perineal tear
9. Classification of perineal tear
10. Cervical tear
11. Rupture uterus-causes
12. Causes of subinvolution of uterus
13. Puerperal sepsis

XIV. Abnormal fetus

1. APGAR score
2. Define LBW baby
3. Causes of LBW baby
4. Causes of IUGR
5. Symmetrical vs asymmetrical IUGR
6. Meconium aspiration syndrome
7. Cephalhematoma
8. Down's syndrome

XV. Miscellaneous

1. Oxytocin
2. Ergometrine
3. PGE_1, PGE_2, PGF_2a
4. Tocolytics
5. Ethacridine lactate
6. Methods of inducing labor
   - Surgical methods
   - Medical methods
7. Artificial rupture of membranes
8. Stripping
9. Eligible couple
10. PEARL index
11. No scalpel vasectomy
12. Reproductive and child health (RCH)
13. Intergrated child development services (ICDS)
14. Maternal mortality rate (MMR)
15. Perinatal mortality
16. Still birth
17. Amniotic fluid embolism
18. High-risk pregnancy

XVI. Operative methods

1. Episiotomy types and procedure
2. Forceps—indications; advantages; disadvantages
3. Vacuum—indications; advantages; disadvantages
4. Cardiotocogram

GYNECOLOGY

Clinical Questions

1. A 44-year-old nulliparous woman, presenting with menorrhagia for 6 months.
   a. What are the possibilities?
   b. Most important investigation. Findings expected.
   c. Medical treatment of menorrhagia.
   d. Important steps of total abdominal hysterectomy.
2. A 44-year-old parous woman on routine cervical cytology screening was found to have Grade III CIN. She is asymptomatic.
   a. Stages of CIN.
   b. Cervical exfoliative cytology.
   c. How will you proceed with the investigation in this patient?
   d. Lymphatic drainage of cervix.
   e. Name any two important symptoms and two important signs of Ca Cx.
   f. Structures removed in radical hysterectomy for Ca Cx.
3. A 53-year-old women, who had menopause at 47-year now complains of vaginal bleeding.
   a. Define postmenopausal bleeding.
   b. Give important causes of postmenopausal bleeding.
   c. What is the most important investigation and give the findings expected in any one condition?
   d. Etiological factors in Ca endometrium.
   e. Management of senile vaginitis.
4. A 55-year-old menopausal woman complains of stress incontinence and mass coming down per vaginum which can be reduced manually.
   a. Classify genital prolapse.
   b. Etiological factors in prolapse.
   c. Give important steps in vaginal hysterectomy.
   d. Urinary problems in prolapse.
   e. How will you differentiate between a decubitus ulcer in a prolapse and a malignant ulcer?
5. A 35-year-old parous woman presents with complaints of severe lower abdominal pain starting 5–6 days before menstruation which is relieved by menstrual flow. There is a history of dyspareunia and menorrhagia. No history of fever. P/V–uterus normal size, tender. B/L adnexal mass, tender nodules in Pouch of Douglas.
   a. What is the most probable diagnosis?
   b. Role of laparoscopy in the condition.
   c. Discuss the possible etiology.
   d. How can you clinically distinguish between adenomyosis and fibroid uterus?
   e. If fever was present, what would have been the immediate diagnosis?
6. A 55-year-old menopausal woman with a history of an asymptomatic swelling in the abdomen since 8 months now presents in the casualty with acute abdominal pain, vomiting and mild pyrexia. O/E tender mass in the abdomen arising from the pelvis.
   a. What is the most probable diagnosis?
   b. Causes of abdominal pain in an ovarian tumor.
   c. Ultrasonography features of a malignant ovarian tumor.
   d. What do you mean by a parasitic fibroid?
   e. Describe the management of this case.
   f. Treatment of malignant ovarian tumor.
7. A young couple married 3 year and having regular sexual intercourse comes to you with complaints of infertility.
   a. How will you assess tubal patency?
   b. Describe two methods for assessment of ovulation.
   c. Describe postcoital test.
   d. Treatment of infertility due to cervical antibodies.
   e. Causes of infertility in fibroid uterus.

Short Notes

I. Anatomy, histology, physiology and gynecological diagnosis

1. Supports of the uterus
2. Lymphatic drainage and blood supply of the uterus
3. Branches of internal iliac
4. Cardinal ligaments
5. Pelvic ureter
6. Female urethra
7. Pelvic diaphragm
8. Graafian follicle
9. Corpus luteum
10. Endometrium
11. LH surge
12. Menopausal symptoms and climacteric
13. Postmenopausal bleeding
14. Pap smear
15. Colposcopy
16. Uses of hysteroscopy
17. D and C
18. Fractional curettage

II. Malformations, intersexuality

1. Hematocolpos
2. Cryptomenorrhea
3. Imperforate hymen
4. Müllerian duct anomalies
5. Hermaphroditism vs Pseudohermaphroditism
6. Turner's syndrome
7. Hirsutism
8. Polycystic ovarian disease (PCOD)
9. Congenital adrenal hyperplasia

III. Vulval and vaginal disease

1. Vulvodynia
2. Molluscum contagiosum
3. Condyloma accuminatum
4. Pruritus vulvae
5. Vulvar dystrophies—types
6. Bartholin's cyst
7. Vulvar intraepithelial neoplasia (VIN)
8. Döderlein's bacilli
9. Vaginal epithelium and pH
10. Cornification index
11. Leukorrhea
12. Trichomoniasis
13. Candidiasis
14. Bacterial vaginosis
15. Senile vaginitis
16. Gartners duct cyst
17. Gonorrhea
18. Lymphogranuloma venereum
19. Granuloma inguinale
20. TB lesion of fallopian tubes
21. Schiller's test

IV. Genital tract injuries/urinary diseases

1. Postcoital tear
2. Complete perineal tear
3. Vaginal fistula
4. Cervical tear
5. Uterine perforation
6. Urethral syndrome
7. Stress incontinence
8. Urethral caruncle
9. Bonney test

V. Pathology of conception

1. Vaginismus
2. Sperm analysis
3. Postcoital test
4. Effective sperm count
5. Artificial insemination
6. ICSI
7. Tests for tubal patency
8. *In vitro* fertilization
9. GIFT, ZIFT
10. Tests for ovulation
11. Ovulation induction
12. Cervical mucus study

VI. Birth control and MTP

1. Natural methods
2. TODAY vagina sponge
3. Femshield
4. Copper containing IUCD and mode of action
5. Progestasert
6. Techniques of IUCD insertion
7. Contraindications of IUCDs
8. Complications of IUCD
9. IUCD-mode of action
10. Femilon
11. Combined oral pills
12. Triphasic pill
13. Mini pill
14. Depo-provera
15. Norplant
16. Centchroman
17. Interceptives
18. Vasectomy
19. Minilap sterilization
20. Pomeroys method and its modification
21. Laparoscopic sterilization
22. Emergency contraception

VII. Trophoblastic disease and ectopic gestation

1. VM-follow-up
2. Check curettage
3. MAC regime
4. Partial vs complete mole
5. Invasive mole vs choriocarcinoma
6. Suburethral nodule
7. Cervical pregnancy
8. Causes of ectopic
9. Sequelae of tubal pregnancy
10. Criteria for ovarian pregnancy
11. Decidual cast
12. Culdocentesis
13. Surgically administered medical treatment (SAM)
14. Rx of ruptured ectopic
15. Medical management of EP
16. Conservative management of EP

VIII. Disorders of menstruation

1. Precocious menstruation
2. Cryptomenorrhea
3. Asherman's syndrome
4. Premature menopause
5. Premenstrual tension
6. Congestive dysmenorrhea
7. Spasmodic dysmenorrhea
8. Causes of menorrhagia
9. DUB-endometrial findings
10. DUB-classification
11. DUB-management
12. Endometrial ablation
13. Metrorrhagia-causes
14. Metropathia hemorrhagica
15. Changes in uterus in metropathia hemorrhagica
16. DoC in ovulatory menorrhagia
17. Medical management of DUB

IX. Hormone therapy

1. Estrogen preparations and uses
2. Adverse effects of estrogens
3. Ovarian hyperstimulation syndrome
4. Tamoxifen
5. Progesterone uses
6. Norethisterone
7. Danazol
8. Antiandrogens
9. Bromocriptine
10. Selective estrogen receptor modulator (SERM)

X. Cervix and endometrium

1. Erosion
2. Nabothian follicle
3. Chronic cervicitis
4. Ectropion
5. Cervical polyp
6. Cervical intraepithelial neoplasia (CIN)
7. Speculoscopy
8. Cone biopsy
9. Large loop excision of transformation zone (LLETZ)
10. Ca cervix-staging
11. Types of abdominal hysterectomy
12. Endocervical Ca
13. Endometrial Ca staging
14. VIA

XI. Prolapse and Displacements of uterus

1. Degree of prolapse
2. Role of pessary in prolapse
3. Decubitus ulcer
4. Fothergills repair
5. Steps of vaginal hysterectomy
6. Le Fortes repair
7. Supports of bladder
8. Cystocele repair
9. Retroversion symptoms

XII. Fibroids

1. Types of fibroids
2. Changes in fibroids
3. Complications of fibroids
4. Myomectomy
5. Laparoscopically assisted vaginal hysterectomy (LAVH)
6. Sarcoma botryoides
7. Cervical fibroids
8. Red degeneration

XIII. Ovarian disease, chemotherapy and radiotherapy

1. Functional vs functioning ovarian tumors
2. Lutein cysts
3. Ovarian tumor WHO classification
4. Low malignant potential (LMP)
5. Serous cystadenoma
6. Mucinous tumors
7. Brenner tumors
8. Meigs and pseudo-meigs syndrome
9. Teratoma ovary
10. Dysgerminoma
11. Granulosa cell tumor
12. Krukenberg tumor
13. Virilizing tumor
14. Complication of ovarian tumors
15. Staging laparotomy
16. 2nd look surgery

17. Twisted ovarian cyst
18. Ca ovary stage 1-management
19. Brachytherapy
20. After loading technique
21. Etoposide, methotrexate, actinomycin D, cyclophosphamide and vincristine (Oncovin) (EMACO) regime

XIV. PID, C/C pelvic pain, diseases of broad ligament, tubes and parametrium

1. Stage of PID
2. Management of PID
3. C/C pelvic pain syndrome
4. Hydrosalpinx
5. Pyometra
6. Post MTP infection
7. Pelvic abscess

XV. Endometriosis and adenomyosis

1. Parovarian tumors
2. Endometriosis-theories
3. Chocolate cysts
4. Management of endometriosis
5. Adenomyosis.

PEDIATRICS

Theory Topics:

One Paper	Whole Subject	40 Marks

Practical Examinations:

Clinical I	Clinical Case	10 Marks
Clinical II	Nutrition Case	10 Marks
Clinical III	OSCE	10 Marks

Oral Examinations: X-rays, Instruments, Drugs, Nutrition. 10 Marks

Clinical Questions

1. A 10-year-old boy presents with fever 10 days with pain and swelling in the knee joint which appeared 2 days after onset of fever, which was followed by similar complaints in the ankle joint 5 days later?
   a. What is the most likely possibility?
   b. What other possibilities will you consider as differential diagnosis?
   c. What are the clinical findings you will look for?
   d. What investigations will you ask for?
   e. Comment on the long-term management.
2. A 5-year-old boy presents to the casualty with tachypnea, tachycardia, wheezing and pedal edema. The child gives history of frequent chest infections in the past, the child looks pale and his extremities are cold.
   a. What is the likely clinical diagnosis?
   b. What are the possibilities to be ruled out that could have resulted in this condition?
   c. What are the clinical signs to look for?
   d. How will you manage the case?
   e. What are the causes of CCF in infants?
3. A 6-year-old child is brought to the casualty in an exhausted state. He is cyanosed. There is history of fever with cough which began 3 days ago which was followed by wheezing. He gives history of attacks of wheezing in the past too.
   a. What is your diagnosis?
   b. What are the immediate differential diagnosis?
   c. How will you manage the case?
   d. Write briefly on the long-term prevention of the condition.
   e. Comment on the drugs used in the treatment.
4. A 10-year-old child presents with fever for the past 2–3 weeks along with severe malaise, and loss of appetite with upper abdominal pain and skin rash. The urine is now high colored O/E : icterus+; hepatomegaly+; spleen tip+
   a. What is the most likely diagnosis?
   b. Discuss the d/d (differential diagnosis)
   c. What are the causative viruses?
   d. What are the investigations to be done?
   e. What are the complications to be kept in mind?
   f. Comment on the preventive measures.
5. After having fever, headache and sore throat for a few days a child presents with weakness of sudden onset of both lower limbs, more on right side with muscle pain and hyperesthesia. Tone of muscle and reflexes are decreased. The child also has some difficulty in breathing.
   a. What is the most important possibility to be kept in mind?
   b. Discuss the important differential diagnosis and compare the clinical features.
   c. How will you proceed with the case ?
   d. Discuss the clinical spectrum of the disease.
   e. Comment on the vaccination measures.
   f. What are the steps in eradication of the disease?
6. A 5-year-old child with fever and cough-5 days; now presents with puffiness of face and pedal edema. The child gives history of two similar episodes in the past 2 years and had taken full medication.
   a. What is your clinical diagnosis?
   b. How will you investigate the case?

c. What are the other possibilities to be kept in mind?
d. Outline the initial and subsequent treatment strategies.
e. What are the complications to be kept in mind?
f. What are the indications for renal biopsy in such a case?

7. A 15-month-old malnourished child, a known case of congenital heart disease presents with fever and cough-3 days. O/E: respiratory rate = 30/min; chest indrawing +; the child is extremely lethargic.
   a. What is your clinical diagnosis?
   b. What are the investigations that can be done?
   c. How will you treat the child?
   d. What are the important etiological agents?
   e. What are the danger signs to look out for?
   f. Write briefly on staphylococcal pneumonia
8. A 11-year-old child presents with fever of moderate intensity, headache and vomiting-10 days duration. For the initial few days, he was constipated, but he is now passing loose stools. O/E: liver + 5–6 cm below the costal margin, spleen also palpable 1–2 cm.
   a. What is the likely diagnosis?
   b. What are the other possibilities to be kept in mind?
   c. What are the important investigations to be done?
   d. How will you treat the boy?
   e. What are the complications that have to be kept in mind?
9. A 10-year-old boy present with 3 weeks duration which was initially continuous, but is now appearing on and off. There is also headache, loss of appetite, loss of weight. O/E: hepatosplenomegaly
   a. What is the likely diagnosis?
   b. What are the important d/d's?
   c. How will you investigate the case?
   d. How will you treat the boy?
   e. What is hyperactive malarial splenomegaly?
   f. What are the features of severe malaria?
10. A 5-year-old child hospitalized after an RTA with multiple injuries develops fever and vomiting followed by convulsions. The child resists examination by light. There is generalized hypertonia. Neck stiffness is present.
    a. What is the most likely diagnosis?
    b. What are the important d/d's?
    c. What are the predisposing factors?
    d. How will you go about investigating the child?
    e. How will you treat the child?
    f. What are the associated complications?
    g. What are the important etiological agents?
11. A 5-year-old girl is brought with bleeding from the gums. She has been having recurrent episodes of fever for the past 1 year, malaise, body pain, tiredness and decreased activity.
    a. What is the most likely diagnosis?
    b. What are the other possibilities to be kept in mind?
    c. How will you go about examining the child?
    d. What are the important prognostic factors?
    e. What are the investigations to be done?
    f. How will you treat the girl?
12. A 13-day-old baby is brought with yellowish discoloration of the skin and eyes.
    a. What are the possibilities to be kept in mind?
    b. What are the causes and clinical features of physiological jaundice?
    c. What all will you specifically ask for in the history and see in the clinical examination?
    d. What is neonatal sepsis?
    e. What are the clinical features of hypothyroidism?

Short Notes

I. Growth and development

1. Define growth and development
2. Laws of growth
3. Periods of growth
4. Primary dentition
5. Define gross motor and fine motor development
6. Developmental delay
7. Deviant development.
8. Developmental regression

9. Developmental quotient
10. Developmental milestones of a 7-month old:
    - 1-year-old
    - 2-year-old
    - 3-year-old
11. Juvenile delinquency
12. Sexual maturity grading
13. Define short stature and classify
14. Primordial dwarf
15. FTT, definition and causes
16. Growth charts
17. Breath holding spells
18. Enuresis
19. Attention deficit hyperactivity disorder
20. Autism

II. Nutrition

1. Essential amino acids
2. Reference proteins
3. Biological value of protein
4. Net protein utilization (NPU)
5. Chemical score of protein
6. Complimentary action of protein
7. Poly unsaturated fatty acid (PUFA)
8. Phrynoderma
9. Omega 3 fatty acids
10. Dietary fiber
11. Balanced diet
12. Iodine deficiency goiter
13. Acrodermatitis enteropathica
14. Role of selinium
15. Endemic fluorosis
16. Plumbism
17. Advantages of breast milk
18. Baby-friendly hospital initiative (BFHI)
19. Contraindication of breastfeeding
20. Expressed breast milk
21. Define weaning
22. Ideal weaning food
23. What is protein-energy malnutrition (PEM)?
24. Classify protein-energy malnutrition
25. Age-independent growth criteria
26. SAT mix
27. Edema pathophysiology

III. Vitamins

1. Sources and functions of vitamin A
2. Classify xerophthalmia (WHO)
3. Treatment of vitamin A deficiency
4. Vitamin A prophylaxis programme
5. Hypervitaminosis A
6. Vitamin D metabolism
7. Classify rickets
8. Clinical features of rickets
9. Radiological changes in rickets
10. Treatment of rickets
11. Vitamin D resistant rickets
12. Rachitic vs Scorbutic rosary
13. Hemorrhagic disease of newborn
14. RDA- Vatamin A, D, B_2, B_{12}
15. Beriberi
16. Clinical features of riboflavin def
17. Pellagra
18. Infantile scurvy

IV. Neonatology

1. LBW, VLBW, ELBW
2. Primary and secondary apnea
3. TABCs of neonatal resuscitation
4. APGAR score
5. Moro reflex and its significance
6. Cephalohematoma
7. Reflexes in breastfeeding
8. Nipple confusion
9. Colostrum
10. Warm chain
11. Problems of LBW babies
12. Problems of pre-term babies
13. Congenital rubella syndrome
14. Congenital syphilis
15. Neonatal sepsis
16. Meconium aspiration syndrome
17. Respiratory distress syndrome
18. Breastfeeding vs breast milk jaundice
19. Prolonged physiological jaundice
20. Clinical estimation of jaundice
21. Kernicterus
22. Phototherapy principles
23. Extrahepatic biliary atresia (EHBA)
24. Neonatal seizures causes
25. Hypoxic ischemic encephalopathy

V. Immunology

1. 10 and 20 vaccine failure
2. Adjuvants
3. Bacillus calmette guerin (BCG)
4. BCG test
5. Mantoux test
6. Vaccine storage

7. Oral polio vaccine vs injectable polio vaccine (OPV vs IPV)
8. DPT vaccine
9. Contraindications of pertussis vaccine
10. Acellular pertussis vaccine
11. Measles vaccine
12. Measles mumps and rubella vaccine
13. Hib vaccine
14. Hep B vaccine
15. Typhoral vaccine
16. Vaccination in splenectomized patients
17. National immunization schedule and its IAP modifications
18. Vaccine protection programme (VPP)
19. Subacute sclerosing panencephalitis
20. Vaccine vial monitor
21. Cold chain
22. Live vaccines

VI. Hematology

1. Causes of microcytic hypochromic anemia
2. Causes of spherocytosis
3. Lab findings in Fe deficiency anemia
4. Fanconi's anemia
5. Hemolytic anemia causes
6. Hemolytic anemia peripheral smear
7. Hereditary spherocytosis
8. Thalassemia clinical features and management
9. Thalassemia peripheral smear
10. Super transfusion vs hypertransfusion
11. Crisis in sickle cell anemia
12. G6PD deficiency
13. Purpura classification
14. Immune thrombocytopenic purpura lab findings
15. Management of ITP
16. Hemophilia
17. Von Willebrand's disease
18. Henöch-Schönlein purpura
19. Hemolysic uremic syndrome
20. Paroxysmal nocturnal hemoglobinuria
21. Acute lymphocytic luekemia (ALL)
22. Sanctuaries of ALL
23. Management of ALL
24. Tumor lysis syndrome
25. Myeloblast vs Lymphoblast

VII. Gastrointestinal tract

1. Hypertrophic pyloric stenosis
2. Define acute watery diarrhea
3. Define dysentry
4. Define persistent diarrhea
5. Rotavirus
6. Signs of dehydration
7. Oral rehydration therapy
8. Oral rehydration solutions
9. Improved ORS
10. Management of diarrhea
11. Causes of malnutrition in diarrhea
12. Causes of seizures in diarrhea
13. Dysentery management
14. Lactose intolerance
15. Milk protein intolerance
16. Indian childhood cirrhosis
17. Portal hypertension in children
18. Neonatal hepatitis

VIII. Cardiovascular system

1. Causes of CCF and management
2. Classify congestive heart disease
3. Features of CCF
4. Jones criteria
5. Rheumatic fever prophylaxis
6. Rheumatic MR/AR
7. Clinical features of infective endocarditis
8. Prophylaxis in IE
9. Fetal circulation
10. NADAS criteria
11. Atrial septal defect (ASD)
12. VSD types
13. Small vs large VSD
14. Complications of ventricular septal defect (VSD)
15. Eisenmenger's syndrome
16. Eisenmenger's complex
17. Patent ductus arteriosus (PDA) clinical features
18. Components of TOF
19. Cyanotic spells management
20. Complications of TOF
21. Fallots physiology
22. Management of tetralogy of Fallot (TOF)
23. CXR in TOF
24. Causes of hypertension in children
25. Rapid oral digitalization
26. Murmurs of aortic regurgitation (AR), Mitral regurgitation (MR), Aortic stenosis (AS), Mitral stenosis (MS), Patent ductus arteriosus (PDA), TOF, ASD and VSD

IX. Respiratory system

1. Respiratory noises
2. Staphylococcal pneumonia
3. Tachypnea
4. Signs of very severe pneumonia
5. Acute respiratory infection (ARI)
6. Bronchiolitis

7. Wheezing causes
8. Oxygen therapy in pneumonia
9. Indications of chest X-ray in pneumonia
10. Bronchial asthma triggering factors
11. Treatment of acute severe asthma
12. Prophylaxis of bronchial asthma
13. Classify asthma (both a/c and c/c)

X. Genitourinary system

1. Causes of hematuria
2. RBC cast, WBC cast
3. Poststreptococcal glomerulonephritis (PSGN)
4. Define proteinuria
5. Define massive proteinuria
6. Complications of AGN
7. Nephrotic syndrome management
8. Complications of nephrotic syndrome
9. Indications of renal biopsy in AGN and nephrotic syndrome
10. IgA nephropathy
11. Define persistent microscopic hematuria
12. Heat and acetic acid test
13. Significant bacteriuria
14. Asymptomatic bacteriuria
15. Management of UTI
16. Vesicoureteral reflux (VUR)

XI. Nervous system

1. Organism causing pyogenic meningitis
2. Complications of pyogenic meningitis
3. CSF findings in pyogenic meningitis:
   - TB meningitis
   - Viral meningitis
4. Management of bacterial meningitis
5. TB meningitis clinical features
6. Reye's syndrome
7. Guillain-Barre syndrome
8. Define AFP
9. Causes of AFP
10. Hydrocephalous types
11. Myelodysplasia
12. Typical vs atypical seizures
13. Febrile seizure prophylaxis
14. Myoclonic seizure
15. Cerebral palsy types
16. Autism
17. Neurocutaneous markers

XII. Musculoskeletal system

1. Duchenne muscular dystrophy
2. Juvenile idiopathic arthritis
3. Causes of floppy infant

XIII. Endocrinology

1. Panhypopituitarism
2. Congenital hypothyroidism
   - Clinical features
   - Management

XIV. Genetic disorders

1. Down's syndrome
2. Turner syndrome
3. Klinefelter's syndrome
4. Craniosynostosis
5. Phenylketonurias
6. Marfan's syndrome
7. Gaucher's disease
8. Wilson's disease
9. Alpha 1 antitrypsin deficiency

XV. Miscellaneous

1. RCH program
2. Universal immunization programme (UIP)
3. ICDS

XVI. Infections

1. Staphylococcal skin scalded syndrome (SSSS)
2. Causes of PUO in children
3. *Measles*: Clinical features complications
4. Atypical vs modified measles
5. Complications of mumps
6. AFP surveillance
7. Pulse polio immunization
8. Poliomyelitis clinical features
9. Infectious mononucleosis (IMN)
10. Enteric fever clinical features diagnosis
11. Diphtheria complications
12. Miliary TB
13. Primary complex
14. TB Management
15. Treatment of malaria
16. Drug choice in cerebral malaria
17. Treatment of hook worm infestation
18. Scabies treatment

Index

Page numbers followed by *f* refer to figure

D

E

F

I

J

K

L

M

N

O

P

Q

R

S

T